T0334619

Computed Tomography

This book acts as a primer for radiographers upon performing computed tomography (CT) examinations. The focus resides in radiation physics, radiobiology, anatomy, imaging protocols and image evaluation. It seeks to provide readers insight into the practical and innovative approaches within CT, backed up with key literature and examples in practice. Recent innovations and the importance of new technology to acquire enhanced quality remain a focal point. These are essential in understanding the importance of dose optimization, patient anatomy and common pathology observed. Patient care will remain central in this book, supported with a dedicated chapter discussing effective communication, patient education, informed consent, coupled with the assessment of laboratory results and vital signs. The editors draw from recent publications and clinical expertise, supported with the growing trend of technological advances utilized within the CT environment. Critically, this volume focuses on the role of CT for an array of audiences but, more specifically, undergraduate and postgraduate radiographers worldwide.

Medical Imaging in Practice

Series Editor:
Christopher M. Hayre,
Senior Lecturer in Medical Imaging, University of Exeter, United Kingdom

Research Methods for Student Radiographers: A Survival Guide
Christopher M. Hayre, Xiaoming Zheng

For more information about this series, please visit: https://www.crcpress.com/Medical-Imaging-in-Practice/book-series/MIIP

Computed Tomography
A Primer for Radiographers

Edited by
Shayne Chau and Christopher M Hayre

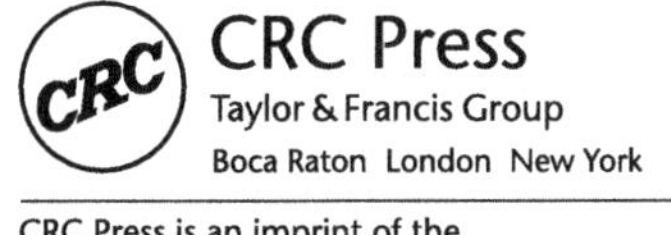

CRC Press is an imprint of the
Taylor & Francis Group, an **informa** business

First edition published 2023
by CRC Press
6000 Broken Sound Parkway NW, Suite 300, Boca Raton, FL 33487-2742

and by CRC Press
4 Park Square, Milton Park, Abingdon, Oxon, OX14 4RN

CRC Press is an imprint of Taylor & Francis Group, LLC

Library of Congress Cataloging-in-Publication Data
Names: Hayre, Christopher M., editor. | Chau, Shayne, editor.
Title: Computed tomography : a practical guide / edited by Shayne Chau and Christopher M. Hayre.
Description: First edition. | Boca Raton : CRC Press, [2023] |
Series: Medical imagining in practice | Includes bibliographical references and index. |
Summary: "This book aims to provide a holistic picture of computed tomography, focusing on the multi-faceted elements of radiation physics, imaging protocols and image evaluation. It will provide readers with insight into practical and innovative technical approaches within the general imaging field, backed up with existing evidence-based research"—Provided by publisher.
Identifiers: LCCN 2022012248 | ISBN 9780367675493 (pbk) |
ISBN 9780367677244 (hbk) | ISBN 9781003132554 (ebk)
Subjects: LCSH: Tomography.
Classification: LCC RC78.7.T6 C64165 2023 | DDC 616.07/57–dc23/eng/20220322
LC record available at https://lccn.loc.gov/2022012248

ISBN: 978-0-367-67724-4 (hbk)
ISBN: 978-0-367-67549-3 (pbk)
ISBN: 978-1-003-13255-4 (ebk)

DOI: 10.1201/9781003132554

Typeset in Times
by codeMantra

Dr Christopher Hayre would like to dedicate this book to Evelynn, with eternal love from Mummy, Daddy, and sisters, Ayva and Ellena.

Shayne Chau would like to dedicate this book to his parents and brother. To his fiancee, Jo, for whom he can find no words that can express his endless affection and gratitude.

Contents

SECTION 4 Cross-Sectional Anatomy

SECTION 5 Imaging Procedures

Acknowledgements

The editors would like to thank the contributing authors. Your commitment to this book reflects the hard work and determination of generating a primer text for radiographers. It has been a pleasure for us to work with you and bring together this collection of highly informative chapters. This work demonstrates the importance of computed tomography within the medical imaging environment. Finally, the editors agree that this has been an exciting and prosperous project, which we hope readers will enjoy and utilize.

Preface

The justification of this edited textbook is the need to focus on the role of computed tomography (CT) for an array of audiences, but more specifically to undergraduate and postgraduate radiographers or CT technologists, the former title will be used throughout. This book draws on the international expertise on important topics such as physical principles of CT, radiobiology, radiation protection and optimization, patient care, cross-sectional anatomy and imaging protocols for body regions and image evaluations of common pathologies. The aim of this book is to not only review innovation and contemporary practice in CT but also cover image evaluations of CT with the goal of delivering high-quality care and safety.

This edited book begins by introducing the foundations, physical principles and patient care in the context of CT. The recent innovation and importance of technologies used to acquire CT images of diagnostic quality are discussed in Section 1. These are essential for understanding the importance of dose optimization to patients worldwide. The patient care aspect will be further supported by evidence-based literature on effective communication methods, patient education, informed written consent, patient education, and assessment of laboratory results and vital signs. The editors draw from recent publications and clinical expertise, supported with the growing trend of technological advances utilized within CT. Each chapter will underscore the multifaceted use and application of each 'sub theme' pertinent to CT to present a single text with critical information for both students and practitioners. Section 4 introduces the readers to cross-sectional anatomy, an integral aspect of the radiographer's role. The cross-sectional anatomy sections in this textbook are intended to be used as a supplementary resource for radiographers. For a full range of cross-sectional images, the reader should refer to other anatomical textbooks. CT protocols vary between each site and between each scanner. As there are no universally accepted protocols, the reader should use the protocols with adjustments made for the individuality of the patient, the type of the scanner and the radiologists' or physicians' preferences. We anticipate this to remain a key text for any undergraduate and post-graduate radiography and/or CT student as it will incorporate a holistic view of the profession transnationally whilst identifying key knowledge and understanding pertinent to the CT practice.

This book aims to provide a holistic picture of CT, focusing on the multi-faceted elements of radiation physics, to imaging protocols and image evaluation. It will provide readers with an insight into both contemporary and innovative technical and practical approaches within the general imaging field, backed up with existing evidence-based research. This is not a text on CT physics and imaging protocols alone but on the application and potential for such technological and radiation protection advances within the CT field. The text, which includes most relevant technical and pathophysiological premises, also clearly signposts to learning points and pitfalls. Throughout the text, there is also an emphasis on image evaluation, with guidance on the recognition of normal, benign, and malignant pathologies and clear instruction on learning points and pitfalls. Given the increasing recognition of advanced scope of practice and professional capabilities in the field of medical radiation science, a focus on CT image evaluation is also a must. It is intended that this text will enhance and offer original discussions surrounding the interconnectivity of the technology, research, and patient care in CT.

Mr Shayne Chau

Dr Christopher M Hayre

Editors

Shayne Chau is a Senior Lecturer in Medical Imaging at the University of Canberra. He is currently an editorial board member of the Journal of Medical Imaging and Radiation Sciences. He has authored and co-authored journal articles in the field of computed tomography, neuroimaging for Parkinson's disease and higher education.

Christopher M Hayre is a Senior Lecturer at the University of Exeter in the United Kingdom and Senior Fellow for the School of Health and Sport Sciences at the University of Suffolk. He has published both qualitative and quantitative refereed papers and brought together several books in the field of medical imaging, health research, technology, and ethnography.

Contributors

Arjun Burlakoti
Lecturer in Anatomy (and Neuroanatomy)
UniSA Allied Health and Human Performance, City East Campus
University of South Australia
South Australia, Australia

Shayne Chau
Faculty of Health
University of Canberra
Canberra, Australia

Rob Davidson
Professor of Medical Imaging
Faculty of Health
University of Canberra
Canberra, Australia

Christopher M Hayre
Senior Lecturer in Medical Imaging
University of Exeter
Exeter, United Kingdom

Lynne Hazell
Medical Imaging and Radiation Sciences
University of Johannesburg
Johannesburg Gauteng, South Africa

Matthew Jarvis
South Australia Medical Imaging
Adelaide, South Australia, Australia

Lars Kruse
Dr Jones and Partners
Medical Imaging
South Australia, Australia

Nicola Massy-Westropp
Senior Lecturer in Anatomy (and Neuroanatomy)
UniSA Allied Health and Human Performance, City East Campus
University of South Australia
South Australia, Australia

Iain M MacDonald
Institute of Health
University of Cumbria
Carlisle, United Kingdom

Gordon Mander
Dept Medical Imaging
Toowoomba Hospital, Darling Downs Health, School of Clinical Sciences
Queensland University of Technology
Brisbane, Queensland, Australia

Tarni Nelson
Charles Sturt University
New South Wales, Australia

Flamur Sahiti
East Kent Hospital Trust
Queen Elizabeth Queen Mother Hospital
Margate, United Kingdom

Euclid Seeram
Monash University
Melbourne, Australia
and
Charles Sturt University
New South Wales, Australia
and
University of Canberra
Australian Capital Territory, Australia

Debbie Starkey
Faculty of Health
Queensland University of Technology
Queensland, Australia

Deb Watson
Sunshine Coast University Hospital
Queensland, Australia

Harsha Wechalekar
Lecturer in Anatomy and Neuroanatomy
UniSA Allied Health and Human Performance, City East Campus
University of South Australia
South Australia, Australia

Section 1

Physics, Principles and Radiobiology in Computed Tomography

1 Computed Tomography in Medical Imaging

Shayne Chau
University of Canberra

Christopher M Hayre
University of Exeter

COMPUTED TOMOGRAPHY (CT) IN THE MEDICAL SETTING SPACE

The list of computed tomography (CT) imaging protocols/examinations being used in clinical settings is arguably endless. This is apparent, especially when radiologists and requesting practitioners have their own special protocols or preferences. The most common CT protocols/examinations ordered across all medical settings (in-patient, out-patient and emergency patient) are

- CT Head without Contrast;
- CT Abdomen and Pelvis with Contrast;
- CT Chest with Contrast;
- CT Abdomen and Pelvis without Contrast (for renal stones);
- CT Angiography Chest for Pulmonary Embolism and
- CT Cervical Spine (for trauma and for pain management).

CT head *without* contrast itself represents nearly 25% of all CT scans performed at most institutions. CT abdomen and pelvis *with* contrast represents approximately 20%. These six scans combined account for about 75% of all CT scans in a calendar year.

CT was clinically introduced in 1971 and was limited to axial imaging of the brain in neuroradiology. CT was then developed into a versatile 3D whole body imaging modality for a wide range of applications, for example, oncology, vascular radiology, cardiology, traumatology and interventional radiology. Nowadays, CT is typically used for (i) diagnosis and follow-up studies of patients, (ii) planning of radiotherapy treatment (performed by our radiation therapy colleagues) and (iii) screening of healthy subpopulations with specific risk factors (such as cardiac scoring, lung cancer screening and bowl cancer screening). For radiotherapy planning, dedicated CT scanners offer extra wide bores allowing CT scans to be performed with a larger field of view. For oncology purposes, integration of a CT scanner with PET or SPECT has allowed for multi-modality imaging applications. This has been a breakthrough in the molecular imaging world. Other new achievements for imaging purposes include dual-source CT (a CT scanner with two X-ray tubes operating at different voltages),

DOI: 10.1201/9781003132554-2

volumetric CT (large row of detectors allowing the entire organ to be scanned within one rotation) and spectral CT (employing two separate X-ray photon energy spectra, allowing visualization of materials that have different attenuation properties at different energies). Below is a summary of historical CT milestones.

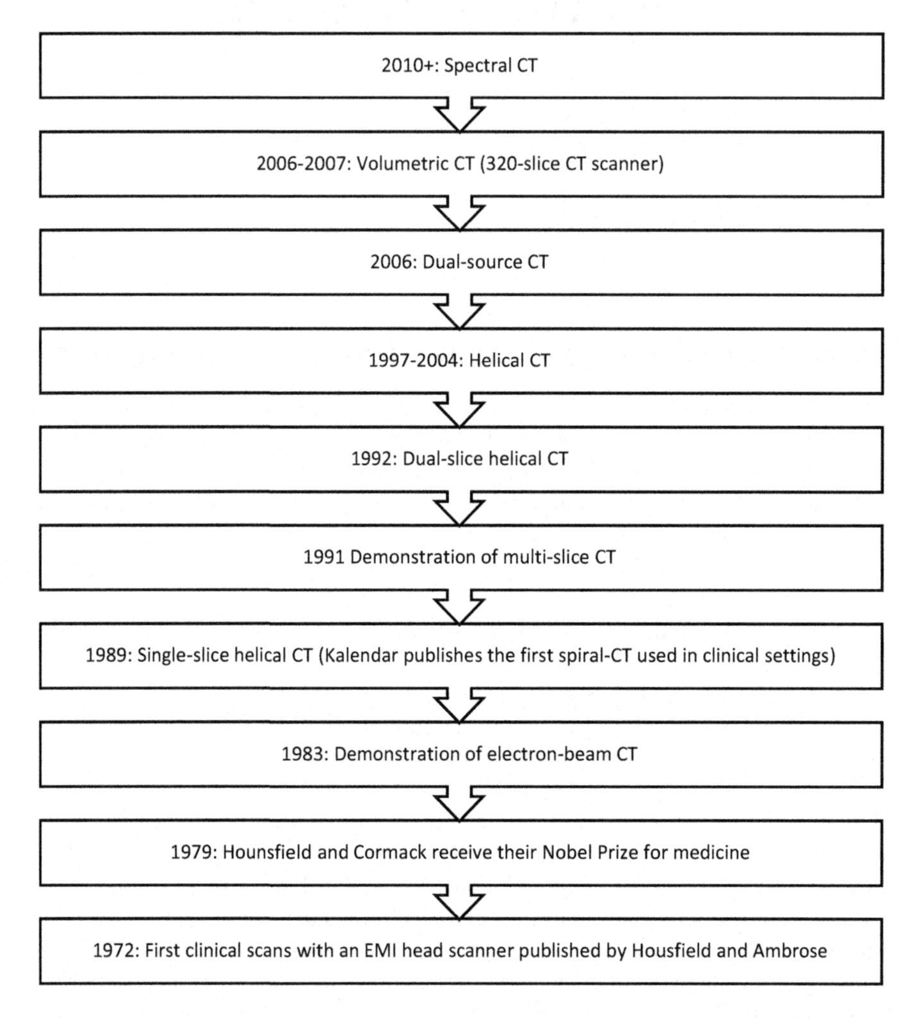

The imaging principles of CT imaging are similar to general radiography whereby differential X-ray attenuation is of interest. As the X-ray beam passes through the patient, a large fraction of the individual X-ray photons is absorbed by the body or scattered out of the scanner. The remaining X-ray photons pass through the body and reach the detector. This therefore creates the digital profile of the patient's internal anatomy. This will be further discussed in the forthcoming chapters. In short, a CT scanner detects and displays different tissues based on their density:

- High-density materials, such as bone and metal, appear as light gray or white on the resultant CT image as they attenuate a significant fraction of the original X-ray beam and appear as light gray or white on the CT image.
- Low-density materials, such as air and fat, on the other hand, appear as dark gray or black as they do not attenuate as much as high-density materials.

The review of physical principles of CT and radiobiology in Section 1 should enable the readers to fully understand the foundation and the clinical use of CT in medical imaging. Section 1 provides an overview of dose optimization in clinical settings and how CT radiographers can optimize their radiation dose while maintaining high-quality images. Section 3 provides a perspective of patient care in CT in the context of Australia. This section explores the multi-facet interaction with patients in the CT department. The readers are then introduced to cross-sectional anatomy in Section 4 with key structures of the head and neck and the thoracic, abdominal, pelvic and musculoskeletal systems. In Sections 5 and 6, the readers will find CT imaging protocols and CT image evaluation for different regions. While there is a rationale to the arrangement of the book, the readers may want to prefer to go to appropriate sections for those questions that may arise about CT cross-sectional anatomy, protocols and image evaluations in their daily practice.

2 Physics and Principles of Computed Tomography

Rob Davidson

CONTENTS

INTRODUCTION

Computed tomography (CT) was invented and developed by Sir Godfrey Hounsfield and Allan Cormack. These two people shared the 1979 Noble Prize in medicine and physiology for their work in developing CT. Since then, both the clinical uses and

DOI: 10.1201/9781003132554-3

technological advances of CT have rapidly grown. CT is now widely recognized as an important clinical imaging tool used in the diagnosis of many patients' clinical conditions and that CT can also assist in the management and treatment of many medical conditions.

This chapter will provide a brief overview of the physical principles and the technical aspects of CT. CT operators, whether diagnostic radiographers/radiological technologists or other clinical users, must have a solid understanding of the physical principles and technical aspects of CT. CT has the potential to deliver high ionizing radiations dose to the patient being scanned and CT, as a diagnostic imaging modality, delivers more radiation dose than any other clinical imaging modality. More details on radiation dose from CT are found in Chapter 3. CT scanning parameters need to be optimized in relation to obtaining the highest possible image quality at the lowest possible radiation dose. Given these important considerations, CT radiographers/radiological technologists and other CT operators must not just be button pushers or blindly follow pre-setup scanning protocols, they must understand how all scanning and image reconstruction parameters link together to enable optimized imaging for the benefit of their patients.

WHY COMPUTED TOMOGRAPHY?

CT acquires axial images or images in the transverse plane of the body. Figure 2.1 shows the orientation of an axial image through a patient that is lying supine on the CT table. More details will follow on how axial images are acquired. However, from

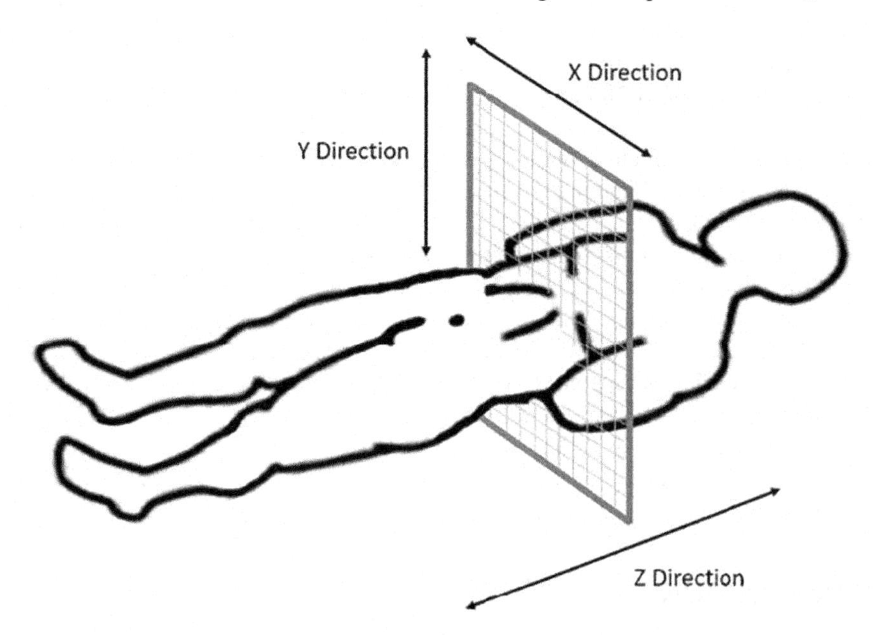

FIGURE 2.1 The axial plane of the body is shown in relation to the long axis of the body. In CT, the acquired axial image will have X and Y dimensions and represent a thickness of anatomy in the Z direction.

these CT axial images, images in other planes and 3D representations of the body can be reconstructed and displayed. CT used to be called computerized axial tomography or CAT scans. Given CT's ability to reconstruct and display images other than axial images, the "axial" or "A" has been dropped from the name (other than in TV programmes and movies that perpetuate the old CAT scan name).

Planar or general X-ray imaging represents three dimensions of the patient's anatomy, though typically the image is of a much larger area of anatomy than a single axial CT image. A planar X-ray image is created by having X-ray photons pass through the patient's anatomy where some photons are attenuated (stopped/absorbed or scatted) by the anatomy and the photons that aren't attenuated exit the patient and are recorded on a detector or image plate. Planar X-ray can be thought of as compressing the three dimensions of the patient's anatomy onto a two-dimensional (2D) image plate or receptor. The 2D X-ray image represents the three-dimensional (3D) anatomy that is irradiated in the X-ray field.

A single axial CT image or slice also represents a 3D section of the patient's anatomy. The third dimension is the width of the CT slice; however, in CT, there will be multiple slices which typically are less than 1 mm in thickness. Multiple thin slices then allow better visualization of the patient's third dimension. Note though, a single CT slice is a 2D representation of a 3D anatomical section, albeit a thin anatomical section. A commonly used analogy for CT slices is a sliced loaf of bread. Figure 2.2 shows a sliced loaf of bread, with a slice when viewed on end representing the X and Y dimensions of the image and the thickness of the loaf's slice being the Z dimension of the image.

It is sometimes stated that the most important aspect of CT is to overcome the issue of planar X-ray where the third dimension of the anatomy is compressed. However, the most important advantage of CT is its vastly improved *contrast resolution* compared to planar X-ray. Simply stated, planar X-ray is not the best imaging for soft-tissue anatomy where a good contrast resolution is needed. The use of CT in medical imaging vastly improves the visualization of soft-tissue anatomy compared to planar X-ray. The first-generation CT scanners were able to visualize the brain and

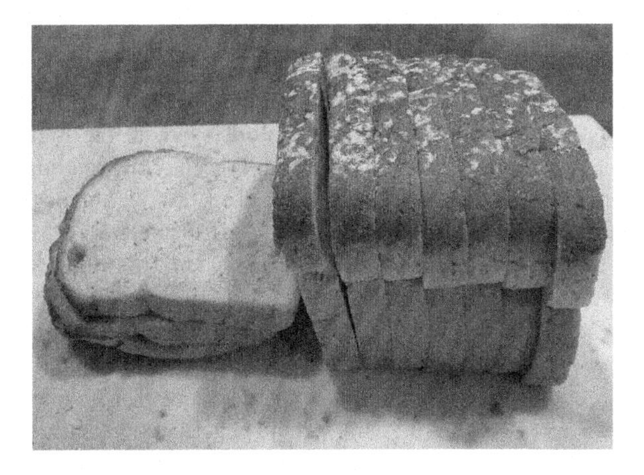

FIGURE 2.2 A loaf of sliced bread, often used as an analogy for CT slices.

fluid in the ventricles of the skull, and these had never been seen previously in X-ray imaging without the aid of some form of contrast agent.

In X-ray imaging, contrast resolution is a measure of the differences in attenuation of the tissues that can be visualized in the image. For tissues to be visualized with differing image densities in planar X-ray imaging, there needs to be approximately a 5% or greater attenuation differences in those tissues. In CT imaging, typically the attenuation differences needed are 0.3%–0.5% or greater. The visualization of such small differences in attenuation of tissues is dependent on many factors, including the amount of X-rays used (the radiation dose), the size of the pixels, the noise of the system scan reconstruction type and other factors that are beyond the discussion in this chapter.

CT does have disadvantages. The radiation dose used to acquire the CT slices, and to be able to provide that level of contrast resolution, is high compared to most other X-ray imaging modalities. As such, optimization of the radiation dose and image quality is an important consideration when establishing and modifying CT protocols and tailoring the exposure parameters for the individual patient's CT examination.

So why CT? CT has improved visualization of tissues in that it only requires a small attenuation difference between the tissues; *and* CT only visualizes a thin section of the patient's anatomy so it overcomes, to a great extent, the 2D compression of a 3D structure. Another advantage that will be briefly mentioned later in this chapter is that these small thickness CT slices can be "stacked" together to create images in anatomical planes other than the original axial plane; and 3D images can be produced.

CT INSTRUMENTS

CT requires some similar instruments to those used in planar or general X-ray imaging. The focus of this section will be to discuss the differences of these instruments used in CT compared to planar X-ray and to briefly introduce the other instruments needed to create a CT image.

MAJOR CT COMPONENTS

As with all X-ray imaging, the three principal components are an X-ray tube, to generate X-ray photons; a high voltage generator, to create the high voltages and electrical current for the X-ray tube; and a means of detecting, reading and recoding the X-ray photons that exist in the patient. These three main components are housed in the X-ray gantry. Figure 2.3 is a photograph of the CT gantry and the table. As will be discussed in more detail later, these three components continuously rotate inside the gantry around the patient.

In CT, the selected X-ray tube voltages used are limited to a few peak kilo-Voltages (kVp), with common kVps of 80, 100, 120 and 140 kVp. The reason for this reduced selection is discussed later in Hounsfield units/CT numbers sub-section. One main difference between a CT scanning and general X-ray is the amount of heat produced by the X-ray tubes. CT scanning requires longer X-ray exposure times, for example, this being multiple seconds for a scan through the patient's abdomen

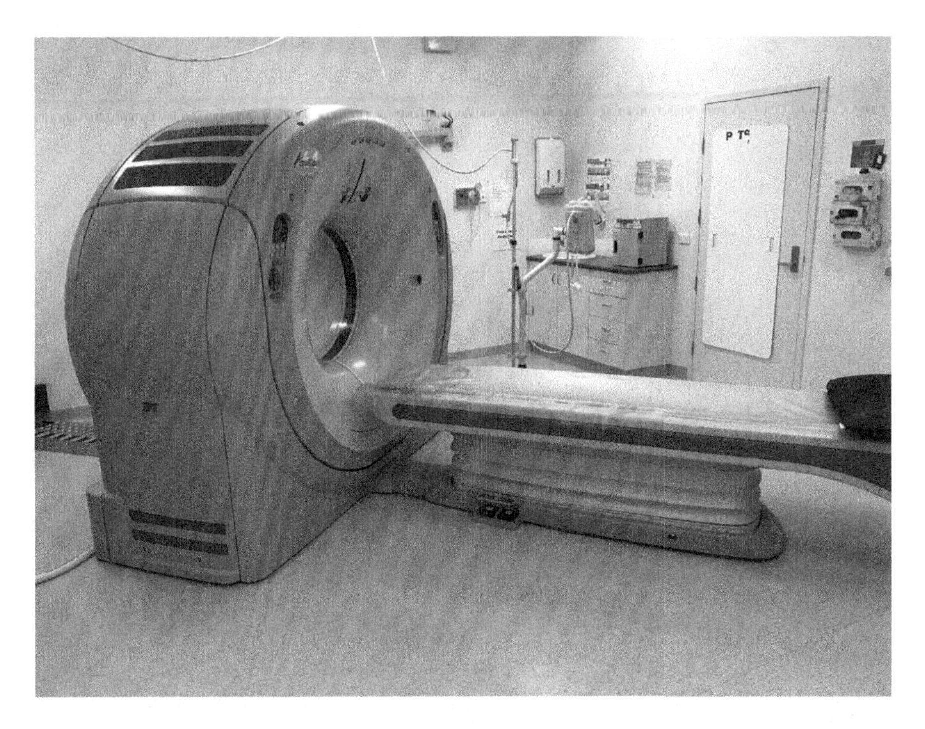

FIGURE 2.3 CT gantry and CT table. (Image with thanks to Mr. Jens Loberg, Goulburn Base Hospital, Australia.)

compared to millisecond exposure times for a planar X-ray image of the same patient. As such, the heat storage capacity and heat dissipation rates for CT X-ray tubes exceeded those of general X-ray tubes. Different CT manufacturers have different approaches to solve the heat issue in CT scanning.

All X-ray tubes produce polychromatic X-ray beams. A polychromatic X-ray beam contains X-ray photons of many different energies, and in CT, this can cause issues and can create artefacts in the image (see the Artefacts section towards the end of this chapter). CT X-ray beams need to have higher levels of filtration to remove lower energy X-ray photons. The filtration, similar to planar X-ray, is achieved by using thickness of aluminium (Al) and/or copper (Cu) materials, though typically in CT these are thicker than that used in planar X-ray.

A further issue in CT is that most cross-sectional areas of the human anatomy, i.e., in the axial plane, are ovate in shape or close to circular. When the X-ray photons have passed through the centre of an ovate object, the distance travelled is greater than that at the edges of the object. Shaped filters, such as bowtie filters, are used to increase the attenuation of the X-ray photons at the edge of the X-ray beam; so an X-ray beam of more uniform exit intensity is created. The use of a bowtie filter helps create a more uniform appearance of the final CT image. The bowtie filter can be removed or inserted into the X-ray beam, depending on the clinical examination. A diagrammatic representation of a bowtie filter can be seen in Figure 2.4.

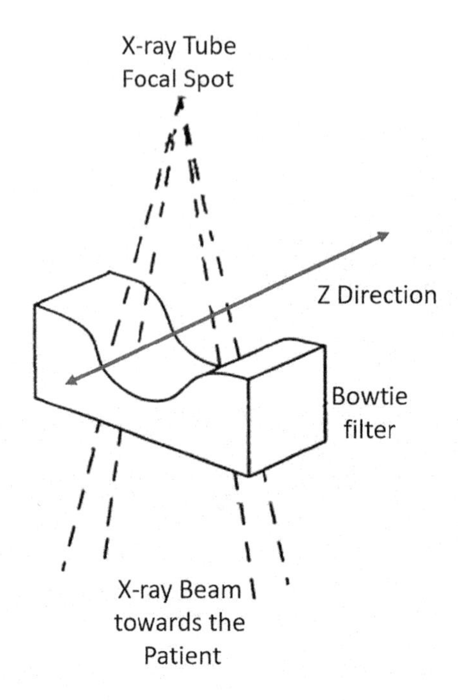

FIGURE 2.4 A diagrammatic representation of a bowtie filter used in CT.

With continuous rotation of the X-ray tube and detectors inside the CT gantry, the high voltage generator must be housed inside the CT gantry and rotated around the patient with the tube and detectors. This means the high voltage generator must be relatively small, and to achieve such size, high-frequency generators are used.

X-ray photons are generated in the X-ray tube, travel through the patient and are attenuated by the patient's anatomy. The X-ray photons exit the patient and are detected and recorded. Unlike planar X-ray imaging plates, CT detectors are a single row of detectors. Multiple rows of detectors are used so as to obtain more than one axial image (slice) per rotation of the X-ray tube and detectors. In a single row of detectors, typically there will be 900+ individual detectors in the row. At each point in time, or more commonly used terminology is at each gantry angle of the X-ray tube and detectors, the row of detectors records the exit beam's intensity at those 900+ points. The 900+ X-ray intensities are converted to an electrical signal which is then digitized and stored in a computer. For every given gantry angle, a row of 900+ digital values are created. These single row or digital values are called a slice profile. More details on slice profiles will be discussed in the section on CT image reconstruction.

CT detectors now have multiple rows of detectors. Early CT scanners mainly had one row of detectors, though some had two rows. With each rotation of the X-ray tube and detectors, one or two images were able to be obtained. CT manufacturers now only produce CT scanners with at least 64 rows of detectors, and now, 512 or more rows of detectors. It is not as simple to state that a CT scanner with 512 rows of detectors will create 512 CT image slices. The reason will be briefly covered later in this section; however, it is due to the patient being moved on the table during the rotation of the X-ray tube and detectors. This is called a helical or spiral acquisition, compared to an axial acquisition when the patient is stationary during the gantry rotation.

An important characteristic of the CT detectors is their detection of the X-ray photons and the conversion efficiency of a photon detection to an electrical signal. Detection and conversion efficiency has been and is a major focus of CT manufacturers. The greater the detection and conversion efficiency of the detectors, the lesser the radiation dose that is needed to create a high signal-to-noise electrical signal, and importantly, less dose to the patient.

Other CT Components

The CT gantry, as shown in Figure 2.3, allows the X-ray tube, detectors and generator to rotate around the patient. Obtaining slice profiles, the row of intensity values at each gantry angle, at 360° around the patient, is a crucial aspect of CT. The mechanism to allow continuous rotation and, at the same time, allow electrical currents to the gantry component and send data back to a computer is achieved using slip rings. Slip rings allow the transfer of an electric signal, and hence data, to and from a stationary to a moving object, in the case of rotating objects. The advent and use of slip rings in CT scanning have reduced the scanning time per rotation from seconds to now 0.3 seconds or less per rotation. With this rotation time and the use of multiple detectors, CT scanning examination time for most CT scans is a few minutes duration compared to 30–60 minutes scan times. Patient's comfort and imaging efficiency is improved.

The conversion of the number of X-ray photons being received at the detector and then converted to digital information that can be used in a computer is achieved with a CT component called the digital acquisition system (DAS). The DAS is essentially an analogue to digital conversion (ADC) system and process. An ADC takes the analogue electrical signal from each detector and converts it to a digital value that can be used to create a digital CT image. The DAS components are the detectors, the ADC and the connection to the computer for data storage and image reconstruction via the slip rings.

The CT unit also includes a CT table. The table has to be able to support a large patient, and importantly, must not attenuate the X-ray beam at a significant level. Carbon fibres are often used in the manufacture of the CT table as they have both strength and low attenuation characteristics.

The computer: The CT scanner incorporates the word "computer" in its name. The CT scanners were developed and used in the late 1960s and throughout the 1970s when revolutionary medical equipment with the computer was incorporated into the system. As will be discussed in more detail later, the computer is needed to do the mathematical calculations that are needed to turn the scan profiles, the data captured by the detectors and converted to digital data, into a digital image. Typical CT computers now have additional functions. Some of these are

- review, display and manipulation of the CT images;
- local storage of the CT images;

- connection to the picture archive and communication system to store the images so that they can be retrieved with patient images and information, and then be able to transfer the images around the hospital or potentially, anywhere in the world;
- convert the thin axial CT slices into images that represent other planes of the body or 3D images or cine images.

DIGITAL IMAGES AND DISPLAY

Digital Images – A Brief Overview

A digital image can be thought of as 2D array of numbers, as shown in Figure 2.5. The numbers are the pixel (picture element) values. The pixels in a CT image are called Hounsfield units (HU) or CT numbers. A single HU or CT number in a CT image represents an amount of X-ray attenuation at a location in the patient's body. In CT, a pixel represents a 3D volume of anatomy in the patient and is known as a volume element of voxel. The depth of the voxel is the slice thickness.

100	101	105	110	113	113	111	108	112	114	113	114	120	133	143
98	103	106	104	107	113	117	113	123	131	136	138	143	152	162
109	114	115	114	122	135	148	144	145	155	167	168	163	165	174
137	139	139	139	146	160	169	161	161	167	175	180	179	178	178
155	163	171	176	176	172	170	190	186	181	175	181	187	189	184
166	163	166	171	180	183	184	172	182	187	183	174	162	140	118
188	189	193	195	187	174	160	173	159	124	80	48	41	40	40
173	168	162	152	129	100	80	40	40	42	40	40	40	40	40
102	72	48	40	40	40	40	47	44	42	42	44	40	43	48
40	40	41	40	42	41	40	47	40	40	42	43	40	40	41
40	40	40	41	40	40	40	41	40	40	40	40	40	40	40
40	41	40	40	40	40	41	40	40	40	40	40	41	40	40
40	40	41	40	41	40	40	40	40	40	40	40	40	40	40
40	40	40	40	40	40	41	40	40	40	40	40	40	40	41
40	40	41	41	40	40	40	40	40	40	40	41	40	40	40

FIGURE 2.5 A digital image array of number. The pixel values are located in rows and columns to provide spatial information of the pixels. The arrows represent that there are more rows and columns not displayed. A typical CT image will have 512, or sometimes 1,024, rows and columns.

A digital image is always rectangular; however, the acquired CT images are square – reconstructed or reformatted CT images can be rectangular. An acquired CT image will typically have 512 rows and 512 columns or 1,024 rows and 1,024 columns of pixels. The size of each pixel is determined by XY dimensions of the X-ray beam as it rotates around the patient. This is called the scan field of view (SFOV). SFOV will be discussed in more detail later in this chapter.

Each pixel value is an integer, that is, it must be a whole number and cannot have a decimal point value as part of the number. Most CT pixels have a maximum value of 3,071 and a minimum value of 1,024. That is, they are 12-bit depth and are signed (meaning both positive and negative integer values are possible). Twelve-bit depth means two raised to the power of 12 (i.e., 2^{12} or 2 multiplied by 2, 12 times) and there are 4,096 possible CT number values for each pixel. The ability to have negative values, not common in digital images, is important in CT and will be discussed more later.

Display of Digital Images

A CT scan can be considered as an array or matrix numbers stored in a computer. To be meaningful, the scans' values, the HU or CT numbers, must be displayed so that the viewer can perceive what the numbers represent. In a CT scan, the HU or CT numbers represent an amount of X-ray attenuation in the voxel. A voxel is a volume of tissue in the patient determined by the pixel's X and Y dimensions and the scan/slice thickness in the Z direction. HU or CT numbers have a linear scale from no or very little X-ray attenuation, e.g., air, to a large amount of X-ray attenuation, e.g., dense bone or metal. Due to this, the HU or CT numbers scale then needs to be displayed using a linear scale.

A possible way of displaying an array of values is using a 3D plot. An example of a CT scan being displayed using a 3D plot is shown in Figure 2.6. In this plot, the HU or CT numbers are represented by a height on the Z-axis of the plot. The Z-axis then represents X-ray attenuation and would have values from −1,024 to 3,071.

Figure 2.6 is not the best way to represent and display HU or CT numbers. A small change of HU values from one anatomical location to an adjacent anatomical location will be lost in the large Z-axis scale. A better way to display HU or CT numbers is an image. Figure 2.7 shows the same CT values as in Figure 2.6, however displayed as an image. A single CT axial scan then can be best displayed and considered as a CT image.

The display colours used in a CT image need to have a linear scale. The best approach for displaying linear scale of values in images is using a grey scale. For CT and X-ray images, white represents a high amount of attenuation and black represents no or very little attenuation. The white to black scale is then easy to visualize and understand what the whites, greys and blacks represent.

An issue in displaying CT values in an image is that HU or CT numbers can have values of −1,024 to 3,071. In a digital image, displaying all of these values then would mean the displayed image contrast would be very low. An example of this using the same images as in Figure 2.7 can be seen in Figure 2.8.

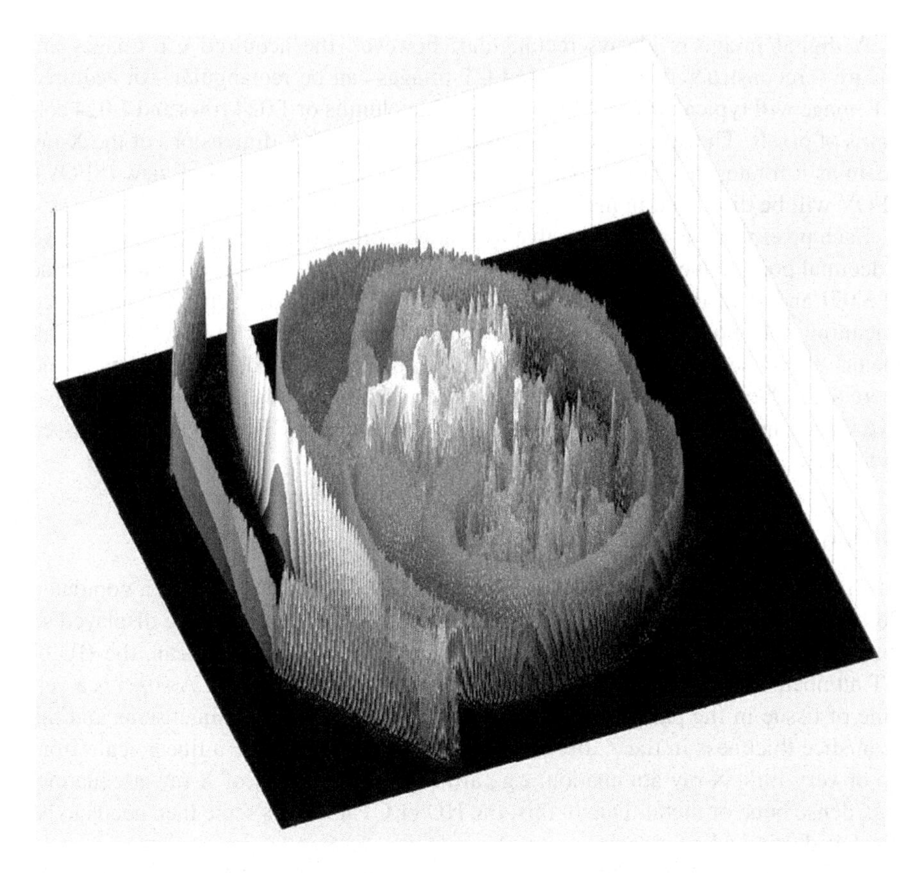

FIGURE 2.6 A CT scan displayed using a 3D plot.

Window Width/Window Level

CT images need to be able to be displayed so that the user can alter the displayed image contrast and brightness. This will aid the user to see differences in X-ray attenuation as depicted by shades of grey in the image. Changing image brightness and contrast is done using a computer function called look-up tables (LUTs). In CT, the LUT process used is known as window width (WW) and window level (WL) or window centre (WC). By altering the WW/WL, the user sets the upper and lower HU value boundaries. At and above the upper boundary, all HU values will appear white in the displayed image. At and below the lower boundary, all HU values will appear black. The HU values in the image between the upper and low boundaries will be in various shades of grey.

The more common way of describing WW/WL use is that the WW sets the range of displayed HU values between white and black, and the WL (or WC) value is the HU number midway between the upper and lower boundaries, that is, the value at the centre of the WW range. These two numbers then describe the displayed image contrast and brightness. For example, a WW/WL of 100/40 would display the CT image with a relatively high contrast and a WW/WL of 1,000/40 would display the

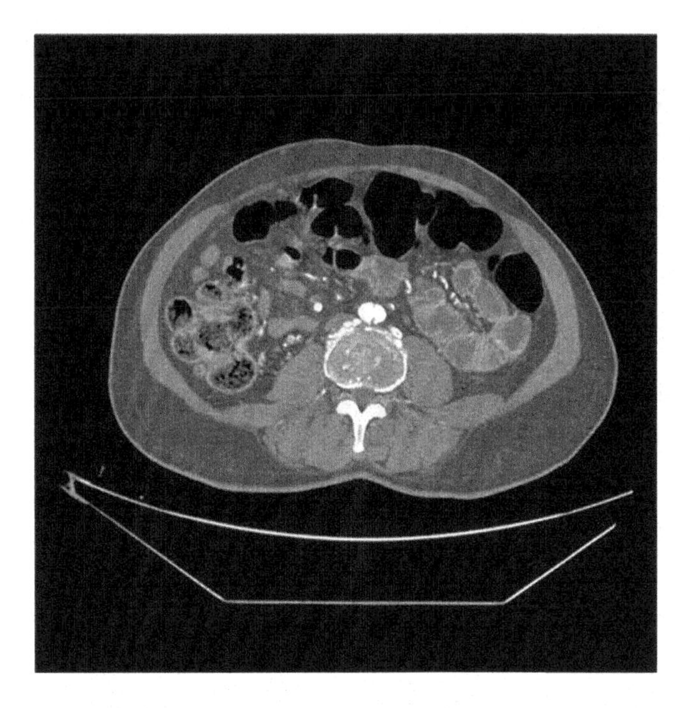

FIGURE 2.7 A CT scan displayed as an image.

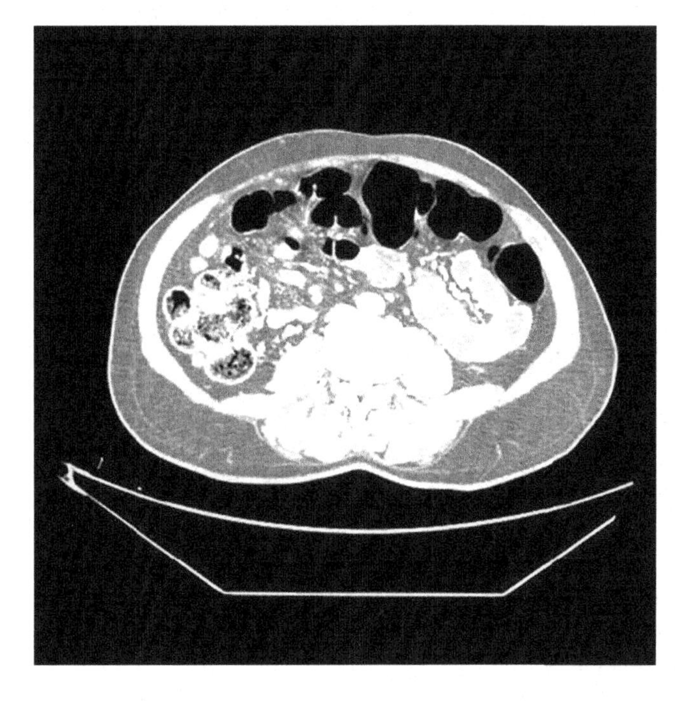

FIGURE 2.8 A CT scan displayed with low contrast. Subtle differences in X-ray attenuation are lost.

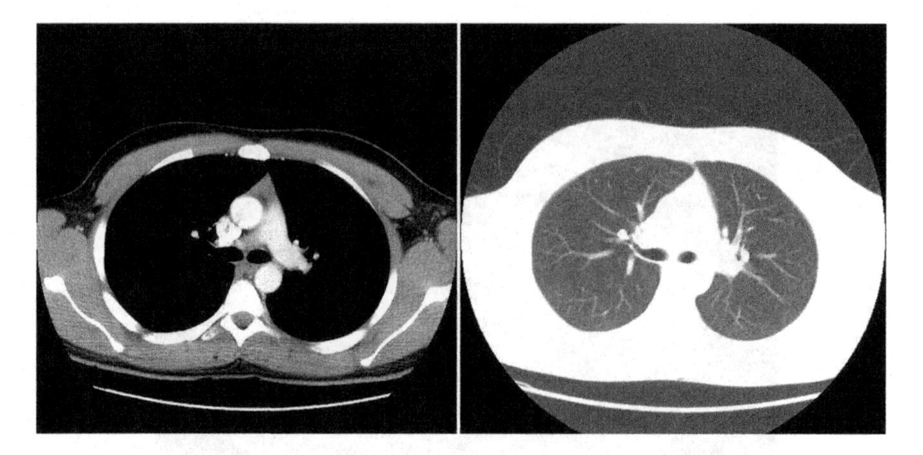

FIGURE 2.9 The same CT scan is displayed with two different WW/WL settings. The WW/WL on the left is 300/40 and shows the mediastinum and muscles. The WW/WL on the right is 1,000/-750 and shows the lungs.

CT image with a relatively low contrast. A CT image displayed with a WW/WL of 100/200 would have more high HU values displayed in the range and the image would appear more white or brighter. A comparison of the same CT image at differing WW/WLs can be seen in Figure 2.9.

Figure 2.10a–c shows the plots of the LUTs at differing levels of WW and WL. The HU values of the CT image are plotted on the X-axis and how those values will be displayed from black to white is plotted on the Y-axis. In Figure 2.10a, HU values in the CT image below −150 will be displayed as black and the HU values above 250 will appear white in the displayed image.

Radiologists and other clinicians may need to measure the HU unit values, for example, of an ovate appearance in the liver to help determine the type of lesion. An important understanding is that changing the WW/WL levels of the displayed image does not change the image HU values.

IMAGE CAPTURE AND RECONSTRUCTION

CT Image Capture

In CT, as with other X-ray imaging modalities, the initial number of photons exiting the X-ray tube is dependent on the setting of the kVp, the tube current measured in milliAmps (mA) and the filtration used in the X-ray beam. As will be discussed later in this section, this is the original X-ray intensity (I_0). The time of a single 360° rotation of the X-ray tube and detectors around the patient, the scan time, will provide seconds value of the milliAmpere-seconds (mAs) of the single scan slice. Typical current scan times are less than 0.5 seconds.

CT image capture is achieved by irradiating the patient with a narrow beam, in the Z direction, of X-ray photons of intensity I_0. The X-ray beam has an XY direction width to cover the detectors and is known as a fan beam. Some of the X-ray photons

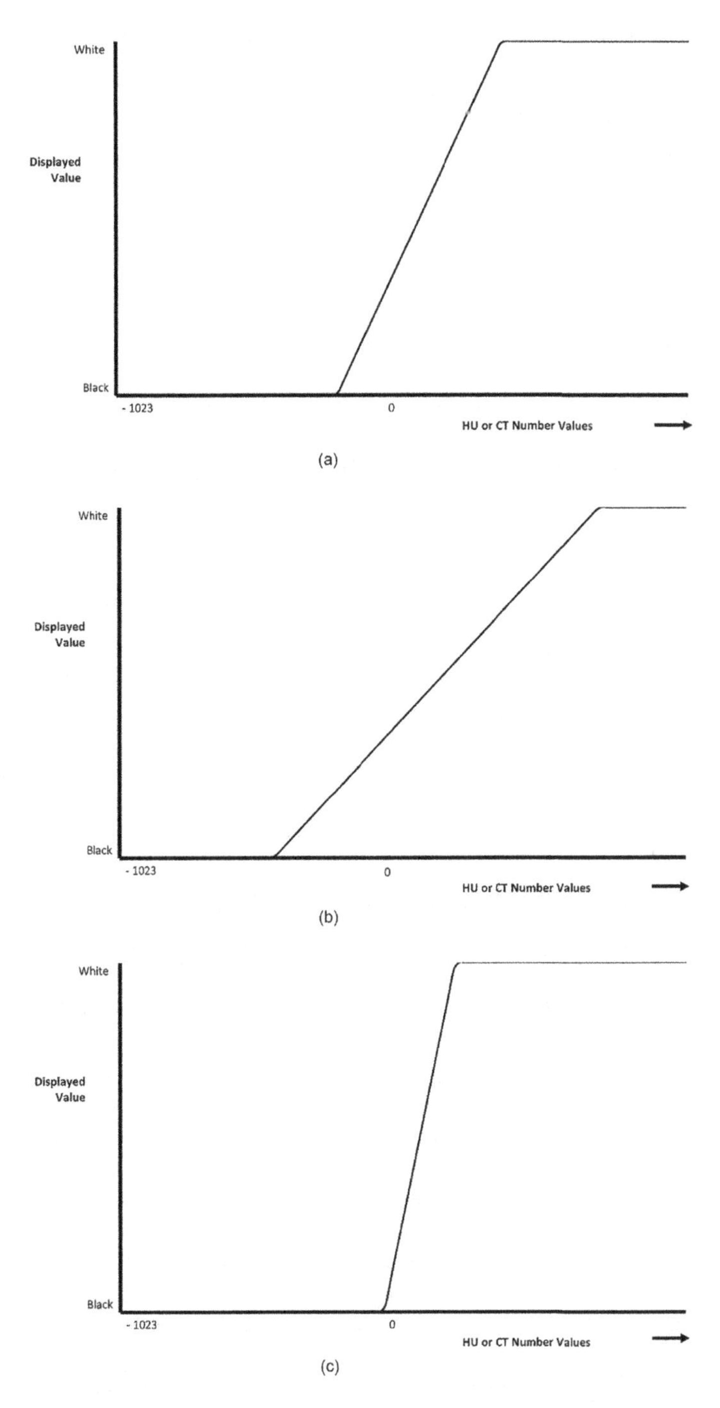

FIGURE 2.10 (a) WW/WL of 400/50. It would provide a moderate displayed contrast and may be used for displaying soft tissue. (b) WW/WL of 1,000/-450. It would provide low displayed contrast and could be used for displaying lungs. (c) WW/WL of 70/40. It would provide high displayed contrast and could be used for a uniform organ such as liver.

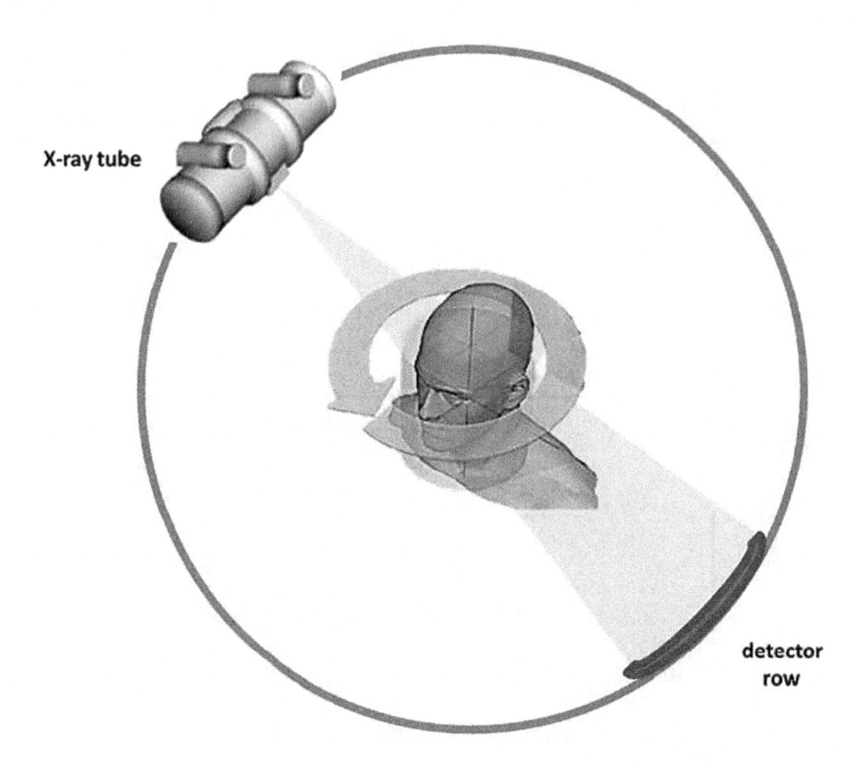

FIGURE 2.11 The X-ray tube and a single row of detectors shown rotating around a patient's head. (Image with thanks to Dr Haney Alsleem, Imam Abdulrahman Bin Faisal University, Saudi Arabia.)

will be attenuated in the patient and others will exit the patient. The exiting photons will be measured and recorded by each detector in the row of detectors. Figure 2.11 depicts the rotation of the tube and a single row of detectors around a patient's head. The measured intensity at each detector is given the notation of the letter *I*. A row of intensity values, *I*, is called a scan profile.

In the current CT scanners, multiple rows of detectors are now used. As such, multiple scan profiles are captured at each gantry angle during a single 360° rotation of the X-ray tube and detectors around the patient. Figure 2.12 depicts the rotation of the tube and multiple rows of detectors around a patient's head. Note in this figure, the X-ray beam is wider in the scanner's Z direction to cover the greater number of detectors. All rows of detectors will have 900+ single detectors per row.

CT scans are performed in two ways, with the patient stationary and with the patient moving during the rotation of the X-ray tube and detectors. When the patient is stationary, this is called "axial" CT scanning. When the patient is moving, it is called "helical" or "spiral" scanning.

In axial scanning, the patient does not move. The rotation of the X-ray tube and detector through the 360° creates multiple scan profiles. As the patient does not move, these scan profiles are all from the same anatomical region in the patient. As such, the X-ray intensity measurements, *I*, at each detector and for each scan profile

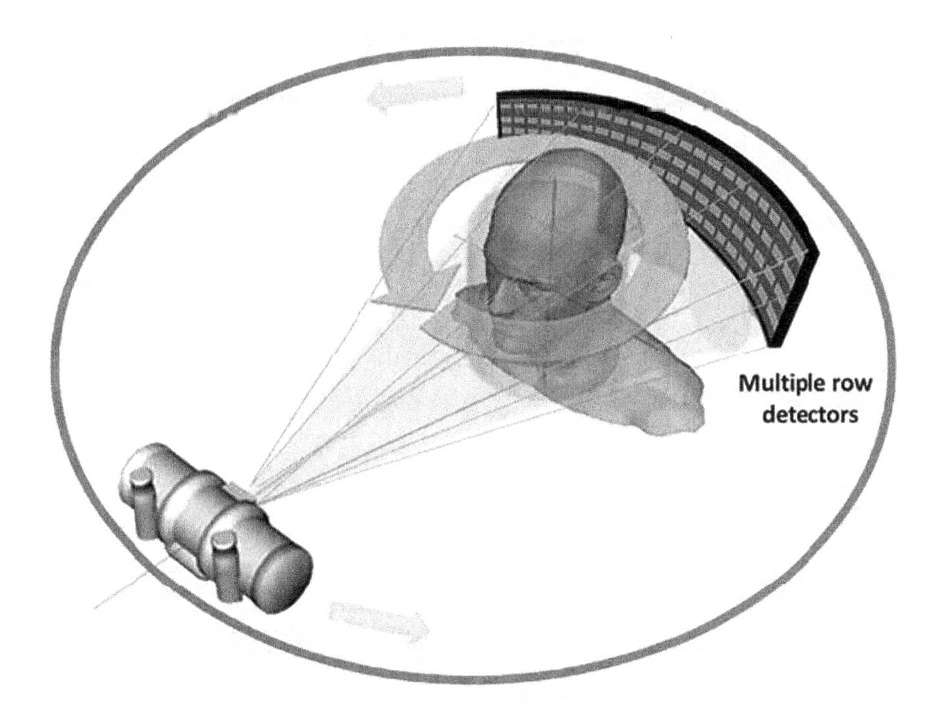

FIGURE 2.12 The X-ray tube and multiple rows of detectors shown rotating around a patient's head. (Image with thanks to Dr. Haney Alsleem, Imam Abdulrahman Bin Faisal University, Saudi Arabia.)

can be fully attributed to the same attenuation characteristic of the scanned anatomy. In helical scanning, this is not the case and adjustments need to be made.

Firstly, consider the scan profiles in axial scanning. At each angle of the gantry, each detector in a row of detectors (900+ detectors) records an intensity of the X-ray beam. Figure 2.13 shows the first aspect of the reconstruction problem and the intensities recorded at each detector.

The Beer–Lambert law, also known as the Lambert–Beer law, is seen in the following equation:

$$I = I_0 e^{-\mu x} \tag{2.1}$$

where I is the measured X-ray intensity at each detector, I_0 is the original X-ray intensity, μ is the total attenuation along the X-ray beam's path and x is the distance travelled by the X-ray beam.

The Beer–Lambert law simply states that the measured intensity, I, will decrease exponentially depending upon the attenuation characteristics of the object in the X-ray beam's path and the length of the path. In Figure 2.13, the X-ray beam's path is divided into 512 small objects each with their own attenuation coefficient, μ, and of known size.

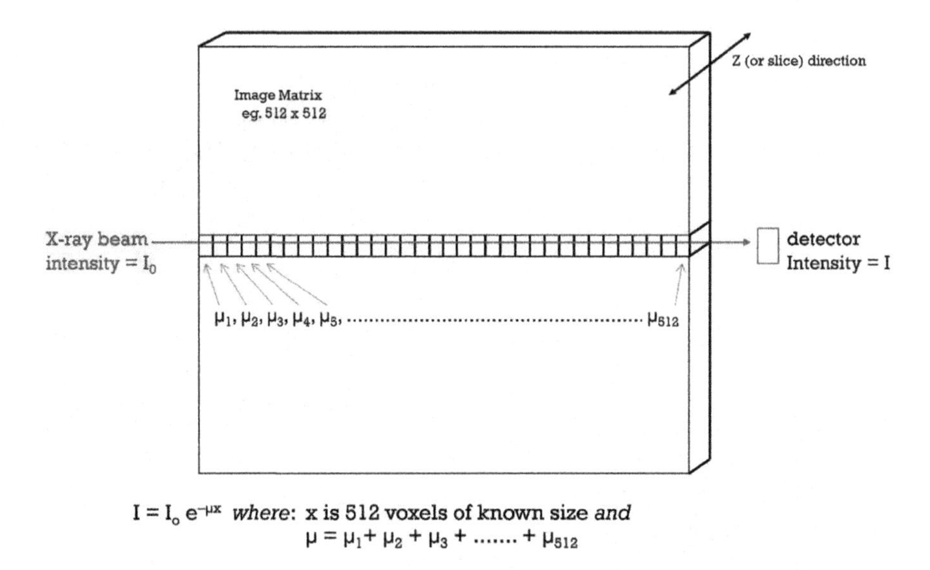

FIGURE 2.13 Beer–Lambert law for recorded X-ray intensity based on the attenuation characteristic (μ) and the distance the X-ray beam travels through the object.

CT Image Reconstruction Problem

The CT image reconstruction problem then is used to calculate the linear attenuation coefficients, μ, for each voxel in the CT slice. For example, in Figure 2.13, along one line of the X-ray beam, reconstruction of 512 μ values is needed. For the entire image, a total of 262,144 voxel values of μ need to be calculated. The original X-ray intensity, I_0, is known or can be measured. The X-ray beam intensity, I, is measured by the detector. The voxel depth is set by the X-ray beam's collimation or the detector width in the Z direction. The voxel's X and Y size is the pixel size. Pixel size is determined by the SFOV and the number of rows and columns in the final image. CT images consist of 512 rows and 512 columns (or 1,024 × 1,024) of pixels so the pixel size in SFOV/512 in the X and Y directions and the final pixel value represent the voxel depth. As such, x of the distance of the path of X-ray beam is known.

From each detector in the row of detectors, all intensities, I, can be measured and the row of I values is the slice profile. A scan profile is simply a row of numbers that represent the X-ray beam's intensity. A scan profile is depicted in Figure 2.14. Multiple scan profiles are obtained at each gantry rotation angle. For this example, let's consider that a slice profile is collected at every degree of rotation around the gantry. That is, 360 slice profiles are collected in 1 rotation of the X-ray tube and detectors around the patient.

Scan profiles from the 360° rotation around the patient can be collectively displayed as a sinogram. The data from the sinogram, the scan profiles, are then used in the image reconstruction. In Figure 2.15, the scan profile numbers have been put in rows of 900+ columns, corresponding to the number of detectors and hence the number of values in each scan profile. The numbers then have a grey scale assigned so the matrix can be perceived as an image. In the example in the figure, the first

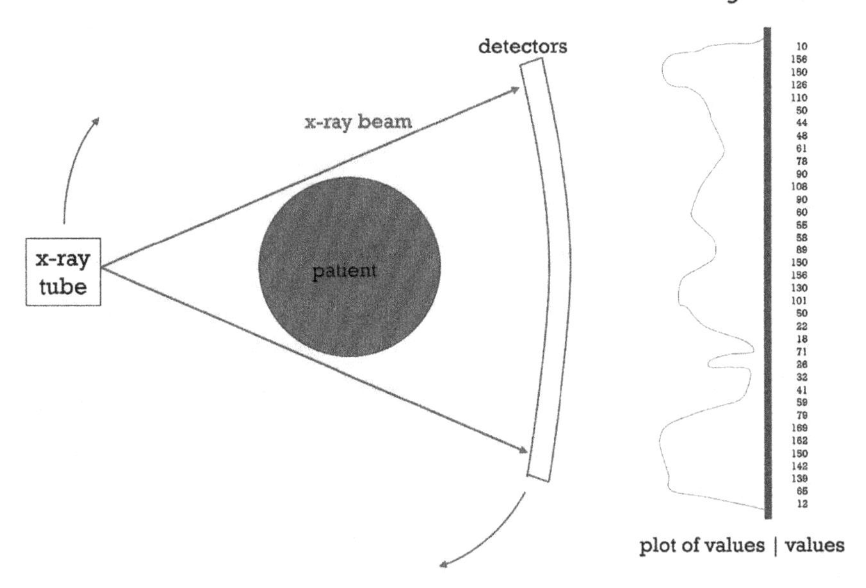

FIGURE 2.14 A scan profile is a row of numbers that represent the X-ray intensity measured by each detector in the row of detectors. Scan profiles are collected at each angle of rotation of the gantry. The beam's width in the Z direction is not shown.

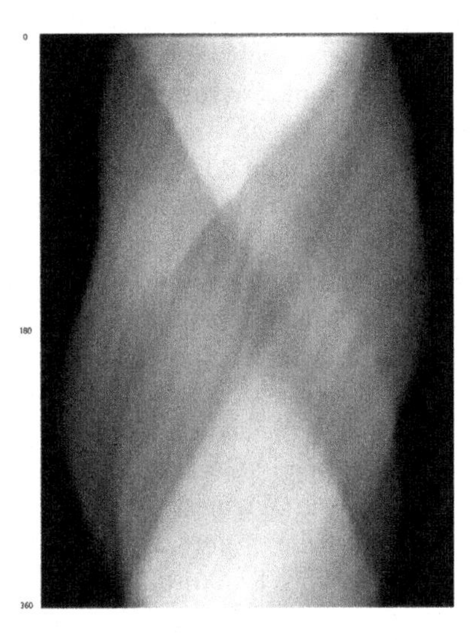

FIGURE 2.15 A representation of a sinogram that consists of all the scan profiles during the 360° rotation of the gantry. Each line across the image represents values in an individual scan profile.

scan profile that was captured is a gantry angle of 0° so the top row of the sinogram is those values. As the scan profiles are acquired during the rotation from 0° through 180° then back to 0° or 360°, the scan profiles' numbers are added to each row of the matrix.

Helical/Spiral Scanning

There are many reconstruction methods for converting CT scan profiles into a CT image. Over the last 10 years, CT manufacturers have placed a lot of emphasis on developing new reconstruction algorithms. The result of these endeavours are new iterative reconstruction techniques that have significantly reduced the noise in the CT images. By reducing noise in the image, the CT scan parameters of mA and time can be reduced, with which earlier reconstruction methods would have produced a noisy image of low quality and may not have had any diagnostic value. The iterative reconstruction techniques overcome noise and allow less radiation to be used. As such, radiation dose to the patient during the scan is reduced. This is discussed in more detail later in this chapter. The 2020 article by Dr. Euclid Seeram, *Computed Tomography Image Reconstruction*, in Radiologic Technology, Vol. 92, No. 2, which provides a good overview of reconstruction methods.

The focus of the section will be to provide an overview of an early CT reconstruction method, which is still used, called filtered back projection (FBP).

The back projection process in FBP can be explained using Figure 2.16. In this figure, "X-ray" beams have passed through an unknown object with two different attenuation characteristics. In this example, only four scan profiles have been collected. The four scan profiles were created by the "X-ray" beam passing through the object at four angles, 45°, 90°, 135° and 180°, from the vertical position of the gantry. The coloured lines represent some of the paths of the "X-ray" beam.

Four 5×5 arrays, the same size as the final image array, were placed at the same angle location at which the scan profiles were collected. For example, scan Profile 1 was collected when the detectors were 45° from the vertical positions; scan Profile 2 was collected when the detectors were 90° from the vertical positions. The scan profile values are then back projected over each corresponding array. For example, in Profile 2, the top scan profile value is 5. The array and the final image are a 5×5 matrix. As there are 5 pixels along the top row of that matrix, each profile value is divided by 5 (the number of pixels) and the result is placed in each of the matrix's pixels along that top row. Note, this is an example created using Microsoft Excel® so the approach is modified slightly to suit Excel use and the low number of scan profiles.

In this example, the four back projected matrices are then added together into a final 5×5 matrix and the total pixel values are then divided by a constant. The resultant output "image" can be seen in Figure 2.17. Using Microsoft Excel®, the cells or "pixels" were colourized to a shade of grey depending on their final value – the same process of using LUTs or WW/WL in displaying a CT image. Given this final "image" was created using only four scan profiles, the "image" is a reasonable representation of the unknown object. Try this yourself using Microsoft Excel® or similar software.

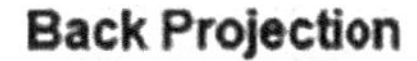

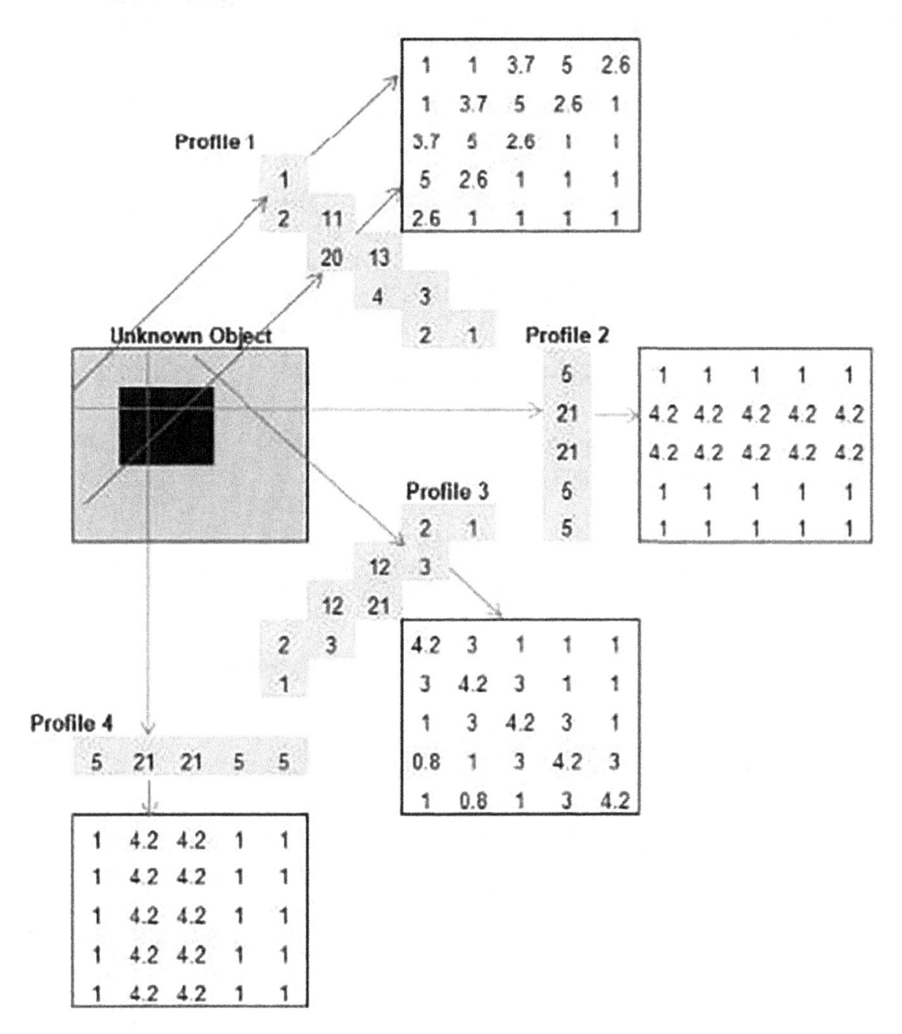

FIGURE 2.16 A diagram of the back projection method.

The back projection method described above shows the scan profiles being projected parallel to each other over the matrix. However, the X-ray beam that creates CT scan profiles starts at a point source and fans out across the width of the detectors, as seen in Figure 2.14. Additional mathematics is needed to correct this in the back projection method.

The main issue with the simple back projection method is that it creates a star pattern around objects which then gives the object a blurred appearance. Figure 2.18 is a representation of a circular object that has been created using the simple back projection method. The grey lines in the image represent the values of the multiple

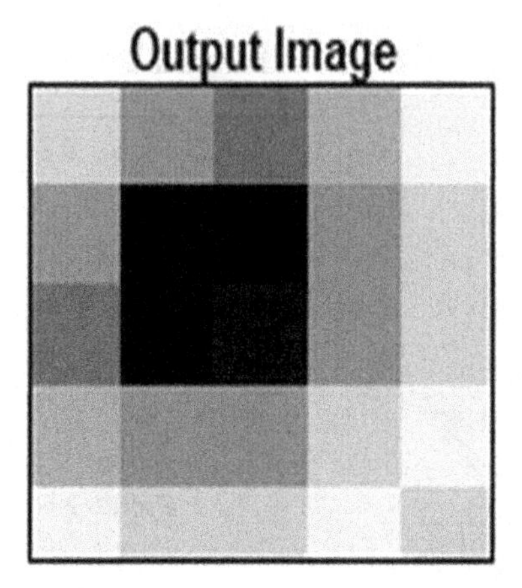

FIGURE 2.17 The output image from unknown object using the Microsoft Excel® back projection method is shown in Figure 2.16.

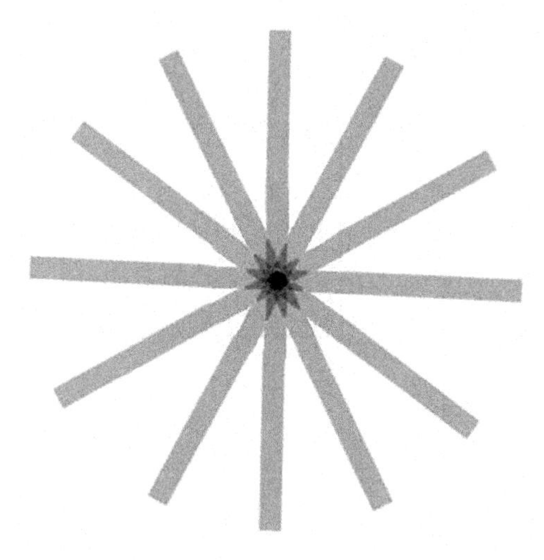

FIGURE 2.18 A circular object that has undergone simple back projection. The simple back projection method creates a star pattern around the object with the result that the object appears blurred.

scan profiles, as shade of grey from the object. The multiple scan profiles have been back projected over the final image leaving a star pattern around the object.

To overcome the star pattern that results from the use of the simple back projection method, the scan profiles are filtered, hence the name FBP. The alternate name for a filter is a convolution kernel. The filtering or convolution is undertaken on each scan profile and can be considered as an edge enhancement process of that scan profile. The result of the edge enhancement/filtering/convolution of the scan profile can be seen in Figure 2.19. The filtered scan profiles are used in the back projection

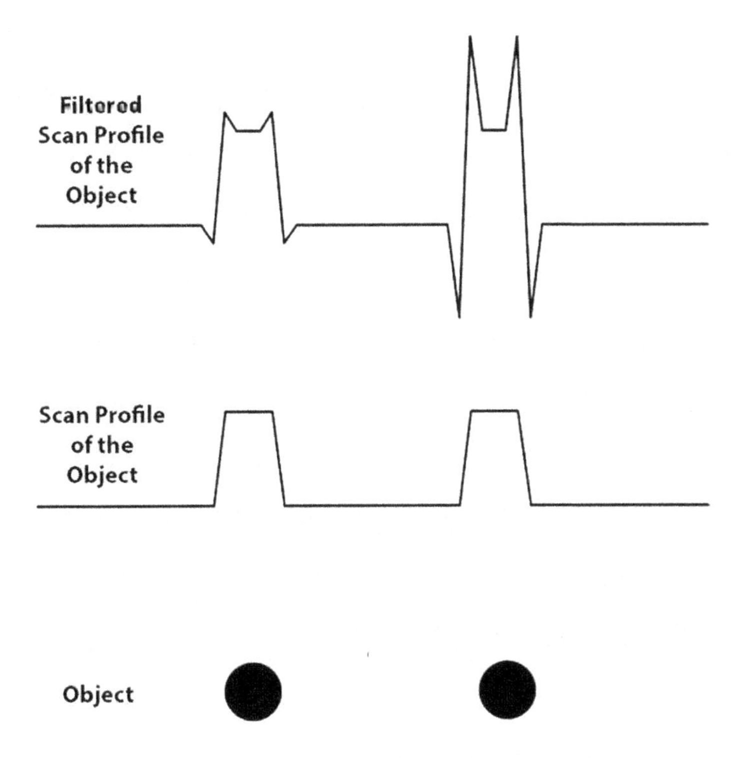

FIGURE 2.19 A circular object with its resultant plot of the scan profile (middle) and filtered scan profile (top). The right filtered scan profile has used a different filter algorithm or convolution kernel and would provide greater edge enhancement. It could be used in a "bony" reconstruction algorithm.

method and the result of using the filtered profiles is the removal of the star artefact and blur of the object.

Altering the filter or convolution used on the scan profiles can change the appearance of the reconstructed image(s). Once the scan profiles are captured and stored, a new image can be created from the existing scan profiles using a different filter or convolution than that used in the original image(s). For example, a CT examination might require visualization of both soft tissue and bone. The "standard" reconstruction algorithm may be used for image reconstruction to best show soft tissue and an "edge" or "bony" reconstruction algorithm could then be used for image reconstruction to best show the bone. Differences in the filter algorithms can be seen in Figure 2.19, with the "bony" filter algorithms shown on the right. Other reconstruction algorithms are typically available. For example, a "lung" reconstruction algorithm is often used in thin slice CT scanning of the lungs with resultant enhancement of the bronchioles and alveoli (see Figure 2.29d for a phantom and compare that with the image in 2.28a). As a result, multiple sets of images can be reconstructed from the same scan profiles without rescanning the patient and enhancing different parts of the anatomy in the image.

CT Image Reconstruction

Helical, or spiral, CT is achieved by moving the patient while the X-ray tube and detectors are emitting radiation and rotating around the gantry. The gantry and patient movement are depicted in Figure 2.20.

The path that the X-ray beam would create is a helical shape around a cylindrical object, noting that the X-ray beam has a width in the Z direction. The path of the X-ray beam is depicted in Figure 2.21.

In axial scanning, the X-rays must be turned off during patient movement to the next scan location, adding to the overall scan time. Helical scanning reduces the scan time for the patient. The helical pitch is the relationship of the table movement per 360° rotation of the gantry to the beam collimation. A pitch of 1 means the table moves the same distance as the width of the beam's collimation in the Z direction. A pitch of greater than 1 means the table moves a greater distance that the width of the beam. Some examples are shown in Figure 2.22.

When using a helical approach, the patient on the table moves in the Z direction during a 360° rotation of the gantry. The resultant slice profiles that are created during the 360° rotation means the X-ray beam has not passed through the same anatomy. Without some means to overcome this issue, there would be movement artefact in the reconstructed image. The method to overcome this is a process called interpolation. Prior to reconstruction of the slice profiles into an image, the slice

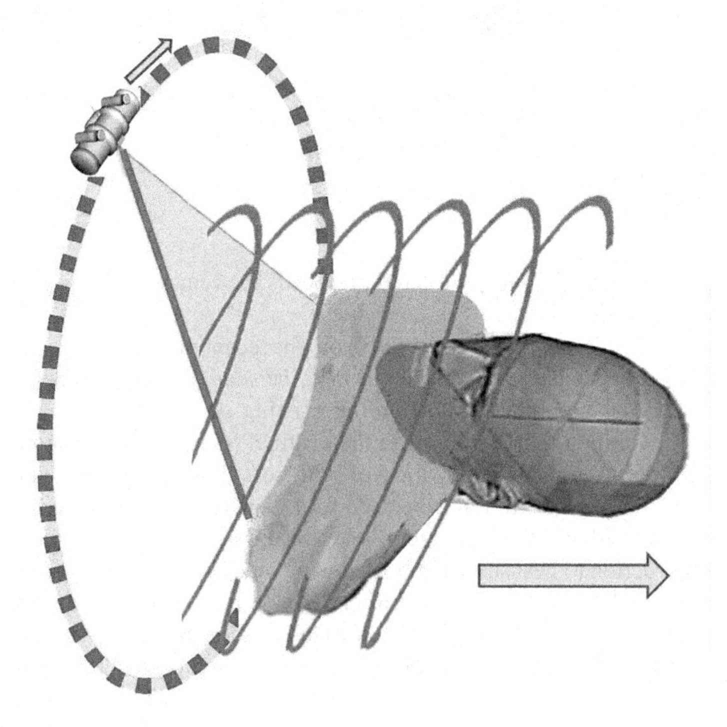

FIGURE 2.20 Helical or spiral scanning showing the X-ray tube and detectors shown rotating around a patient's head while the patient is moving through the gantry. (Image with thanks to Dr. Haney Alsleem, Imam Abdulrahman Bin Faisal University, Saudi Arabia.)

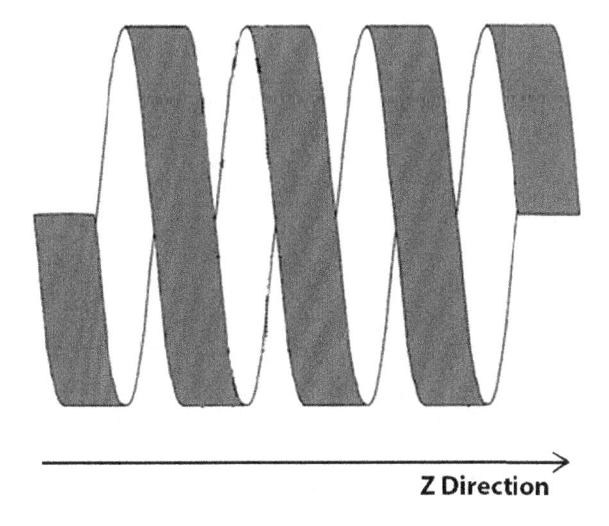

FIGURE 2.21 Helical or spiral path of the X-ray beam around a cylindrical object.

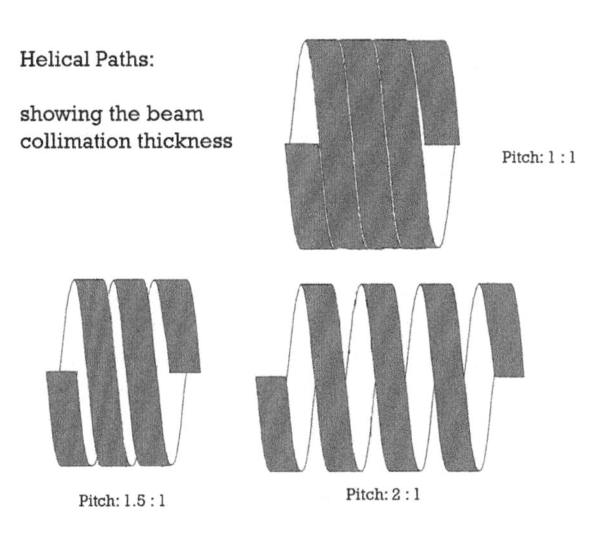

FIGURE 2.22 Helical paths of the X-ray beam around a cylindrical object at differing pitches.

profiles must undergo interpolation to create "stationary" scan profiles. The "stationary" scan profiles are used in the image reconstruction process.

Interpolation is essentially determining an unknown value from two (or more) known points each with a known relationship (in the case distance) to the location of the unknown value. The calculated interpolated value is also known as the weighted average of known values.

An example of its use is seen in Figure 2.23. In helical reconstruction, X-rays have passed through the patient the entire length of the helical CT acquisition. As such, the plane or Z location of the CT slice reconstruction can be chosen at any point along the pathway of the helix.

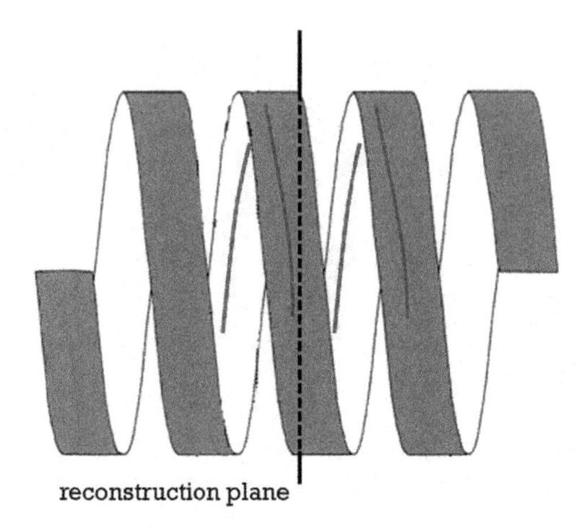

FIGURE 2.23 The selected reconstruction plane in the helical paths of the X-ray beam. The two blue and two red lines represented the slice profiles at the same angle in the gantry rotation, with the second of these profiles obtained after another 360° rotation of the gantry and table movement in the Z direction.

In axial imaging, the location of the reconstructed slice must be where the X-rays passed through the anatomy. In axial imaging, if a single row of detectors is 5 mm in thickness and an axial single slice scan is taken at a 55 mm superior to a zero-reference point and the next single slice scan is taken at 65 mm superior to the same zero-reference point, then there is a 5 mm gap in the patient's anatomy that cannot have a CT image created. No axial image can be created at 50 mm superior to a zero-reference point without rescanning the patient at that location. Helical imaging leaves no gap in the patient's anatomy where X-ray has not passed through. In the same example, in helical CT scanning, it is possible to reconstruct CT images at every 1 mm distance between 55 and 65 mm superior to the zero-reference point.

In Figure 2.23, let's assume that the desire reconstruction plane is 50 mm superior to the zero-reference point or +50 mm (note, this is not possible in the previous axial imaging example without rescanning the patient at that location). Let's further assume that at +50 mm Z location, the gantry angle during the rotation was at 90°. In this example, the table is moving superiorly, that is, the Z location numbers are increasing. An early scan profile was collected at location +48 mm where the gantry was at 280° rotation, in the image, the left-sided red line. After a further rotation of 360°, the gantry is again at 280° rotation and the table had moved from 5 to +53 mm Z location. The two red lines represent slice profiles 360° apart and they were on either side of the selected location for the reconstruction of the CT image. The two blue lines also have similar criteria. The 2 red and 2 blue slice profiles are known data and have known distances away from the reconstruction plane. Each of the intensity values, I, in the two slice profiles at the same gantry angle are being used to give an interpolated value at the location of the reconstruction plane.

All slice profiles, at the same gantry angle on either side of the desired Z slice location selected for the reconstruction of the axial image, are used to create 360° of "stationary" scan profiles. The "stationary" scan profiles are used to reconstruct the

CT image at that location. In the above example, using +50 mm location to create an axial slice at +51 mm, the process re-uses the existing or real slice profiles to create "stationary" scan profiles suitable to create an image at +51 mm.

The disadvantage of helical reconstruction is that the slice profile data are obtained over a longer Z-direction distance than when the data are obtained in axial imaging, i.e., when the patient is stationary. In axial imaging, the slice thickness is essentially the width of the detector row or narrower and there is some slight broadening of the *slice* profile of the image; however, this can be ignored. A slice profile can be considered as a side on view of the CT image. In axial imaging, if the X-ray beam was collimated to 5 mm thickness in the Z direction, then the slice profile can be considered as being 5 mm in thickness. Using the above discussed helical interpolation method, the so-called 360° interpolation method, to obtain the slice profiles and with a pitch of 1, the slice profile increases by approximately 180%. This means that a helical CT image obtained from a 5 mm Z-direction wide detector, the slice profile width would be approximately 1.8×5 mm, and as such, the helical image is essentially 9 mm thick, not 5 mm. The greater the pitch used, the more the slice profiles broaden. To overcome this, the 180° interpolation method is used.

The 180° interpolation method takes into account that from each scan profile an equal but opposite scan profile can be created. An example of this can be seen in Figure 2.24. Here, two scan profiles are shown at 90° gantry angle and at 270°. They have the same intensity, *I*, values however in reverse due to the 180° rotation of the gantry.

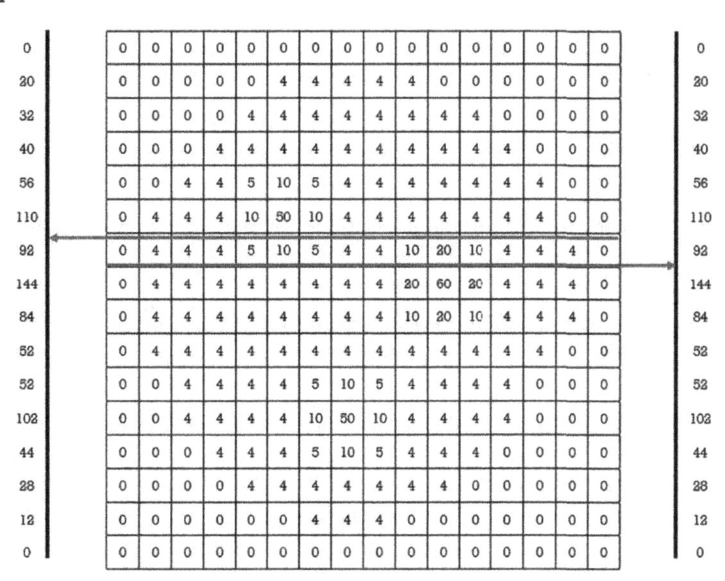

FIGURE 2.24 Equal, but opposite, scan profiles that are 180° gantry rotation apart. The red arrows show the X-ray beam direction to create the two scan profiles.

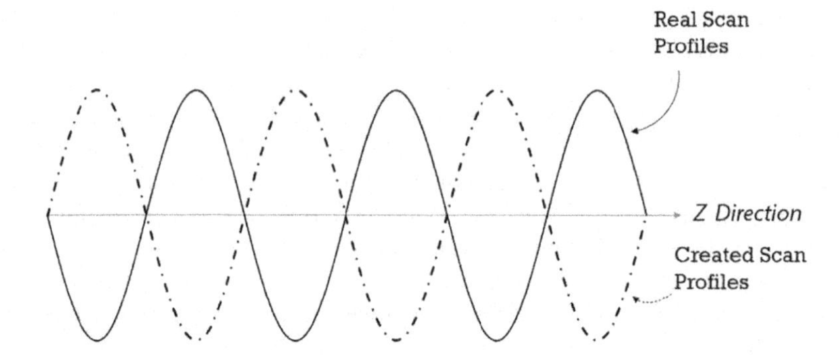

FIGURE 2.25 The gantry angle locations of the real scan profiles and the created or pseudo profiles. At the same Z location, the real and pseudo profiles are at 180° gantry angle rotation apart.

Using this feature, a second helical path of pseudo slice profiles can be created that is equal but opposite to each scan profile. These created scan profiles are 180° gantry angle rotation away from the original scan slice profiles, however at the same Z location of the patient. Creating the pseudo slice profiles for the entire helical path of the CT scan creates a second or pseudo sinogram (see Figure 2.15 for an example of the original sinogram) that is used in the interpolation process. An alternative way of considering this is seen in Figure 2.25. In this figure, the gantry location, in degrees, is represented by a sine wave. The solid line represents the angle where the original scan profiles were created, and the dotted line represented the angle of where the pseudo scan profiles were created.

Using the original and the pseudo-scan profiles in the 180° interpolation process, the so-called 180° helical reconstruction process, the image's slice profile only increases by approximately 130% not 180% of the 360° helical reconstruction process.

Using the 180° helical interpolation, a CT image obtained from a 5 mm Z-direction wide detector, and the slice profile width would be approximately 1.3 × 5 mm being 6.5 mm thick, not 9 mm thick when using the 360° helical reconstruction process. The image slice profile created using the 180° helical reconstruction process is close in thickness to a slice that was obtained using axial scanning techniques.

Irrespective of which scanning method, axial or helical, is used, the results is the creation of scan profiles that are used in the creation or reconstruction of the CT image.

Hounsfield Units/CT Numbers

The result of the image reconstruction process is an array of numbers. The value of each pixel in the array represented the linear attenuation coefficient (μ) of the voxel the pixel represents. There are several issues with using linear attenuation coefficient values as the pixel value. Most images require pixel values to be integers, i.e., whole numbers. The linear attenuation coefficient (μ) of water at an energy of 60 keV is approximately 0.206 cm^{-1} (Hubbell and Seltzer, 2004). While such numbers can be stored in a computer, integers are more appropriate for images. The next issue is that μ of objects varies depending on the energy of the X-ray beam. The linear attenuation coefficient (μ) of water at an energy of 100 keV is approximately

0.170 cm^{-1} (Hubbell and Seltzer, 2004). To make the storage of pixel values easier and more consistent, that is not dependent on the energy of the X-ray beam, HU or CT numbers were devised. The following equation is used to convert values of μ to HU values:

$$HU = \frac{(\mu_{object} - \mu_{water})}{\mu_{water}} \times k \quad (2.2)$$

where HU is the Hounsfield units or CT numbers, μ_{water} is the linear attenuation coefficient of water at that kVp/filtration combination, μ_{object} is the linear attenuation coefficient of each matrix value and $k = 1{,}000$

The μ_{water} is known prior to the scan commencing and stored in the CT's computer. These values are known for every kVp setting and filtration combination that can be used on the CT scanner. This is the reason why there are only a few kVp settings being allowed to be used in CT scanning. The constant, k, allows the result of the equation to be larger than a small number with decimal points. The value of 1,000 means the range of HU values sits within −1,024 to +3,071, or in digital value terms, fits within the range of signed 12-bit values.

The following are the examples of the use of Equation 2.2:

$$\mu\left(\text{cm}^{-1}\right): \text{cortical bone} = 0.604; \text{white matter} = 0.213 \text{ and water} = 0.206$$

(μ values at 60 keV from Hubbell and Seltzer, 2004)

$$\text{HU of cortical} = (0.604 - 0.206) / 0.206 \times 1{,}000$$

$$\text{bone} = 1{,}935(\text{rounded value})$$

$$\text{HU of white} = (0.214 - 0.206) / 0.206 \times 1{,}000$$

$$\text{matter} = 39(\text{rounded value})$$

It can also be seen from Equation 2.2 that the HU value of water will be zero. Any object with attenuation characteristics of less than water will have negative HU values and any object with attenuation characteristics of greater than water will have positive HU values. From the relationship of μ_{water} to μ_{object} and that μ will each change at a similar rate depending on the energy of the X-ray beam, the HU unit for the object will be approximately the same no matter what kVp and filtration combination was used in the scan. For example, the HU value obtained using 120 kVp for a type soft tissue in the body may be 40 and will be similar if 80 or 140 kVp was set. This characteristic of HU values means that CT is one of the few imaging modalities than can provide an objective measure of X-ray attenuation. In CT, it is a relative measure of X-ray attenuation of an object compared to the X-ray attenuation of water.

Thins vs Thicks

Early CT scanner had one row of detectors, not multiple rows. Those CT scanners had detector rows that were wide, e.g., 10mm, and slice thickness was controlled by collimating the X-ray beam in the Z direction from a maximum of 10mm down to the desired slice thickness, e.g., 2mm. The current CT scanner has multiple rows of detectors. Typically, now, the width of each detector row is of sub-millimetre in the Z direction. For example, in some models of CT scanner, the detector rows are 0.5mm and less in Z direction width.

An issue with acquiring such thin slices is the number of images created during a scan. Assuming that there is no slice profile width broadening and that all created images are 0.5mm thick, then for a CT scan of the abdomen from diaphragm to symphysis pubis, approximately 40cm in distance, 800 CT slices will be created.

There are distinct advantages of having thin axial slices. The voxels are isotropic, which means their X, Y and Z dimensions are the same or similar. Having isotropic voxels when images are created in planes from the axial images, such as coronal and sagittal reconstruction, and when 3D images are created, the so-called "stair-step artefact" is not present. However, the disadvantage of thin slices is that for an abdomen CT scan, 800 CT images need to be viewed by radiologists or clinicians. To overcome this issue, "thicks" are created from the "thins". A desired slice thickness for that anatomical region is selected. Multiple "thins" that are added together to create a "thick" of the desired slice thickness. As example, 5mm thickness may be the desired thickness for the abdominal CT scan. If the "thins" are 0.5mm thick, then ten images are added together to create a "thick" of 5mm thickness. The advantage of this is that clinician only view 80×5mm images. If needed, the radiologist can still call up and review the "thins".

An example is in Figure 2.26a–c. Figure 2.26a and b was acquired with "thins" of 0.63mm thickness and 0.5mm apart. These two images and three other images were added together to give the image in Figure 2.26c. This image covers the anatomy of 5×0.5mm, i.e., it is 2.5mm in thickness. Note the apparent loss of detail in c of the maxillary plate; however, the posterior arch of C1 is seen as a complete arch that is not seen in one image of a and b. This effect of loss of detail is called partial volume effect (discussed more in the later Artefact section) and results from the voxel thickness (the slice thickness) being wider. This effect is seen irrespective of how the images were created, either as "thicks" created from "thins", and in older CT scanners, when the X-ray beam was collimated wider. Partial volume effect will always occur to some extent as voxels must have a finite thickness. The wider the voxel depth, the greater the likelihood that tissues with two or more different μ will be in the same voxel. If this occurs, the multiple μ values will be averaged into a resultant single HU value. Note, partial volume effect can also occur if pixel size, i.e., in the XY direction, is too large.

One of the advantages of CT discussed in the "Why CT" section above is overcoming the compression of 3D anatomy into a 2D image. In planar X-ray images, the partial volume effect is the thickness of the anatomy that the X-ray beam passes through and is much greater than in CT.

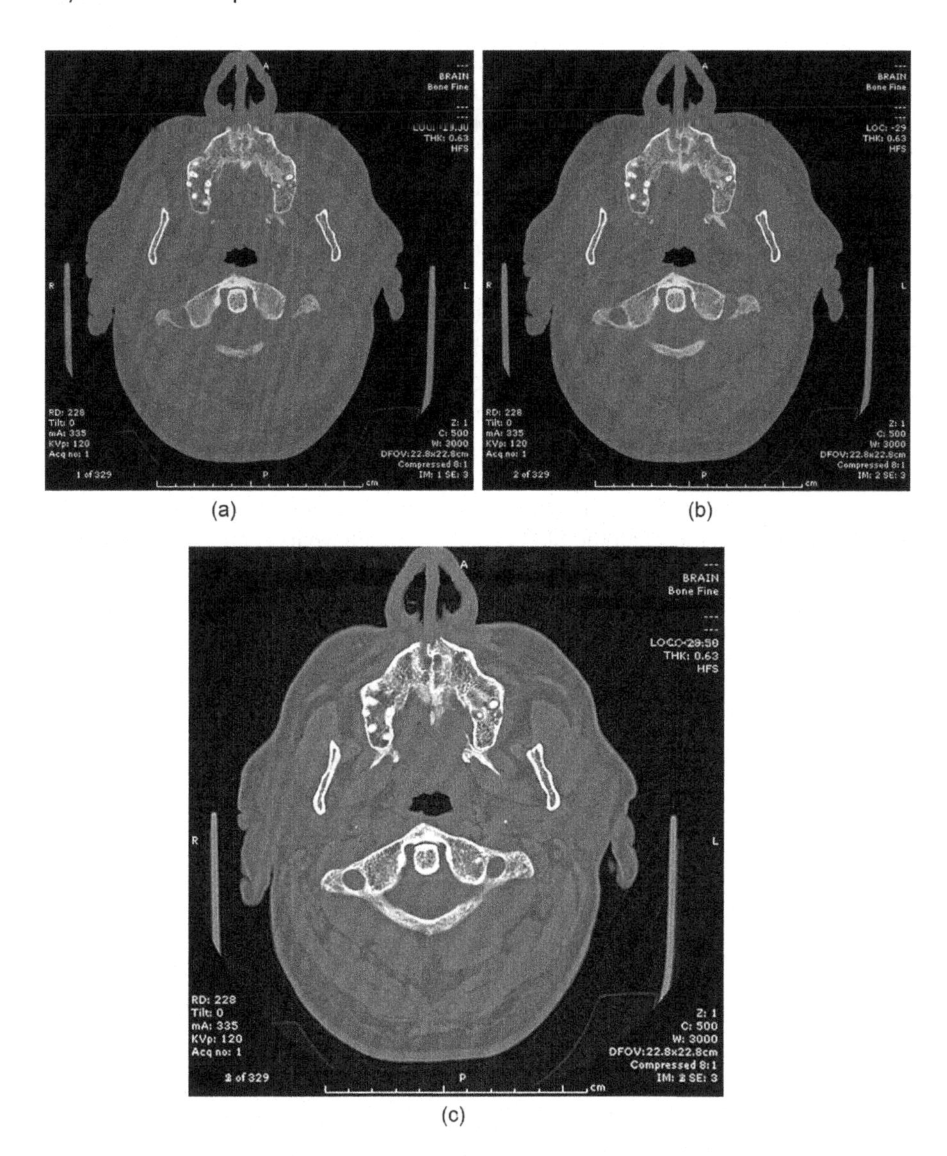

FIGURE 2.26 (a) and (b) Thins that were acquired 0.5 mm apart. (c) 5×thins added together to create a 2.5 mm thick CT image.

Scan and Display Field of View

Anatomical coverage in the XY direction of each CT axial slice is controlled by the gantry size; the distance between the X-ray tube focal spot and the detectors and the angle of the fan of the X-ray beam. The SFOV describes the anatomical coverage. Typically, most CT scanners will have two SFOVs, one to cover larger anatomical regions, e.g., the chest or abdomen and a smaller SFOV for heads, paediatrics, and the other to cover small anatomical regions. To reduce the SFOV size from the largest size, the X-ray fan beam is collimated sideways in the XY direction, i.e., the angle of the fan beam is reduced, and as such, less detectors in each row are being used during the CT scan acquisition.

The X-ray tube and detectors rotate around a central point in the gantry called the isocentre. The isocentre then is the centre of the SFOVs. Figure 2.27 shows the relationship of the scanner's isocentre and SFOV. The aperture is the hole in the gantry and is larger than the largest SFOV.

The images, once acquired and displayed, can be magnified so that the objects in the image appear larger. This is changing the display field of view (DFOV). One method is a simple zoom in or enlargement of the digital image. The DFOV is reduced compared to the SFOV. While the appearance of an object in the image will be larger, the actual scan pixel sizes will not change.

The alternate method is commonly called retrospective reconstruction. Retrospective reconstruction will create a new image or a new series of images. The DFOV is set so as to be smaller than the SFOV and does not have its centre at the isocentre of the gantry, i.e., the new image's centre can be offset from the isocentre. This retrospective reconstruction method uses the original scan profiles; however, using a smaller selected DFOV not all of the scan profile data is needed in the reconstruction. Also, an alternate filter algorithm or convolution kernel can be applied to the scan profiles to give the new images an alternative appearance. From this reconstruction method, selecting a smaller DFOV than the SFOV can be done prospectively, i.e., before the axial scans are started, from the scout/topogram/planning scan.

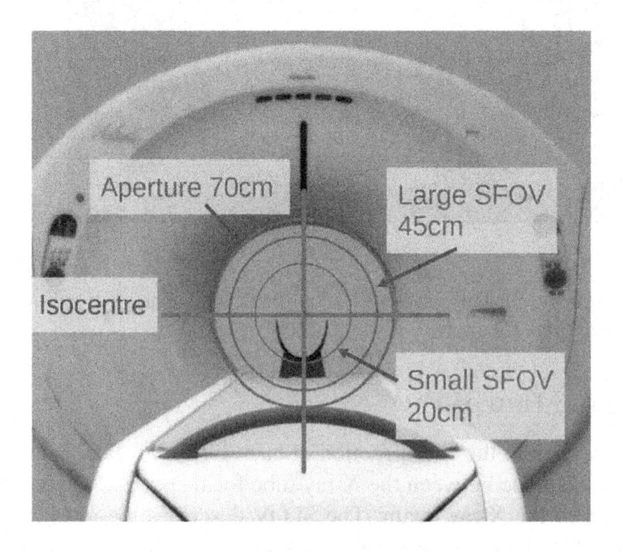

FIGURE 2.27 CT gantry showing the isocentre and the SFOVs. Note that the aperture and SFOV sizes will vary depending on the manufacturer and model of the CT scanner. (Image with thanks to Mr. Jens Loberg, Goulburn Base Hospital, Australia.)

Scouts/Topograms/Planning Scans

A scout/topogram/planning scan is used, as the latter name suggests, for planning the axial scans location and coverage of the anatomy. The X-ray tube and detectors are kept stationary, the X-rays turned on and the patient moves to the desired distance through the X-ray beam. The resultant image is similar to a digital planar X-ray image. The patient moves in or out of the gantry through the beam starting at the set top or bottom table location. The image is then created in a row, or a few rows, at a time, until the end table location is reached. Some examples can be seen in Figure 2.28. With the patient lying supine and the gantry at 0°, the image will be AP; with the gantry at 180°, the image will be PA; and with the gantry at 90° or 270°, the images will be lateral.

The scout/topogram/planning scans are used to set the upper and lower table range or Z direction limits for axial scans. This then ensures the appropriate anatomical coverage in the Z direction of the axial images in that series of scans.

By viewing both an AP and lateral scout images, the DFOV can be set smaller than the SFOV to provide anatomical coverage in the AP and lateral directions and ensure the smallest pixel size for that anatomical coverage. As well, if images are needed with smaller DFOV than the SFOV, the software will allow the user to offset the DFOV from the isocentre. For example, using the scout images in Figure 2.28, a small offset DFOV could be used to image the lumbar vertebra.

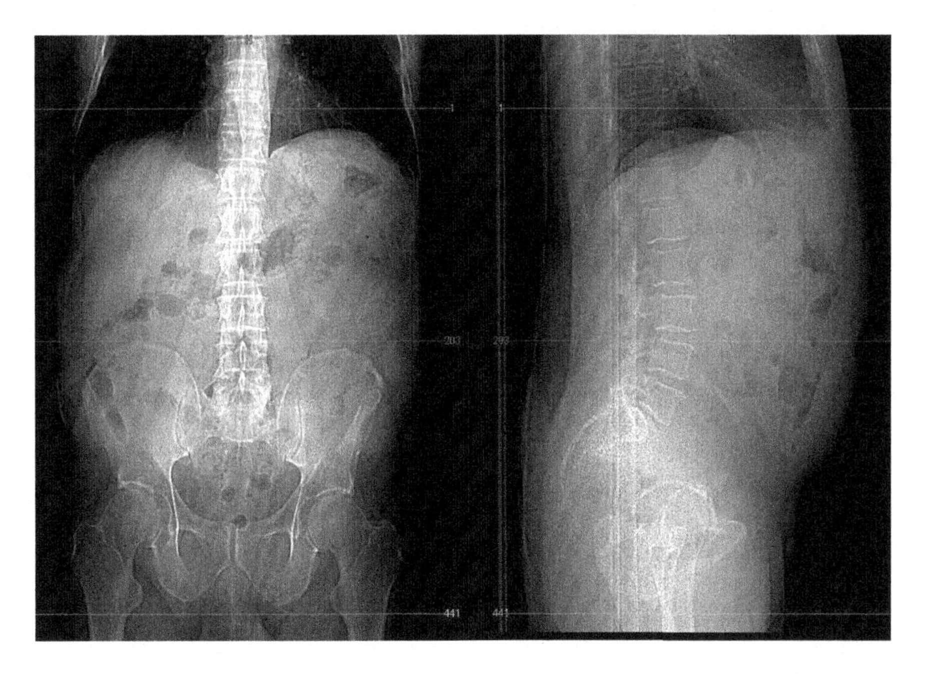

FIGURE 2.28 Scouts/topograms/planning scans of the abdomen. The scout on the left was acquired with the gantry at 0° and the scout on the right was acquired with the gantry at 90°. The images show the head end (H) of the patient and table locations of 1, 203 and 441 mm which are inferior to the zero-reference point of the table.

The scout/topogram/planning scan is also used for ensuring the patient's anatomy that is located in the centre of the gantry both vertically and laterally. Dose, image quality and HU accuracy issues can occur in the patient's anatomy that is not centrally located around the isocentre of the gantry.

IMAGE QUALITY IN CT

Image quality in CT needs to be considered in the four main areas: contrast resolution, spatial resolution, noise and artefacts. With CT being used more in dynamic imaging such as CT angiography, temporal resolution is also an important consideration. A detailed review of temporal resolution is beyond the scope of this chapter; however, an appropriate level of temporal resolution means that images of moving objects, such as iodinated contrast in blood vessels, depict the motion accurately.

Contrast Resolution, Spatial Resolution and Noise

Spatial Resolution

Spatial resolution is sometimes called high contrast resolution in CT imaging. Spatial resolution is a measure of the accuracy of the detail seen in the image. When measuring spatial resolution in CT, small objects with large HU value differences, or with high contrast, are used. Spatial resolution in CT must be considered in three dimensions. In CT, spatial resolution needs to be considered in the plane of the axial image, that is in the XY direction, and is called in-plane resolution. In the Z direction or in the slice direction, spatial resolution is called cross-plane resolution. Spatial resolution has been discussed in other sections above. Cross-plane resolution is the thickness of the slice or the depth of the voxel in the cross-plane or Z direction spatial resolution of the CT image. The in-plane or XY spatial resolution is controlled by the reconstruction FOV of the image and the image matrix size. For example, if the reconstruction of DFOV is 25 cm in diameter and the image matrix is 512×512 rows and columns, then each pixel has dimensions of 250 mm/512, approximately 0.5×0.5 mm. Note, CT images are square with equal number of rows and columns, whereas planar X-ray images may be rectangular with an unequal number of rows and columns.

Other factors that can affect spatial resolution are the filter algorithm or convolution kernel used to filter the scan profile. An example of the differences is seen in Figure 2.29a and c where the images were acquired with the same kVp, mA, scan time and slice thickness; however, Figure 2.29a was reconstructed with a "standard" filter algorithm and Figure 2.29c was reconstructed with a "lung" filter algorithm. There is a visible difference in the displayed details of objects in the image.

Other factors that can affect detail in a CT image are the focal spot size and ray sampling method used in the back projection method, however, these are not fully discussed in this chapter.

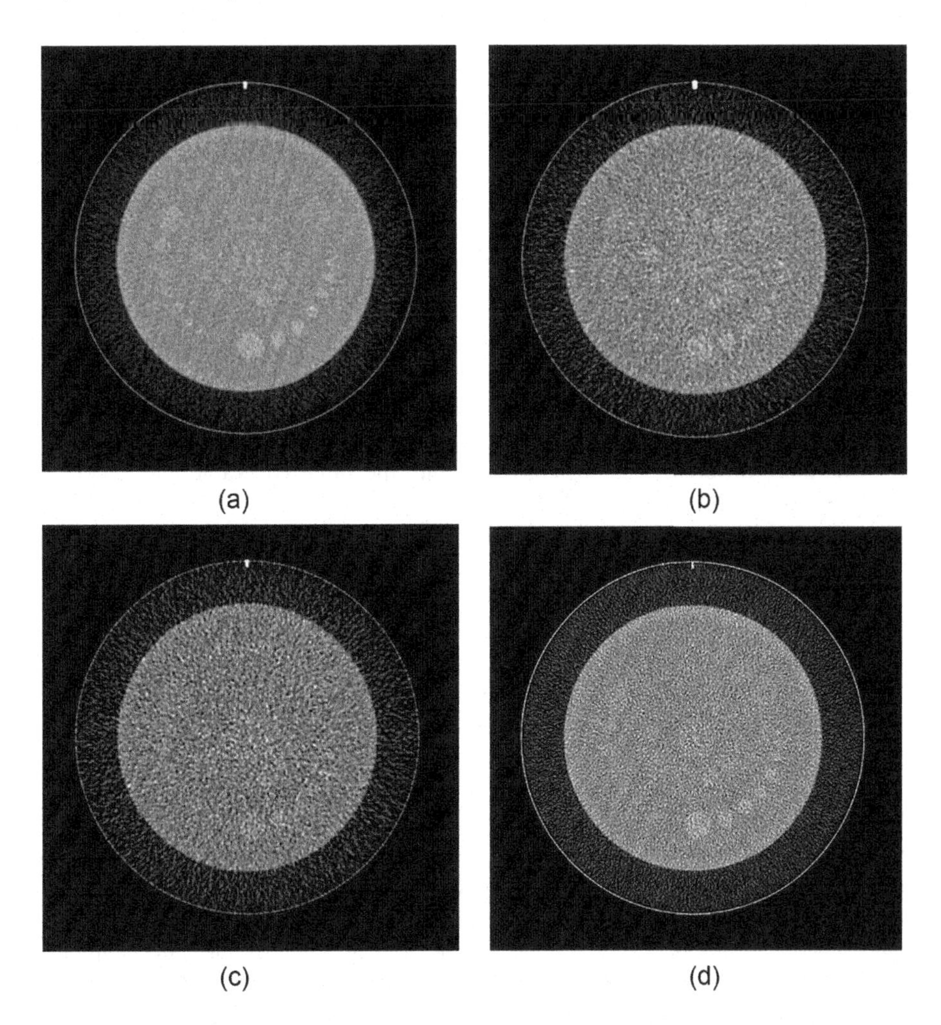

FIGURE 2.29 CT phantom (Catphan 500, Phantom Laboratory, Cambridge, NY) low-contrast module images obtained at different CT settings. (a) 120 kVp, 200 mA, 5 mm slice thickness, standard reconstruction algorithm. (b) 120 kVp, 200 mA, 1 mm slice thickness, standard reconstruction algorithm. (c) 120 kVp, 20 mA, 5 mm slice thickness, standard reconstruction algorithm. (d) 120 kVp, 200 mA, 5 mm slice thickness, lung reconstruction algorithm.

Contrast Resolution

As discussed previously, contrast resolution in CT is the major reason for the use of CT over other X-ray imaging modalities. Contrast resolution is also known as low-contrast resolution in CT. Contrast resolution in X-ray imaging, and hence in CT, is the ability to distinguish two objects from each other due to the object's ability to attenuate X-ray photons. In CT, if two different objects have the same HU values, even though they are different types of objects or different organs, the observer of the CT image is not able to differentiate the two objects apart. The two objects with the same HU will be displayed with the same grey scale level as each other.

Factors that affect contrast resolution have been discussed in other sections above, however, they are as follows:

- The kVp and filtration used for the scan. The kVp and filtration setting will determine the mean energy of the X-ray beam that is used in the reconstruction calculations. While converting these μ values to HU does overcome this to some extent, there will be slight difference in the resulting HU values that are calculated when using different kVp and filtration settings.
- The k value is used in Equation 2.2. The current k is 1,000; however, if this was a smaller value (in the early days of CT k was 500), then there would be more different μ values converted into the same HU value than when $k = 1{,}000$ is used.
- The bit-depth of the pixel values. This is set at 12 bit-depth with the range of possible HU values being −1,024 to 3,071. If the bit-depth was 8, then there would only be 256 possible HU values. When using 8 bit-depth images, the HU values calculated using Equation 2.2 would be "binned" into a smaller number of possible pixel values so that there would be multiple μ values that have the same HU value and there would be a loss of information as the contrast resolution would be reduced.

Noise

Noise in a CT image can be thought of as the variations of the HU that occur in a uniform object such as a water phantom. The measure of noise in CT is the standard deviation of the HU numbers in a uniform or homogeneous object. The image appearance of noise can be described as a "salt and pepper" appearance and examples of noise are seen in the uniform areas of the CT phantom's (Catphan 500, Phantom Laboratory, Cambridge, NY) low contrast module in Figure 2.29a–d. Noise essentially decreases image quality and is not a desirable feature in any image.

There are many CT scanning parameters that affect noise in a CT image, and as such, it can be a complex issue to reduce noise. Some of the parameters are

- kVp,
- mA,
- scan time,
- slice thickness,
- helical pitch and interpolation method
- and many others.

One of the easiest ways to overcome noise in an image is to increase the amount of X-ray photons reaching the detectors, for example, by increasing the mA. Noise is proportional to 1 divided by the square root of the number of X-ray photon, which in turn is proportional to the mAs (the multiplication of mA and scan time). This relationship is shown in the following equation:

$$\text{Noise} = \frac{1}{\sqrt{\text{mAs}}} \tag{2.3}$$

For example, if the scan mAs is increased by a factor of 4, the noise will be halved. However, the dose to the patient is proportional to the mAs, and in this example, the patient's dose would increase by a factor of 4 for an improvement of the image quality by reducing the noise to a half. This approach may not be in alignment with the image optimization, which is an approach ensuring that patient dose is minimized to a level where the resultant image will still have diagnostic value.

New iterative reconstruction algorithms that are being used as the iterative process of these algorithms can reduce noise in comparison to FBP reconstruction methods using the same scan profiles, and as such, the same scanning parameters of kVp, mA, scan time and slice thickness.

Contrast Resolution, Spatial Resolution and Noise Relationship

There is an integral relationship between contrast resolution, spatial resolution and noise. This relationship is depicted in Figure 2.30 and sometimes called the image quality triangle. If one of these three factors of image quality is adjusted, it can affect one or both of the other two. The effect can be positive or negative. When trying to maintain one of these factors, altering another will have implications on the radiation dose delivered to the patient.

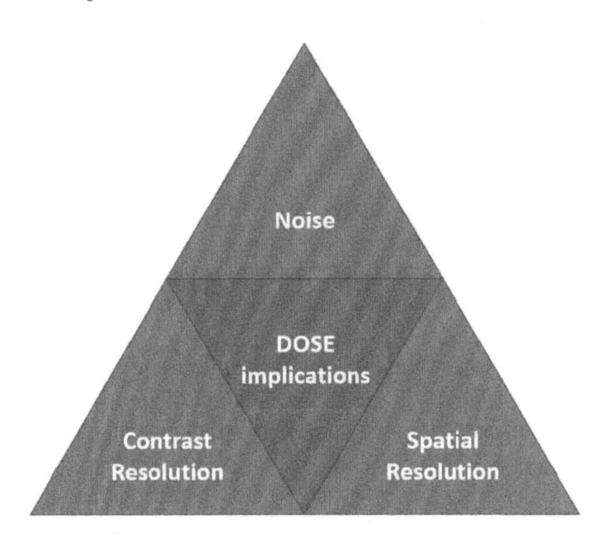

FIGURE 2.30 The relationship of noise, contrast resolution and spatial resolution, and their interdependence on image quality. These also have implications on the radiation dose delivered to the patient.

For example:

- if spatial resolution is increased so that the pixel or voxel size becomes smaller to visualize more details in the image, noise will increase. While trying to improve the visible detail in the image, overall image quality will decrease.
- if noise is decreased, contrast resolution will improve. The ability to differentiate between two objects with similar HU values will be increased.

Noise can be decreased by increasing the mAs and hence radiation dose to the patient. An increase in radiation dose is not desirable.

Noise can also be decreased by using an iterative reconstruction algorithm instead of a FBP algorithm.

A method of reducing patient radiation dose and increasing the contrast resolution is to lower the mAs and use an iterative reconstruction algorithm. Often iterative reconstruction algorithm will allow users to set their desired noise level.

Some examples are provided in Figure 2.29a–d. Compared to three images, b, c and d against a, Figure 2.29a was created using 120 kVp, 200 mA, 5 mm slice thickness and a standard reconstruction algorithm. Figure 2.29b has a thinner 1 mm slice thickness than a. Noise is more apparent in b than in a as less photons reach the detectors. Figure 2.29c was using 20 mA though with the same 5 mm thickness. Noise is more apparent in b than in a as less photons reach the detectors. Figure 2.29d was created using a lung filter or convolution on the slice profiles. While noise is more apparent in b than in a, the detail visible in the image is greater due to the edge enhancement effect of the lung filter.

Detailed discussions on the relationship between detail visible in the image and image contrast can be found in the article by Alsleem and Davidson (2013) and in the textbooks in the reference and bibliography of this chapter.

ARTEFACTS

Artefacts are appearances in an image that do not represent the object or objects being imaged. In CT, as with most medical imaging modalities, artefacts can be generally grouped into three main categories of patient-related artefacts, physics-based artefacts and hardware-based artefacts. In this chapter, only a brief review of artefacts will be undertaken.

The more common patient-related artefacts are patient movement and the presence of clothing and jewellery in the image. Patient movement artefacts can result from voluntary movement or from involuntary movement. The patient's voluntary movement can be reduced by reducing scan times or by having the patient hold their breath. With scan times such as 0.25 or 0.33 seconds per rotation and multiple rows of detectors, larger anatomical areas can be covered in one breath hold. Involuntary movement, such as heart or pulsatile movement, can be harder to control. When imaging the blood vessels in the heart during cardiac CT angiography (CCTA), gating, which is turning on and off the X-ray beam, can be used. In CCTA, the X-ray beam is turned on during diastole and turned off during systole.

Administration of drugs such as beta-blockers can help control the patient's heart rhythm during CCTA scanning.

Physics-based artefacts including noise, which can result from a low number of photons reaching the detectors, have been discussed above. Other physics-based artefacts are the following:

- Beam hardening artefacts. These artefacts result from a phenomenon called beam hardening, which is based on the average energy of the X-ray beam that increases as it passes through an object. Low energy photons in the beam will be attenuated in the early part of the beam's path through the object, and as such, the average photon energy increases on its travel through the object.

  The reconstruction method in CT is based on a prior understanding of the average energy of the beam, and hence setting of the linear attenuation coefficient, μ, of water, at the kVp and filtration level used in the scan. If the average energy of the X-ray beam increases, then in one area of the anatomy, it can result in beam hardening artefacts. A typical example of this in CT scan of the head. The scan is set up for the entire head using the same kVp and filtration factors. Scan coverage includes all the head. In the inferior aspect of the head, there is a greater amount of bone versus the superior part of the head and artefacts result.
- Partial volume effect. This effect results from the finite size of the voxel. Typically, this occurs when the slice thickness or the Z dimension of the voxel is large, however, it can occur if pixel size, in the XY direction, is also large.

  A large voxel located in the patient may have more than one type of anatomy with differing linear attenuation coefficients, μ. The resulting HU value of the pixel that represents the voxel will be an average of the μ values in the voxel.

  A common way to reduce the partial volume effect is to scan the patient using thin slices. With current multi-slice CT scanner, this is now the routine CT acquisition method:
- Photon starvation. This is typically caused by metal objects that completely stop the X-ray photons reaching the detectors. The resultant slice profiles have some detector intensity values that are zero. Zero values in the slice profile cause image reconstruction issues, and the result is streaked across the image. This is typically seen with large metal objects, such as hip replacements. Metal artefact reduction software is used to replace the zero values in the scan profiles with a prediction of the expected scan profile values as if the metal was not present in the scan. New iterative reconstruction methods also overcome this issue.

Hardware-based artefacts are becoming less as the engineering of CT scanners is overcoming such problems. As an example, early CT scanner used high-pressure gas-filled detectors. If one of the detectors lost pressure, then its ability to detect the X-ray photons was lost. This resulted in a so-called ring artefact which has an appearance of a ring around the isocentre of the image. The current CT scanner uses solid-state detectors, and as such, ring artefacts are now very rarely seen.

CONCLUSION

This chapter section on the physical principles of CT has only provided an overview of these principles. CT operators must have a solid understanding of the physical principles and technical aspects of CT. Without such an understanding, radiation dose and image quality cannot be optimized for the benefit of the person at the centre of their focus, the patient.

REFERENCES

AAPM Report No. 233, 2019, Performance Evaluation of Computed Tomography Systems - The Report of AAPM Task Group 233, https://www.aapm.org/pubs/reports/detail.asp?docid=186, viewed on 12 Feb 2021.

Alsleem, H and Davidson, R, 2013, Factors Affecting Contrast-Detail Performance in Computed Tomography: A Review, *Journal of Medical Imaging & Radiation Sciences*, Vol 44, 62–70.

Hubbell, J and Seltzer, S, 2004, X-Ray Mass Attenuation Coefficients: NIST Standard Reference Database 126, National Institute of Standards and Technology, https://www.nist.gov/pml/x-ray-mass-attenuation-coefficients, viewed on 12 Feb 2021.

Seeram, E, 2020, Computed Tomography Image Reconstruction, *Radiologic Technology*, Vol 92, No 2, 155CT–169CT.

BIBLIOGRAPHY

Kalender, W, 2011, *Computed Tomography: Fundamentals, System Technology, Image Quality, Applications*, 3rd edn, Publicis, Erlangen.

Seeram, E, 2016, *Computed Tomography: Physical Principles, Clinical Applications, and Quality Control*, 4th edn, Elsevier, St Louis.

3 Radiobiology

Iain M MacDonald
University of Cumbria

CONTENTS

INTRODUCTION

COLLECTIVE EFFECTIVE RADIATION DOSE AND THE CONTRIBUTION OF COMPUTED TOMOGRAPHY (CT) DOSE

According to the Organisation for Economic Co-operation and Development (OECD, 2021), there are 101 computed tomography (CT) examinations per year per 1,000 inhabitants in the United Kingdom (data from hospitals), 141 CT examinations in Australia (data from hospitals and ambulatory care providers) and 279 in the United States of America (data from hospitals and ambulatory care providers). This is a large number of examinations and, as CT uses X-rays, a form of ionising radiation, there needs to be an understanding of the potential harmful effect of this radiation on the population.

When considering the radiation risk from CT examinations, it is important to place it in the context of other doses found in everyday life from ionising radiation – both naturally occurring radiation and artificial. Natural ionising radiations are received by the whole population, examples include radon gas from rocks and some building materials which occur in homes and workplaces. By far, the largest proportion of artificial radiation that the population is exposed to is irradiation for medical purposes. It has been estimated that the global per caput effective dose is 3 mSv in the year 2000, where 2.4 mSv was from natural background radiation and 0.34 mSv from medical

DOI: 10.1201/9781003132554-4

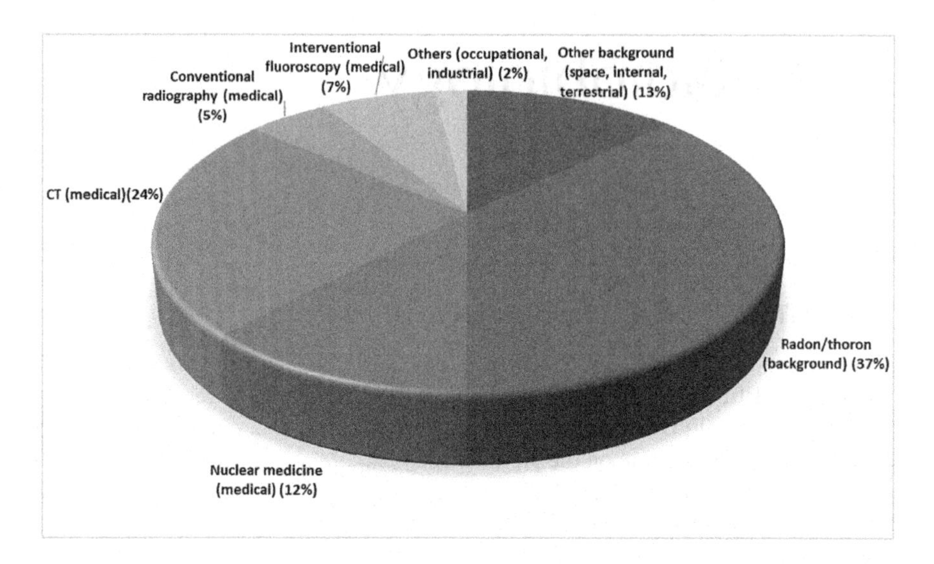

FIGURE 3.1 The collective effective dose in USA as a percentage of all exposure categories. Note that CT provides almost a quarter of the collective effective dose of the population. (Adapted from Schauer and Linton (2009).)

radiation procedures with the rest from other artificial sources (Ron, 2003). On average, people in the UK are exposed to 2.7mSv of ionising radiation per year, which includes both naturally occurring radiation and artificial medical exposures (Public Health England, 2011). The question arises for the purpose of this book: How much of the medical irradiation of the population is due to CT? A report issued in 2009 by the National Council on Radiation Protection and Measurements (Schauer and Linton, 2009) demonstrated that, of the collective effective dose in the USA, almost a quarter (24%) of the radiation exposure to those in the USA from all sources was due to CT, increasing from 15% in the early 1980s (Figure 3.1).

The Effects of Radiation on the Human Body

The two types of ionising radiation effects on the human body, defined by the International Commission for Radiation Protection (ICRP,1977) are deterministic and stochastic effects. When cells are damaged, or destroyed, leading to a loss in the functioning of tissue and if sufficient cells are affected by the radiation, this is called a deterministic effect. Examples of these range from skin reddening to lethal effects if the dose reaches such a threshold level. At very low levels of radiation dose, deterministic effects have a very low probability, but will move towards a probability of 1 if dose reaches a threshold level of dose for that effect to occur. The other effect of radiation on the body is the stochastic effect, which is the biological state where the cell acquires genetic mutations (DNA changes) due to the effect of the radiation, potentially causing the development of cancer over time by the damage to chromosomes. Stochastic effects may happen at much lower doses than deterministic effects, and the greater the dose, the greater the probability of cancer occurring. However, an

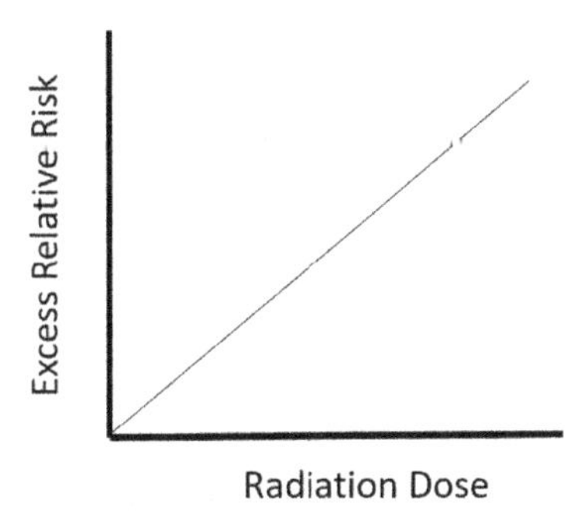

FIGURE 3.2 The linear no-threshold relationship between radiation dose and relative risk associated with stochastic effects of radiation.

important point is that it is generally considered that there is no absolute threshold dose for inducing cancer, so there is no minimum dose for the stochastic effect of radiation to be manifested. The linear no-threshold (LNT) model of stochastic effects assumes that the incidence of cancer is directly proportional to dose (Figure 3.2). This simple concept is easy to apply, but it can lead to the presumption that no radiation dose is safe, even if it is small, as in naturally occurring background radiations. Low doses of radiation, typically used in imaging procedures, have been demonstrated to have stochastic effects on genetic material (see the section on the evidence for radiobiological damage from low-dose X-rays). For CT procedures, the deterministic threshold limits for effects of radiation on the body are far above those used in CT, with the biggest concern being stochastic effects (Smith and Webb, 2010).

MEASUREMENT OF CT DOSES

As CT uses ionising radiation, it is important to understand how the dose of radiation is calculated. There are three principal methods of measuring the dose from ionising radiations in general:

1. The most basic of the three definitions is the *absorbed dose* (D), which is the amount of energy due to the X-rays absorbed (E), measured in Joules per kg of tissue. The unit of grays (Gy) where 1 Gy is equal to 1 J/kg. This is a less useful measurement of radiation dose in CT. For example, consider patient 'A' had a scan that consisted of ten slices, and patient 'B' received a scan of 20 slices with all other factors remaining identical. The absorbed dose per unit mass to the tissue in patient A is approximately the same as in patient B. This is due to the dose of the additional ten slices being absorbed in a different area. However, the total energy imparted by the ionising radiation for patient B is twice that of patient A.
2. The *equivalent* dose (H_T) is the absorbed dose multiplied by a weighting factor for the type of radiation. Conveniently for the X-rays used in CT, this weighting factor is 1. Therefore, the unit of H_T is J/kg, though this is typically given in Sieverts (S_V) or more usually millisieverts (mSv) for the doses in CT.

3. There is recognition that some tissues are more sensitive to damage from the effects of radiation than others, and this leads to the concept of *effective dose*. This is the equivalent dose (H_T) multiplied by the tissue weighting factor for that particular organ (w_T). These weighting factors are given in Table 3.1. These values are important as they represent the fraction of the total stochastic radiation risk for the different organs and tissues that make up the body. The gonads risk points to the induction of hereditary conditions, while in the other organs there is a risk of inducing cancer with the radiation used.

The most relevant quantity for estimating the risk of cancer from a CT procedure is the effective dose (US Food and Drug Administration, 2017). However, typical values for effective dose should be seen as estimates that are not able to be precisely associated with a particular CT system or patient. The actual effective dose could be two or three times larger than the estimate with the effective dose from diagnostic CT procedures ranging from 1 to 10 mSv per scan.

Dose may be measured in CT in a number of different ways and is complicated by the fact that the X-ray beam profile across each slice is not uniform and slices that are adjacent receive dose from each other (Smith and Webb, 2010). Computed tomography dose index (CTDI) is the most fundamental measurement of dose. For a nominal 14-slice CT examination, CTDI is defined as follows:

$$CTDI = \frac{1}{T}\int_{-7T}^{+7T} D_z \, dz$$

where T is the slice thickness and D_z is the absorbed dose at position z.

This has quickly become obsolete, as the number of slices is large in a modern CT scanner. The adapted measure is therefore CTDI_{100}, measured over a 100-mm-long ionisation chamber, where N is the number of slices acquired and T is the nominal width of each slice:

$$CTDI_{100} = \frac{1}{NT}\int_{-50\,\text{mm}}^{+50\,\text{mm}} D(z)\,dz$$

TABLE 3.1

Tissue Weighting Factors Used to Calculate Effective Dose

Tissue	Tissue Weighting Factor
Bone-marrow (red), colon, lung, stomach, breast and remainder tissues[a]	0.12
Gonads	0.08
Bladder, oesophagus, liver and thyroid	0.04
Bone surface, brain, salivary glands and skin	0.01

Source: Adapted from the 2007 Recommendations of the ICRP Commission on Radiological Protection publication 103 (2007).

[a] The remainder tissues number 14 in total: Adrenals, Extrathoracic region, Gall bladder, Heart, Kidneys, Lymphatic nodes, Muscle, Oral mucosa, Pancreas, Prostate, Small intestine, Spleen, Thymus and Uterus/cervix. The weighting factor (0.12) is divided equally between these: 0.0086 for each remainder tissue.

Further refinement occurs when it is recognised that the $CTDI_{100}$ value is dependent upon positioning within the scan plane: dose varies depending on the position. Therefore, the weighted CTDI, $CTDI_w$, is defined as follows:

$$CTDI_w = \frac{1}{3}(CTDI_{100} \text{ centre}) + \frac{2}{3}(CTDI_{100} \text{ periphery})$$

In measuring this value, one of the two test objects is used that approximates either the head or the body (Figure 3.3). They are made from clear cast acrylic and both are 15 cm in length. An ionisation chamber detector is inserted into the circular cut-outs, denoted as black in the diagrams, measuring dose at the centre and the periphery of the test objects for the calculation above.

When helical scans are performed, the measurement $CTDI_{vol}$ is given by $CTDI_w$/pitch and is measured in gray (mGy, cGy). Pitch is the ratio of the table feed (d) per rotation of the X-ray tube to the slice thickness (S), and in most clinical scans, lies between 1 and 2:

$$Pitch = \frac{d}{S}$$

$$CTDI_{Vol} = \frac{CTDI_w}{pitch}$$

These measurements of dose are quite crude approximations and simulations for CT dose for real patient situations are an area of active research (Smith and Webb, 2010). $CTDI_{vol}$ is a commonly used dose descriptor. It is particularly important to note that $CTDI_{vol}$ is *not* the dose to that particular patient, even though this is presented to the operator on the scanner console before the scan is initiated and may be recorded as part of the information about the examination. In fact, the dose is directly dependent on the size and shape of the patient, while $CTDI_{Vol}$ is calculated in standard conditions using the acrylic phantom measuring radiation output for a particular scanner and protocol. It allows comparison of protocols and scanner radiation outputs, but not *individual* patient doses (McCullough et al., 2011). There has been work on size-specific dose estimation (SSDE) in CT which gives a more accurate representation of the dose a patient receives. This takes into account the patients size based on the anteroposterior and lateral dimensions of the patient and provides a coefficient which can be used to transform $CTDI_{Vol}$ into a radiation dose for that particular patient's volume of tissue that has been irradiated (American Association of Physicists in Medicine, 2011). Using this formula, an approximate dose for organs can be obtained in the centre of the scan range using $CTDI_{Vol}$ and measurements of patient sizes.

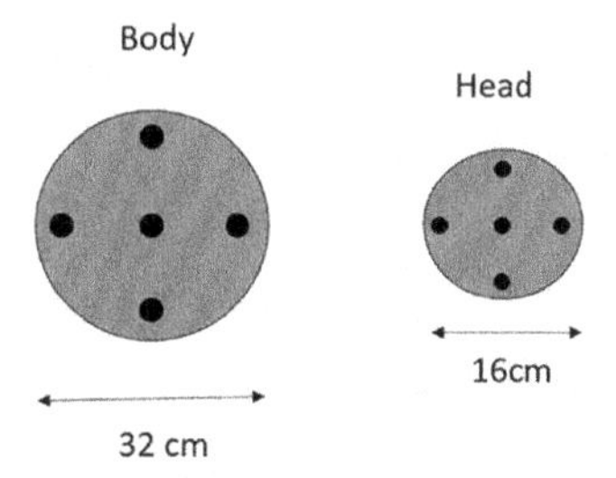

FIGURE 3.3 Diagrammatic cross-section of the CTDI dose phantoms.

TABLE 3.2
Examples of CT Doses

Examination	Clinical Indication	Scan Region/ Technique	$CTDI_{vol}$ Per Sequence (mGy)	DLP Per Complete Examination (mGy cm)
Head	Acute stroke	Post fossa	80	
		Cerebrum	60	
		Brain (whole)	60	
		All sequences		970
Cervical spine	Fracture	All sequences	21	440
Chest	Lung cancer	All sequences	12	610
Chest – high resolution	Interstitial lung disease	Axial	4	140
		Helical	12	350
Chest-abdomen-pelvis	Cancer	All sequences		1,000
CT Angiography (CTA)	Abdominal aorta/blood vessels	All sequences	15	1,040
CT Pulmonary Angiography (CTPA)	Pulmonary embolism	All sequences	13	440
Abdomen	Liver metastases	All sequences	14	910
Abdomen and pelvis	Abscess	All sequences	15	745
Virtual colonoscopy	Polyps/Tumour	All sequences	11	950
Kidneys-ureters-bladder	Stones/Colic	All sequences	10	460
Urogram	Tumour/Stones/Colic	All sequences	13	1,150
Coronary CT angiography (CTA)		Prospective, no padding		170

Source: Adapted from National Diagnostic Reference Levels (NDRLs) from August 2019 (Public Health England, 2019).

For example, using this formula, the brain absorbed dose is 50–60 mGy and the effective dose, however, is 1.5 mSv.

Another commonly used dose descriptor is the dose length product (DLP). This is a measure of the energy absorbed per unit length of scan (in the z-axis). And it adapts $CTDI_{vol}$ by including a measure of the scan length:

$$\text{DLP} = CTDI_{\text{Vol}} \times \text{Scan length during exposure}$$

Conventionally, DLP is measured in milligray centimetres (mGy cm). Scanners show the $CTDI_{vol}$ and DLP indices both before and after a scan is carried out. This dose report is sent with the images to PACS. Table 3.2 shows some example values for $CTDI_{vol}$ and DLP in common CT examinations.

POTENTIAL RADIATION RISKS FROM CT EXAMINATIONS

One of the main risks associated with them is the increased possibility of cancer induction from X-ray exposure (US Food and Drug Administration, 2017). The FDA state that, when used appropriately, the benefits of a CT scan far outweigh the risks.

However, the possibility of cancer induction is reflected by McCullough et al. (2015) when considering articles in the popular press and scientific literature. These often imply that CT may cause cancer and the authors identify that the magnitude of the concern in the press that CT scans increase cancer risk is unreasonably high.

It is important to appreciate that some CT examinations may need more than one scan, i.e. multiple scans of the same area, and this adds to the cumulative dose. An example may be to observe tissue vascularity, when a scan using iodinated contrast media may be undertaken in the venous and arterial phases. These scans may add up to 20 or even 30 mSv effective dose in total (McCullough et al., 2015). Sadetzki and Mandelzweig (2009) state that 2 or 3 CT scans may be commonly carried out, which may involve 30–90 mSv of effective dose. They suggest this is comparable to a subgroup of 25,000 studied atomic bomb survivors who had a statistically significant increase in solid cancers with doses of 5–150 mSv. However, radiation doses with a cumulative dose up to 100 mSv are referred to as 'low dose' radiations (Vaiserman et al., 2019). There has been concern that patients can undergo CT exams with cumulative effective dose greater than 100 mSv over a 5-year period (Rehani et al., 2020). In their study, 1.33% of patients in 324 hospitals received a cumulative effective dose $\geq$ 100 mSv, with around 20% of the patients being less than age 50, thus having more time for the oncologic effects of the radiation to become apparent. The minimum time for an individual patient to reach 100mSv was 1 day. These figures are concerning as they put patients out of the low-dose radiation category into a higher dose category. This serves to emphasise the need to justify requests for CT examinations which takes account of previous imaging and clinical need, balancing the risks and benefits of the study. There should also be emphasis on reducing the dose for examinations by using up-to-date CT equipment that is able to scan with reduced dose to patients and optimised protocols.

Evidence for Radiobiological Damage of X-Rays

There are documented effects of radiation in radiotherapy where X-rays are used in much larger doses, compared to CT, in order to kill cancer cells. For example, dose-related side effects of the radiation include potential damage to the heart in breast cancer radiotherapy, primarily due to damage to cardiac macro- and microvasculature. This can affect some individuals more than others, i.e. individual variability (Sardaro et al., 2012). Individuals react to ionising radiation in ways that are not equal (Foray et al., 2012), leading to the phrase 'individual radiosensitivity', though this historically refers to the risk from radiotherapy tissue reactions (deterministic effects) rather than radiation-induced cancers (stochastic effects). There have been efforts recently to look at the detection of DNA damage at much lower doses of radiation similar to, and in some cases, lower than that used in CT. Inter-individual responses can be seen even with doses as low as 1 mGy with immunofluorescence techniques where individual DNA damage in nuclei may be seen (Rothkamm and Löbrich, 2003). Further, in low-dose exposures that range from 2 to 500 mGy, inter-individual differences in response have emerged. For example, in X-ray exposures in mammography-like conditions, ex vivo epithelial mammary cells, cells from women with high familial risk of cancer, had an excess of unrepaired DNA double-strand breaks and enhanced low and repeated dose effects (Colin et al., 2011b). Unrepaired and misrepaired DNA double-strand breaks are the key events in radiation-induced toxicity (radiosensitivity) and genomic instability, and the individuals' susceptibility to induction of cancer is due to ionising radiation exposure. This is described by Colin et al. (2011a) as 'cancer-proneness'. Their findings suggest that in these relatively low doses, there was a threshold for radiation-induced genomic instability amongst some individuals which they defined as hyper-radiosensitivity at low doses. This would lead to the assertion that individual factors related to radiosensitivity are important even at low doses of radiation such as CT. However, it must be stated that these experiments were not carried out in patients where the cells form parts of tissues and organs and were purely ex vivo. These findings of varying levels of radiosensitivity in individuals may have implications in CT and research in this area will be of great interest to the CT community.

RADIATION HORMESIS

The concept that biological systems are able to respond in a positive manner to a low dose of some agent than at higher doses where they respond negatively as it becomes toxic is termed hormesis (Calabrese and Baldwin, 2000). In terms of CT, this may mean that the dose of radiation considered in general as 'low' as it is under 100 mSv which may actually be of benefit to health (Vaiserman et al., 2018). This is because there is evidence that low doses of ionising radiation can stimulate adaptive responses in organisms, and therefore, the LNT concept of ionising radiation stochastic effects whereby even small doses of radiation that can cause cancer can be challenged (Cuttler, 2018). This effect is shown diagrammatically in Figure 3.4. The decreased biological effect is seen as the portion of the graph below the *x* axis.

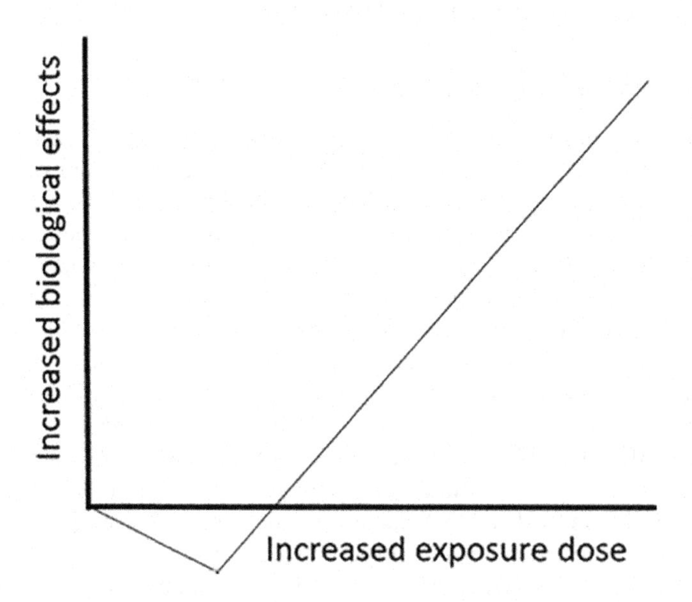

FIGURE 3.4 The hormetic model of ionising radiation exposure and biological effect. (Adapted from Baldwin and Grantham (2015).)

This low-dose exposure helps the body, and as the dose increases, this benevolent effect decreases (Baldwin and Grantham, 2015).

As an example of the positive effects of low-dose radiation, pain relief properties of radon therapies have been described for centuries in rheumatic disease (Rühle et al., 2017). This use of alpha particle radiation emitted from inert radon gas is used in treatment spas in Europe and is believed to provide analgesic and anti-inflammatory effects for rheumatic disease (Annegret and Thomas, 2013; Rühle et al., 2017). There is evidence for changes in the body due to the exposure to the radiation: blood tests reveal modulation of peripheral immune cells after the radon therapy in concordance with reduction of inflammation (Rühle et al., 2017). Annegret and Thomas (2013) also found that pain relief from radon spa therapy can last for 9 months post-treatment. The effect of natural background radon gas on lung cancer prevalence was studied by Cohen (1995). He examined lung cancer rates in different areas of the USA and concluded that there was a strong tendency for lung cancer rates to *decrease* with *increasing* radon exposure due to background radiation. This again is in contradiction to the LNT model which would have predicted the opposite effect for inhaled radon decay products. In another study based in the USA, states were grouped into high-impact states and low-impact states depending on their proximity to nuclear weapons testing sites (Lehrer and Rosenzweig, 2015). Lung cancer rates were lower in high-impact states than in low-impact states. Again this study would appear to contradict the LNT model. In terms of radiations used for medical purposes, Scott, Haque and Di Palma (2007) consider responses to low-LET (low linear energy transfer) ionising radiations such as X-rays and gamma radiations. This type of ionising radiation may stimulate the removal of cells that exist with genomic instability such as neoplastically transformed cells. They suggest that, for example, long-term smokers (with pre-cancerous lung lesions) and alcoholics (with pre-cancerous liver lesions) may have some pre-cancerous cells removed by diagnostic X-rays and CT scans, though caution that more research is needed to validate these claims.

The emphasis on radiation hormesis is away from the DNA focussed view of radiation damage to a more systemic view, that is, low doses of radiation can trigger adaptive responses that can prevent environmentally induced health effects including neoplasms that are malignant (Vaiserman et al., 2018). DNA damage rises with increasing dose, but certain cell defence mechanisms are more efficient at lower doses. Below a single tissue dose of approximately 0.1 Gy, the net benefits tend to be greater than the detriment. This can stimulate mechanisms that repair the initial damage and protect from subsequent irradiation that may initiate cancer, including at a whole body level (Feinendegen et al., 2007). At a biochemical level, low-dose radiation may stimulate unscheduled DNA repair and induce free radical detoxification and repair systems; at the cellular level, it may stimulate the immune response (Macklis and Beresford, 1991).

The hormetic effect of low doses of radiation challenges the widely adopted LNT hypothesis, and therefore, currently lies outside the mainstream of opinion. According to Shibamoto and Nakamura (2018), there is a steady increase in the number of laboratory studies of low-dose radiation effects, and conclusions about whether low-dose radiation has harmful or beneficial effects should be made soon. This will allow further discussion of the appropriateness of the LNT model and should have important implications for the use of CT.

CT RADIATION DOSE IN CHILDREN

The use of ionising radiation in diagnosis of children in particular has raised concern about the iatrogenic damage that may be caused (Sadetzki and Mandelzweig, 2009). They suggest that the susceptibility of children to this damage is entirely plausible from a biological perspective, as tissues are still growing and dividing cells become more susceptible to somatic damage. There is also the fact that children have a longer life expectancy than adults who have CT scans during which time oncologic effects may be able to become apparent: they have a longer life expectancy in which to develop radiation-induced cancer (Shah and Platt, 2008). A number of studies have been carried out in evaluating the excess relative risk (ERR) of inducing cancer in children as a consequence of their age. In a study of atomic bomb survivors, the ERR per Gray of absorbed dose decreased with increasing age at the time of exposure, particularly for thyroid cancer (Preston et al., 2007): so as children mature, it appears that the ERR of radiation-induced cancer decreases. This pattern of ERR decreases as patient age increases: in the case of children who have radiotherapy for cancer of the head, neck or upper thorax when measuring their increased risk of thyroid cancer (Sigurdson et al., 2005), with doses in their study being up to 20–29 Gy. Over 30 Gy, a decrease in the dose–response model was seen due to the cell-killing effect of the radiotherapy.

According to Goodman et al. (2019) since the turn of the millennium, there has been increased emphasis on the risks from radiation using CT scans, particularly the potential risks with children. This has also spread into the adult community and led to debates, particularly in the USA, to keep radiation as low as reasonably achievable and the ‘Image Gently’ campaign to child-size the amount of radiation used (Goske et al., 2008). Due to the concern of dose in CT with children, Strauss et al. (2010) suggest that radiation doses for children should be differentiated from adult doses by (i) ‘child sizing’ CT scanning parameters; (ii) optimising paediatric examining parameters; (iii) scanning only the indicated area (scan once) and (iv) preparing a child-friendly and expeditious CT environment. This advice appears to be a rational response to concerns over paediatric CT radiation dose.

Turning to studies based on CT in children and the possibility of inducing cancer, a recent study from the Netherlands looked at CT scans of almost 200,000 children from 1979 to 2012 (Meulepas et al., 2019). They concentrated on leukaemia and brain tumours, the most frequently encountered radiogenic malignancies, potentially being induced by CT scans. They found a statistically significant relationship between dose and effect for brain tumours, though not for leukaemia. For perspective, they indicate that there are around 10,000 brain CT scans carried out every year on Dutch children with the estimate of one brain tumour case per annum being attributed to the radiation from the CT scan. This may vindicate somewhat the assertion of Brenner and Hall (2007) that the risks to one individual are not great, but the increasing exposure to radiation in the population may become a public health issue. An earlier UK-based study also identified an increased cancer risk in children who have had CT scans. Pearce et al. (2012) found that in children who had their first CT scan at age less than 10 years, cumulative dose of 50 mGy may increase the risk of leukaemia by 3 times and 60 mGy may triple the risk of brain cancer. However, as these diseases are relatively rare in the population of children, the absolute risk is one extra case of leukaemia and one extra case of brain tumour per 10,000 head CT scans. Goodman et al. (2019) suggest that paediatric CT dose optimisation is work in progress though it is hampered by difficulties in measuring *actual* dose to patients. They also argue that a cohort of 5 million participants would be needed to accurately quantify cancer risk for doses of 10 mSv. The balancing of image quality and patient dose has been happening since the millennium, resulting in partnerships between the various bodies interested in this area. This concern for the CT radiation dose given to children will continue to benefit patients, both small and large.

A detailed study of literature around paediatric dose from radiological imaging (including CT) was carried out by Marcu, Chau and Bezak (2021). This considered literature published from 2010 to 2020, with 45 studies included in their evaluation and provided some very useful findings of the agreements across studies (Table 3.3). This table considers all examinations using radiological imaging; however, their findings are applicable to CT examinations except 2.

More specifically, Marcu, Chau and Bezak (2021) provided findings based on exposed anatomy in the paediatric population. In the head and neck, their review identified no association with brain tumour development (medulloblastoma) after a CT scan for head injury. CT of the chest in the paediatric population revealed that the chest diameter was a stronger predictor of CT dose than the patients weight and total scan length. Chest organ dose and cancer risk with CT decrease exponentially with increasing average diameter of the chest, and cancer risk also decreases with patient age. Plain radiography is preferred over CT of the traumatic injuries to the thoracic spine in female paediatric patients due to a significantly lower dose to the breast

TABLE 3.3
General Agreements from Review of the Literature around Paediatric Exposure

Key Findings across the Literature Reviewed
1. Dose reduction by using non-imaging modalities, wherever possible, or plain radiographs
2. Dose reduction by protection of radiosensitive organs (e.g. thyroid shield and breast shield)
3. Use of CT imaging selectively rather than routinely – whole body CT (panscan) should be justified
4. Use of dedicated scan protocols for each imaging modality and device
5. Recording of specific exposure parameters for each patient during the procedure (particularly fluoroscopy)
6. Creation of dose registries for paediatric exposure
7. Cumulative dose monitoring for long-term risk analysis
8. Comparative dose-risk analysis amongst the imaging modalities for different conditions in order to evaluate the optimal choice for each case

Source: Adapted from Marcu, Chau and Bezak (2021).

tissue. Chest radiography for blunt trauma has a good correlation with CT information with a greatly reduced radiation dose. Partial body (thorax-abdomen-pelvis) doses from CT depend heavily on acquisition parameters of pitch and tube current together with the patients' size. The organs that have the greatest risk of cancer incidence are the ovaries in females and the liver in males. These findings of Marcu, Chaua and Bezak (2021) are particularly relevant as their systematic review of the literature is comprehensive and current at the time of publishing of this chapter.

The question of inducing cancer in the unborn child as a result of a CT scan was the subject of study in Ontario, Canada (Ray et al., 2010). Here, comparison was made between those children whose mothers had undergone 'major radio diagnostic testing', defined as either a CT scan or a radionuclide study in pregnancy (5,590 mothers) compared to 1,829,927 who had not from 1991 to 2008. Their findings indicated that 73% of mothers underwent CT scans in pregnancy, the rest having radionuclide studies with an overall proportion of 3.0 per 1,000 pregnant women having a major radio diagnostic test at a mean gestational age of 15.7 weeks. After a median follow-up time of 8.9 years, the study found that the overall prevalence of cancer in the children who were in utero at the time of the procedure was around 1 in 10,000, the relative risk being 1.8 times that of an unexposed pregnancy. The research would indicate that, though children are at increased risk of developing stochastic effects due to their biological risk to the radiation used in CT, the individuals risk is generally low. However, it is right to recognise that all CT examinations must be fully justified before they are undertaken and to 'image gently'.

CONCLUSION

This chapter has explored a number of facets of the radiobiology of CT, ranging from the contribution of CT to the general ionising radiation doses of the population to specifics of measuring CT dose and the biological effects of radiation. Although there are disadvantages of the use of CT in that ionising radiation is used that can cause stochastic radiation effects on the body, the benefits of a CT examination, assuming that it is adequately justified, should greatly outweigh the disadvantages.

REFERENCES

American Association of Physicists in Medicine, 2011. Size Specific Dose Estimates (SSDE) in pediatric and adult body CT examinations. Report of the AAPM Task Group 204, College Park, MD, 2011.

Annegret, F. and Thomas, F., 2013. Long-term benefits of radon spa therapy in rheumatic diseases: Results of the randomized, multi-center IMuRa trial. *Rheumatology International*, *33*(11), pp. 2839–2850.

Baldwin, J. and Grantham, V., 2015. Radiation hormesis: Historical and current perspectives. *Journal of Nuclear Medicine Technology*, *43*(4), pp. 242–246.

Brenner, D.J. and Hall, E.J., 2007. Computed tomography—An increasing source of radiation exposure. *New England Journal of Medicine*, *357*(22), pp. 2277–2284.

Calabrese, E.J. and Baldwin, L.A., 2000. Radiation hormesis: Its historical foundations as a biological hypothesis. *Human & Experimental Toxicology*, *19*(1), pp. 41–75.

Cohen, B.L., 1995. Test of the linear-no threshold theory of radiation carcinogenesis for inhaled radon decay products. *Health Physics*, *68*(2), pp. 157–174.

Colin, C., Devic, C., Noël, A., et al., 2011a. DNA double-strand breaks induced by mammographic screening procedures in human mammary epithelial cells. *International Journal of Radiation Biology*, *87*(11), pp. 1103–1112.

Colin, C., Granzotto, A., Devic, C., Massart, C., Viau, M., Vogin, G., Maalouf, M., Joubert, A. and Foray, N., 2011b. MRE11 and H2AX biomarkers in the response to low-dose exposure: Balance between individual susceptibility to radiosensitivity and to genomic instability. *International Journal of Low Radiation*, *8*(2), pp. 96–106.

Cuttler, J.M., 2018. Treating neurodegenerative diseases with low doses of ionizing radiation. In Rattan, S. and Kyriazi, M. eds., 2018. *The Science of Hormesis in Health and Longevity* (pp. 1–17). Elsevier Science and Technology, San Diego, CA.

Feinendegen, L.E., Pollycove, M. and Neumann, R.D., 2007. Whole-body responses to low-level radiation exposure: New concepts in mammalian radiobiology. *Experimental Hematology*, *35*(4), pp. 37–46.

Foray, N., Colin, C. and Bourguignon, M., 2012. 100 years of individual radiosensitivity: How we have forgotten the evidence. *Radiology*, *264*(3), pp. 627–631.

Goodman, T.R., Mustafa, A. and Rowe, E., 2019. Pediatric CT radiation exposure: Where we were, and where we are now. *Pediatric Radiology, 49*(4), pp. 469–478. doi:10.1007/s00247-018-4281-y.

Goske, M.J., Applegate, K.E., Boylan, J., Butler, P.F., Callahan, M.J., Coley, B.D., Farley, S., Frush, D.P., Hernanz-Schulman, M., Jaramillo, D. and Johnson, N.D., 2008. The image gently campaign: Working together to change practice. *American Journal of Roentgenology*, *190*(2), pp. 273–274.

International Commission on Radiological Protection, 1977. *Recommendations of the International Commission on Radiological Protection* (No. 26, pp. 1–80). Elsevier Science & Technology.

Lehrer, S. and Rosenzweig, K.E., 2015. Lung cancer hormesis in high impact states where nuclear testing occurred. *Clinical Lung Cancer*, *16*(2), pp. 152–155.

Macklis, R.M. and Beresford, B., 1991. Radiation hormesis. *Journal of Nuclear Medicine*, *32*(2), pp. 350–359.

Marcu, L.G., Chau, M. and Bezak, E., 2021. How much is too much? Systematic review of cumulative doses from radiological imaging and the risk of cancer in children and young adults. *Critical Reviews in Oncology/Hematology*, *160*, p. 103292.

McCollough, C.H., Bushberg, J.T., Fletcher, J.G. and Eckel, L.J., 2015. Answers to common questions about the use and safety of CT scans. In *Mayo Clinic Proceedings* (Vol. 90, No. 10, pp. 1380–1392). Elsevier.

McCollough, C.H., Leng, S., Yu, L., Cody, D.D., Boone, J.M. and McNitt-Gray, M.F., 2011. CT dose index and patient dose: They are not the same thing. *Radiology*, *259*(2), pp. 311–316.

Meulepas, J.M., Ronckers, C.M., Smets, A., Nievelstein, R., Gradowska, P., Lee, C., Jahnen, A., van Straten, M., de Wit, M.Y., Zonnenberg, B., Klein, W.M., Merks, J.H., Visser, O., van Leeuwen, F.E. and Hauptmann, M., 2019. Radiation exposure from pediatric CT scans and subsequent cancer risk in the Netherlands. *Journal of the National Cancer Institute*, *111*(3), 256–263. doi:10.1093/jnci/djy104.

OECD, 2021. *Computed Tomography (CT) Exams.* Available at: https://data.oecd.org/healthcare/computed-tomography-ct-exams.htm (Accessed on 14 March 2021).

Preston, D.L., Ron, E., Tokuoka, S., Funamoto, S., Nishi, N., Soda, M. and Kodama, K., 2007. Solid cancer incidence in atomic bomb survivors: 1958–1998. *Radiation Research*, *168*(1), 1–64.

Public Health England, 2011. *Ionising Radiation: Dose Comparisons.* Available at: https://www.gov.uk/government/publications/ionising-radiation-dose-comparisons/ionising-radiation-dose-comparisons (Accessed 14th March 2021).

Public Health England, 2019. *National Diagnostic Reference Levels (NDRLs) from 19 August 2019.* Available at: https://www.gov.uk/government/publications/diagnostic-radiology-national-diagnostic-reference-levels-ndrls/ndrl#national-drls-for-computed-tomography-ct (Accessed 15th March 2021).

Ray, J.G., Schull, M.J., Urquia, M.L., You, J.J., Guttmann, A. and Vermeulen, M.J., 2010. Major radiodiagnostic imaging in pregnancy and the risk of childhood malignancy: A population-based cohort study in Ontario. *PLoS Medicine*, *7*(9), p. e1000337.

Rehani, M.M., Yang, K., Melick, E.R., Heil, J., Šalát, D., Sensakovic, W.F. and Liu, B., 2020. Patients undergoing recurrent CT scans: Assessing the magnitude. *European Radiology*, *30*(4), pp. 1828–1836.

Ron, E., 2003. Cancer risks from medical radiation. *Health Physics*, *85*(1), pp. 47–59.

Rothkamm, K, Löbrich M., 2003. Evidence for a lack of DNA double-strand break repair in human cells exposed to very low x-ray doses. *Proceedings of the National Academy of Sciences of the USA*, *100*(9), pp. 5057–5062.

Rühle, P.F., Wunderlich, R., Deloch, L., Fournier, C., Maier, A., Klein, G., Fietkau, R., Gaipl, U.S. and Frey, B., 2017. Modulation of the peripheral immune system after low-dose radon spa therapy: Detailed longitudinal immune monitoring of patients within the RAD-ON01 study. *Autoimmunity*, *50*(2), pp. 133–140.

Sadetzki, S. and Mandelzweig, L., 2009. Childhood exposure to external ionising radiation and solid cancer risk. *British journal of Cancer*, *100*(7), pp. 1021–1025.

Sardaro, A., Petruzzelli, M.F., D'Errico, M.P., Grimaldi, L., Pili, G. and Portaluri, M., 2012. Radiation-induced cardiac damage in early left breast cancer patients: Risk factors, biological mechanisms, radiobiology, and dosimetric constraints. *Radiotherapy and Oncology*, *103*(2), pp. 133–142.

Schauer, D.A. and Linton, O.W., 2009. NCRP report No. 160, ionizing radiation exposure of the population of the United States, medical exposure—Are we doing less with more, and is there a role for health physicists? *Health Physics*, *97*(1), pp. 1–5.

Scott, B.R., Haque, M. and Di Palma, J., 2007. Biological basis for radiation hormesis in mammalian cellular communities. *International Journal of Low Radiation*, *4*(1), pp. 1–16.

Shah, N.B. and Platt, S.L., 2008. ALARA: Is there a cause for alarm? Reducing radiation risks from computed tomography scanning in children. *Current Opinion in Pediatrics*, *20*(3), pp. 243–247.

Shibamoto, Y. and Nakamura, H., 2018. Overview of biological, epidemiological, and clinical evidence of radiation hormesis. *International Journal of Molecular Sciences*, *19*(8), p. 2387.

Sigurdson, A.J., Ronckers, C.M., Mertens, A.C., Stovall, M., Smith, S.A., Liu, Y. and Inskip, P.D., 2005. Primary thyroid cancer after a first tumour in childhood (the Childhood Cancer Survivor Study): A nested case-control study. *The Lancet*, *365*(9476), pp. 2014–2023.

Smith, N.B. and Webb, A., 2010. *Introduction to Medical Imaging: Physics, Engineering and Clinical Applications* (pp. 1–283). Cambridge University Press.

Strauss, K.J., Goske, M.J., Kaste, S.C., Bulas, D., Frush, D.P., Butler, P., and Applegate, K.E., 2010. Image gently: Ten steps you can take to optimize image quality and lower CT dose for pediatric patients. *American Journal of Roentgenology*, *194*(4), pp. 868–873.

The 2007 recommendations of the international commission on radiological protection. ICRP publication 103. 2007. *Annals of the ICRP*, *37*(2–4), pp. 1–332.

US Food and Drug Administration, 2017. *What are the Radiation Risks form CT?* Available at: https://www.fda.gov/radiation-emitting-products/medical-x-ray-imaging/what-are-radiation-risks-ct. Accessed 14th March 2012).

Vaiserman, A., Koliada, A., Socol, Y., 2019. Hormesis through low-dose radiation. In Rattan, S. and Kyriazi, M. eds., *The Science of Hormesis in Health and Longevity* (pp. 129–138). Elsevier Science and Technology, San Diego, CA.

Vaiserman, A., Koliada, A., Zabuga, O. and Socol, Y., 2018. Health impacts of low-dose ionizing radiation: Current scientific debates and regulatory issues. *Dose-Response*, *16*(3), pp. 1–27.

Section 2

Dose Optimization

4 Dose Optimization

Euclid Seeram
Monash University
Charles Sturt University
University of Canberra

CONTENTS

INTRODUCTION

The double-edged sword of medical radiation refers to the benefits of imaging vs the risks associated with patients' exposure to ionizing radiation. Weighing the value of diagnostic medical imaging against potential cumulative radiation risk

DOI: 10.1201/9781003132554-6

often is referred to as the *risk–benefit ratio*. The benefits of medical imaging are well known based on the work of several investigators (Handee and O'Connor, 2013). For example, diagnostic medical imaging advances have led to more effective surgical treatments and negated the need for some invasive exploratory procedures. Technological advances have helped decrease inpatient hospital stays; improve cancer, stroke, cardiac, and trauma diagnosis and treatment; and enabled rapid diagnosis of life-threatening vascular conditions (Hricak et al., 2011). The risks of radiation also have been studied extensively, and Hendee and O'Connor recently summarized the kinds of injuries seen (Handee and O'Connor, 2013). The authors drew attention to Radiation Effects Research Foundation data and models based on Japanese atomic bomb survivors that form the basis of the Biological Effects of Ionizing Radiations VII (BEIR VII) report (National Research Council, 2006).

Hendee and O'Connor (2013) did not dispute fact-based reports such as BEIR VII but cautioned that the literature and media often extrapolate BEIR radiation risk factors without placing them in context. Hendee and O'Connor (2013) accepted the additional patient exposure from computed tomography (CT) and other medical radiation but cautioned that reports on the effects of radiation dose would be better explained with facts about the effective dose to avoid alarming the public regarding appropriate diagnostic imaging procedures (ibid).

Dauer et al. (2010) reviewed 200 peer-reviewed studies on radiobiology research and epidemiological studies, which did not consider the BEIR VII report. The authors reported that mechanisms of action for radiation effects at low doses likely differ from those at high doses, although high-dose exposures form the basis for estimates of radiation risk at low doses. The Radiation Effects Research Foundation data demonstrate that at high doses (100 mSv and higher), the evidence of increased cancer is statistically significant (Hendee et al., 2013). Because patient doses from diagnostic medical imaging examinations are much lower, several dose–response models have been proposed to extrapolate cancer risks from a high-dose situation to the risks of the low doses used in diagnostic imaging. These models fall into two categories: linear dose–response models and nonlinear dose–response models (ICRP, 2007).

Linear dose–response models essentially comprise two types: a linear dose–response model without a threshold and a linear dose–response model with a threshold. The *linear dose–response model without a threshold* shows that no amount of radiation is considered safe and that any dose, no matter how small, carries some degree of risk. The *linear dose–response model with a threshold* proposes that no adverse effect from radiation below a certain level, known as the threshold dose, is observed. A biological response occurs only when the threshold dose is reached (ICRP, 2007).

Hendee and O'Connor (2013) stated that the linear dose–response model without a threshold is more commonly used because it is a simpler and conservative approach, which is more likely to overestimate cancer risk at low doses than to underestimate the risk of cancer induction. The authors further stated, however, that because medical imaging doses are so low, there is no evidence that the no-threshold model is effective at estimating cancer induction risk.

BIOLOGICAL EFFECTS OF RADIATION EXPOSURE

Biological effects of radiation fall into two broad categories: stochastic effects and deterministic effects. *Stochastic effects* are random, and the probability of their occurrence depends on the amount of radiation dose an individual receives. The probability increases as the dose increases, and there is a no-threshold dose for stochastic effects. Any amount of radiation, no matter how small, has the potential to cause harm. If harm occurs, the damage generally becomes apparent years after exposure; therefore, stochastic effects also are called *late effects*. Examples of stochastic effects include cancer and genetic damage (Brennan and Hall, 2007). Stochastic effects are considered a risk from exposure to the low levels of radiation used in medical imaging, including CT examinations.

Deterministic effects are those for which the severity of the effect (rather than the probability) increases with radiation dose and for which there is a threshold dose. Examples of deterministic effects include skin burns, hair loss, tissue damage, and organ dysfunction. Deterministic effects are also referred to as *early effects* and involve high exposures that are unlikely to occur in medical imaging examinations. A notable exception, however, is the high doses used in fluoroscopy for image guidance in interventional procedures. These doses have been known to cause skin burns. Since the early use of fluoroscopy in interventional procedures, dose management has improved considerably through better dose-monitoring technology and operator education. This type of approach is an important strategy leading to optimization of the benefit–risk ratio, a major goal of medical imaging.

RADIATION PROTECTION PHILOSOPHY

In diagnostic medical imaging, practitioners purposefully expose patients to a low dose of ionizing radiation as a means to improve or restore patients' health. The goal of radiation protection is to prevent deterministic effects by ensuring that doses remain well below relevant threshold doses and to minimize the probability of stochastic effects. To accomplish this goal, radiation protection in medical imaging is guided by national clinical society research and recommendations and frameworks such as those established by the International Commission on Radiological Protection (ICRP), national radiation protection organizations such as the National Council on Radiation Protection and Measurements, and the U.S. Food and Drug Administration (FDA), along with individual state guidelines and regulations (ICRP, 2007; U.S. Food and Drug Administration, 2014).

ICRP System

Three fundamental principles guide the ICRP System for Radiation Protection in medical imaging:

- Justification,
- optimization, and
- application of dose limits.

The principles of justification and optimization address individuals who are exposed to radiation, and the principle of dose limits deals with occupational and environmental exposures and excludes medical exposure.

Justification

The principle of justification specifically deals with the notion that any exposure to a patient should do better than harm. Justification essentially falls within the domain of the patient's referring physician and radiologists who are educated on the risks of radiation exposure. In general, the patient's physician orders the radiography examination based on a clinical assessment of the patient's condition. Once an examination has been justified, or deemed appropriate, the principle of optimization becomes important in the conduct of the examination.

Optimization

The ICRP principle of optimization is intended to protect the patient from unnecessary radiation by using a dose that is as low as reasonably achievable (ALARA). The ultimate goal of optimization is to minimize stochastic effects and to prevent deterministic effects.

The ICRP recommends approaches to dose optimization associated with radiography equipment and daily operations. *Equipment optimization* refers to the manufacturer's design and construction of the imaging unit, and *operations* refers to the options radiologic radiographers choose that enable them to follow the ALARA principle during the examination.

IMAGE QUALITY

Optimization also must address image quality. Specifically, dose optimization strategies must not compromise the image quality required by physicians to diagnose diseases and conditions. Dose optimization is a responsibility of the radiologic radiographer's clinical practice (Mahesh, 2009). According to Matthews and Brennan, the ultimate responsibility for applying optimal technique rests with the individual conducting the examination, and the radiographer usually ensures dose optimization (McCollough et al., 2006). In addition, applying ALARA principles to minimize exposure to the patient, along with self and others, is a component of the scope of practice for all CT radiographers.

THE NEED TO OPTIMIZE CT DOSES

The clinical benefits of CT evaluation and diagnosis of disease are numerous and have continued to expand since the introduction of the technology in the 1970s. A significant increase in the use of CT has occurred because of many technical advances in CT scanner design and performance. Several studies have shown, however, that patient doses from CT examinations are high relative to other radiography examinations (Pearce et al., 2012) and that CT doses typically range from 5 to 50 mGy to each organ within the image field (Wallace et al., 2010). As of 2011, CT contributed the highest collective amount of medical radiation exposure in the United States compared with any other medical imaging modality (Hricak et al., 2011). The relatively high doses related to CT examinations, particularly for pediatric patients, have called attention to the risks of cancer associated with CT scanning (Tian et al., 2014).

The literature on cancer risks from CT includes several examples. A retrospective cohort study published in *The Lancet* in 2012 assessed the risk of leukemia and brain tumors in children and young adults following CT scans. According to Pearce et al., the true risk from low-dose radiation exposure from CT scans is uncertain. The authors noted:

> Potential increases in future cancer risk, attributable to the rapid expansion in CT use have been estimated with risk projection models, which are derived mainly from studies of survivors of the atomic bombs in Japan. These studies have been criticized because of concerns about how applicable the findings from this group are to the relatively low doses of radiation exposure from CT scans and to non-Japanese populations. Some investigators claim that there are no risks, or even beneficial effects, associated with low-dose radiation.

Mathews et al. reported the cancer risk in a large cohort of individuals who had been exposed to CT examinations as children and adolescents. Study participants were followed for a mean period of 9.5 years to determine whether they developed a cancer. Although the authors were still following the study population when the report was published, they found an increased risk of cancer in the children and adolescents who had CT scans from 1985 through 2005. The authors stated that radiation doses from CT scans with contemporary units and techniques likely are lower than those their study cohort had received. The authors also suggested that estimating risks from many studies has been difficult because of relatively small study sizes and selection bias (ibid).

Recently, research by Pearce et al. (2012) and Mathews et al. (2013) assessed cancer risk from CT scanning in large cohorts. Pearce et al. assessed the excess risk of leukemia and brain tumors in children and young adults following CT scans. The authors followed up with patients who had CT scans in Great Britain between 1985 and 2002 and were younger than age 22 years at the time of their scans. Pearce et al. found that cumulative doses from CT scanning could be approximately 50 mGy. A dose of 60 mGy can triple leukemia risk. Among the population studied, 74 of more than 178,600 patients had leukemia during the follow-up period and 135 of more than 176,580 patients had a brain tumor.

The authors noted that relative risk for leukemia was associated with a cumulative dose from CT of at least 30 mGy, and for brain cancer, relative risk was associated with a cumulative dose of at least 50–75 mGy. Both cancers are rare, and cumulative absolute risk therefore remains slight. The authors recommended that attention to CT dose be a priority for manufacturers and the radiology community and that alternative imaging methods that do not use ionizing radiation be considered for children when appropriate (Pearce et al., 2012).

Mathews et al. (2013) estimated cancer risk in more than 680,000 individuals who had received CT scans when aged 0–19 years old were one of the first large studies to derive direct estimates of cancer risk from CT instead of extrapolating risk from high-dose exposures. The authors have continued to research possible lifetime risk from CT scanning in the study population (ibid). Although long-term follow-up of patients exposed to CT scans continues and some risk estimates have yet to be determined, the literature clearly makes the case for dose optimization in CT. In recognition of these potential risks, several authors have emphasized the need to apply principles of the dose–image quality relationship in CT. To understand dose optimization in CT, however, it is essential to thoroughly understand CT dosimetry and CT image-quality metrics.

CT DOSIMETRY FUNDAMENTALS

The nature of CT dosimetry is complex and challenging because of the continuous technological evolution of CT scanners. Dosimetry involves the measurement of the dose to the patient and is characterized by several metrics. These metrics refer to radiation dose quantities and their associated units.

Metrics Display

Of the three-dose metrics commonly used in CT, two of which are shown on the dose report that displays on the CT scanner console. These include the *computed tomography dose index* (CTDI) and the *dose-length product* (DLP). The third dose metric of importance in CT, and in any imaging modality using ionizing radiation, is the *effective dose*. The International System of Units quantity for the CTDI and the DLP is expressed in milligrays (mGy); it is expressed in millisieverts (mSv) for the effective dose. The effective dose relates the radiation exposure to risk and is considered the best method available to estimate stochastic radiation risk (ICRP, 2007). Still, an effective dose is an estimate only, based on weighting factors applied to the body's tissue or the organ being irradiated (Berrington de Conzalez, 2009).

Dose Metrics Calculation

The CTDI, DLP, and effective dose are essential for CT dose optimization. The CT scanner directs a fan-shaped or cone-shaped beam toward an array of detectors. The X-ray tube and detectors rotate 360° around the patient to collect attenuation data. The X-ray tube collimator determines the beamwidth. The typical dose distribution is a bell-shaped curve, as shown in Figure 4.1. The dose distribution is given by the function D(z), where *D* is the dose and *z* is the longitudinal axis of the patient. D(z) is extremely important for the CT dose because this is the dose distribution, or dose profile, that is measured.

Measurement of the dose distribution requires estimation based on at least two types of phantoms (one that simulates the patient's head and a larger one that simulates a patient's body.) The phantoms have several holes (a central hole and four peripheral holes) to accommodate a pencil dosimeter; see Bushberg et al. (2012) and Seeram (2009) for an expanded discussion on CT dose measurement.

The CTDI initially was conceptualized only as an index. The metric was not intended to serve as a method to assess patient radiation dose. Nevertheless,

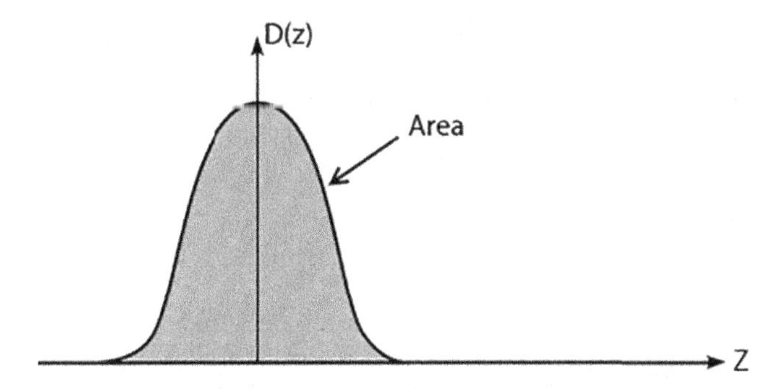

FIGURE 4.1 The width of the X-ray beam is determined by the collimator near the X-ray tube. An ideal dose distribution along the z-axis has a flat top and steep sides and is the same width as the X-ray beam. A more realistic bell-shaped dose distribution curve, as illustrated here, is typical of most CT scanners.

CTDI-based dosimetry is the current international standard for estimating CT radiation.

The FDA first developed a definition of the CTDI, which was referred to as the $CTDI_{FDA}$ and defined as:

$$\text{CTDI}_{\text{FDA}} = \frac{1}{n * sw} \int_{-7\text{mm}}^{+7\text{mm}} D(z)dz \tag{4.1}$$

In the formula, n is the number of distinct planes of data collected per revolution of the tube and detectors, sw is the nominal slice width, and z represents the longitudinal patient axis. For multislice CT scanners, n is the number of active detector rows (e.g., $n = 64$) during the scan. The integral sign in the equation above is numerically equal to the area under the dose distribution curve (the shaded region) as shown in Figure 4.1.

The CTDI_{FDA} is limited to only 14 sections of 7-mm thickness. Therefore, this limitation led to the development of CTDI_{100} to extend the length of the scan measurement to 100 mm. This dose index is expressed mathematically as follows:

$$\text{CTDI}_{100} = \frac{1}{nT} \int_{-50\text{mm}}^{+50\text{mm}} D(z)dz \tag{4.2}$$

Within this formula, nT is equal to the nominal colimited slice thickness.

Yet another dose index was introduced following CTDI_{100}. The weighted CTDI, expressed as CTDI_{W}, addresses the average dose in the x–y axis of the patient. The CTDI_{W} is expressed mathematically as follows:

$$\text{CTDI}_{\text{W}} = \left(\frac{1}{3}\right)(\text{CTDI}_{100})_{\text{center}} + \left(\frac{2}{3}\right)(\text{CTDI}_{100})_{\text{periphery}} \tag{4.3}$$

The use of a weighted CDTI was subsequently followed by yet another change to account for the pitch in multislice CT scanners. This CTDI is referred to as the $CTDI_{vol}$ audit and is expressed mathematically as follows:

$$\mathrm{CTDI_{vol}} = \frac{\mathrm{CTDI_w}}{\mathrm{pitch}} \tag{4.4}$$

When the pitch is 1, the $\mathrm{CTDI_{vol}}$ equals the $\mathrm{CTDI_W}$.

The $\mathrm{CTDI_{vol}}$ is the index displayed on the CT scanner console before scanning begins. This is because the CT manufacturer has measured the $\mathrm{CTDI_{vol}}$ over the range of kilovoltage (kV) values for the specific scanner before shipping the scanner. The stored value is scaled appropriately, according to selected milliampere second (mAs) and pitch, and displayed on the console.

The value of the $\mathrm{CTDI_{vol}}$ is the same whether a radiographer scans a 1-mm or 100-mm length of tissue. The DLP was introduced to provide a much more accurate representation of the dose for a defined length of tissue. The DLP provides a measure of the total dose for a CT examination and can be expressed algebraically as follows:

$$\mathrm{DLP} = \mathrm{CTDI_{100}} \times L \tag{4.5}$$

In this formula, L equals the length of the scan (in centimeters) along the patient's z-axis.

DLP is expressed in mGy-cm. Although the $\mathrm{CTDI_{vol}}$ does not depend on scan length, the DLP is directly proportional to the scan length. This is illustrated in Figure 4.2.

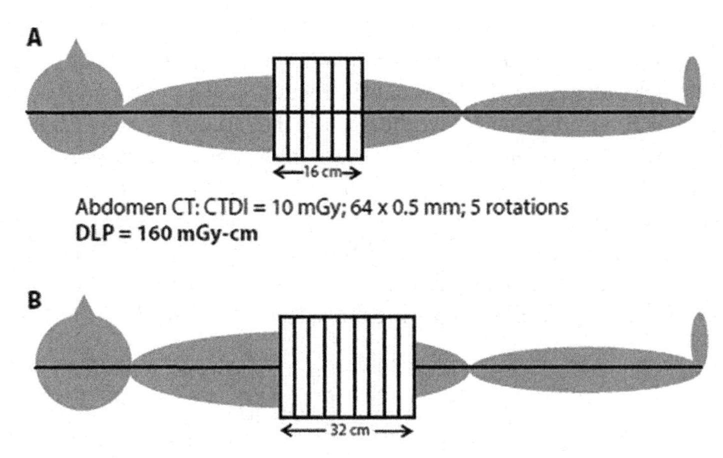

FIGURE 4.2 Hypothetical dose-length product (DLP) values for 2 CT scans of the abdomen. A. The scan length is 16 cm, and the DLP is 160 mGy-cm. B. The scan length is 32 cm, and the DLP is 320 mGy-cm. The DLP is directly proportional to the scan length.

The next stage in this area of patient dose assessment is to address the risk of a CT examination. This requires the use of the effective dose. Effective dose is used in radiation protection to relate exposure to risk, and it takes into account that different tissues have different radiosensitivities. For example, the gonads are more radiosensitive than the brain. As only parts of the body (rather than the entire body) are exposed in medical diagnostic imaging, risk of stochastic radiation response is proportional to the effective dose rather than to the tissue dose. The effective dose is expressed by the following equation:

$$\mathrm{ED} = \sum W_T H_T \tag{4.6}$$

In this formula, H_T is equal to the organ or tissue dose and W_T is the tissue weighting factor.

The DLP can provide only a rough estimate of effective dose. In clinical practice, the DLP is approximately proportional to the effective dose. For simplicity, the effective dose is obtained by multiplying the DLP by constants referred to as *k values* which have been previously established. For example, the *k* value (mSv/mGy-cm) for a CT scan of the head is 0.0021; the *k* value for a CT scan of the pelvis is 0.015. Knowing these *k* values enables calculation of the effective dose as follows:

$$\mathrm{ED} = k \times \mathrm{DLP} \tag{4.7}$$

The effective dose allows for a comparison of the dose received from CT scanning with the dose received from natural background radiation. For example, while the annual effective dose from natural background radiation is reported to be 3 mSv, it is 1.5 mSv for CT and 3 mSv for medical imaging (CT scanning, radiography, interventional, nuclear medicine).

Common radiologic examinations deliver the following effective doses:

- Chest radiograph – 0.02 mSv.
- Radiograph of the abdomen – 1 mSv.
- Barium enema examination – 5 mSv.
- Diagnostic coronary angiogram – 5 mSv.

In contrast, the typical effective doses for common CT scans are higher:

- Head – 2 mSv.
- Chest – 5 mSv.
- Abdomen – 5 mSv.
- Pelvis – 5 mSv.
- Abdomen and pelvis – 10 mSv.
- Coronary angiography – 10 mSv.

TECHNICAL FACTORS AFFECTING THE DOSE IN CT

The optimization principle of the ICRP implies that radiation dose must be kept ALARA. This means that using the lowest possible dose must not compromise the diagnostic quality of an image. CT dose optimization requires an understanding of the factors affecting dose and all image quality factors. Dose and image quality are closely related.

Image quality includes characteristics such as noise, spatial resolution, and contrast resolution. Spatial resolution depends on geometric factors such as focal spot size, slice thickness, and pixel size, but contrast resolution and noise depend on the X-ray beam's quality (energy) and quantity (number of X-ray photons). Bushong presents the following mathematical expression to demonstrate the relationship between CT dose and image quality:

$$\text{Dose} = k * \frac{\text{Intensity} \times \text{Beam Energy}}{\text{Noise}^2 \times \text{Pixel Size}^3 \times \text{Slice Thickness}} \tag{4.8}$$

In this equation, k is a conversion factor.

This expression implies the following about dose and image quality:

- Reducing the noise in an image by a factor of 2 requires an increase in the dose by a factor of 4.
- Improving the spatial resolution (pixel size) by a factor of 2 requires an increase in the dose by a factor of 8.
- Decreasing the slice thickness by a factor of 2 requires an increase in the dose by a factor of 2 (keeping the noise constant).
- Decreasing both slice thickness and pixel size (spatial resolution) by a factor of 2 requires an increase in the dose by a factor of 16 ($2^3 \times 2 = 2 \times 2 \times 2 \times 2$).
- Increasing milliamperage and kilovolt increases patient dose proportionally. For example, a 2-fold increase in milliamperage increases the dose by a factor of 2. Additionally, doubling the dose requires an increase by the square of the kilovolt.

Examples of changes in the CTDI_W values as a function of kilovolt and milliampere seconds have been presented by McKnitt-Gray. At 100 kVp, the CTDI_W for a head phantom is 26 mGy; the CTDI_W increases to 55 mGy at 140 kV. For a body phantom, the CTDI_W is 11 mGy at 100 kV and 25 mGy at 140 kV. In addition to the technical factors (kV, mAs, noise, pixel size, and slice thickness), several other factors influence the dose in CT scans (see Table 2.1.2). These include

- pitch;
- scan field-of-view;
- beam collimation;
- noise-reducing image reconstructive algorithms, particularly iterative reconstruction;
- gantry tilt;

- anatomical coverage;
- automatic exposure control (AEC), such as tube current modulation;
- whether a scanner is a single-detector or a multidetector unit;
- overbeaming and overranging;
- patient centering;
- repeats;
- noise index; and
- improved detection efficiency.

The key factors that radiographers select to optimize dose are exposure technique factors (mAs and kV), pitch, collimation and slices, AEC, noise index, overbeaming and overranging, and noise-reducing image reconstruction algorithms.

Exposure Technique Factors

Exposure technique factors are the milliampere seconds and kilovolt selection. The milliampere seconds are equal to the milliamperage multiplied by the exposure time(s); the exposure value depends on how long it takes the X-ray tube to rotate one full revolution. The milliampere seconds determine the photon flux, which affects the patient's dose and is directly proportional to the milliampere seconds. For example, Cody and McNitt-Gray (2006) found that by scanning a 32-cm body phantom at 220 mAs with a rotation time of 0.5 second, the $CTDI_W$ was 7.4 mGy, and at 440 mAs with a rotation time of 1 second, the $CTDI_W$ was 30.2 mGy. These results are consistent with those reported in 2002 using a single-detector CT scanner (McNitt-Gray, 2002). As mentioned earlier, the dose is proportional to the square of the kilovolt peak (kV^2). This exponential expression poses some difficulty for radiographers in practice because this power (2) can vary from 2.5 to 3.1 and depends on the patient's size. As noted by Maldjian and Goldman (2013), decreasing the kilovolt peak from 140 to 120 kV reduces the dose by 28%–40% for a typical phantom. The authors reported that further decreasing to 80 kV reduces the dose by approximately 65%. Precise adjustment of dose should not be obtained solely through manipulation of peak kilovoltage (ibid).

Pitch

The *pitch* is a parameter that radiographers can select in multislice CT scanning. The pitch is defined as a ratio of the distance the table travels per rotation to the total collimated X-ray beamwidth. The dose and the pitch relationship in CT are calculated as follows:

$$\text{Dose} \propto \frac{1}{\text{pitch}} \tag{4.9}$$

when all parameters (mA and rotation time, for example) remain constant. Therefore, if the pitch increases by 2, the dose is reduced by 0.5 mGy. With all factors held constant at 120 kV, 300 mA, 1 second, and 10 mm using a single-slice scanner, the pitch for a body phantom has been shown to increase from 0.5 with a dose of 36 mGy, while a pitch of 2.0 decreases the $CTDI_{vol}$ to 9 mGy. With the use of AEC, the tube current increases when the pitch is increased, and therefore, it is not best practice to reduce exposure with multislice CT scanners (McCollough et al., 2012).

Collimation and Slices

Collimation in CT defines the beam width and refers to the efficient use of the beam at the detector. For multislice CT, the slice or section thickness (width) is defined by the number of detector elements grouped or binned together in each detector channel (Seeram, 2009). In general, as the collimation width increases (wider beam = thicker section), the dose decreases. As the section thickness decreases, the exposure must increase to maintain the same signal-to-noise ratio as a thick section. A 2.5-mm section requires two times more exposure than a 5-mm section. The relationship for the noise in the image is as follows:

$$\text{Noise} \propto \frac{1}{T} \tag{4.10}$$

In this formula, *T* equals the reconstructed or nominal section thickness.

A thin section measuring 2.5 mm will have increased noise (1.4 times more) than will a 5-mm-thick section. Therefore, if a 2.5-mm-thin section is used in the examination, the technique factors (mAs and kV) must be increased to offset the increased noise associated with thinner sections. McNitt-Gray (2002) reported that when the beam width for a multislice CT scanner increased from 5 mm (4 × 1.25-mm collimation) to 20 mm (4 × 5-mm collimation) and all other factors remained constant, the $CTDI_W$ for a body phantom decreased from 33 to 20 mGy.

Overbeaming and Overranging

Overranging refers to the use of additional rotations before and after the planned length of tissue so that the first and last images can be reconstructed (Kaza et al., 2014). *Overbeaming* is the excess dose beyond the edge of the detector rows per rotation of a multisection (Coakley et al., 2011). Both overranging and overbeaming increase radiation dose to the patient. Adaptive collimation is used in modern CT scanners to reduce patient dose at the beginning and end of scanning. Christner et al. (2010) demonstrated that dynamic collimation can reduce the dose by approximately 40%.

AEC and Image Quality Index

The addition of AEC to CT using *automatic tube current modulation* techniques can be traced back to 1981, and today, all CT scanners feature some form of automatic tube current modulation. The principal objective of automatic tube current modulation is to adjust the milliamperage in either the z-axis (longitudinal), the x–y axis (angular), or both, to reduce patient dose. An important characteristic of AEC systems is a preselected image quality index, also referred to as a *reference* or *target image quality index*. The index is stored in the CT scanner by the manufacturer before shipping. When a radiographer acquires a scan, the unit adjusts milliamperage so that the exposure approximates are used to create the reference image. Various CT manufacturers use different reference image quality models. For example, several CT manufacturers use the following models:

- GE Healthcare – noise index;
- Philips Healthcare – reference image;
- Siemens Healthineers – quality reference milliampere seconds; and
- Canon Medical Systems, formerly Toshiba Medical Systems – CT numbers.

Furthermore, the reference or target image quality index depends on several factors such as tube voltage, patient size, anatomic region, and the diagnostic task. Therefore, the index is an operator-selectable parameter.

It has been demonstrated that automatic tube current modulation can reduce the dose by 20%–40% in adults and up to 26%–50% in adults and children. In addition, and as an illustration of using the GE Healthcare noise index, as the noise index increases, the patient dose decreases but at the expense of a "noisy image". The relationship between the noise index and dose is expressed as follows:

$$\mathrm{NI} \propto \frac{1}{\sqrt{D}} \tag{4.11}$$

In this expression, D equals dose.

Kanal et al. (2007) showed that when the noise index is reduced by 5%, the dose increases by approximately 11%. If the noise index is increased by 5%, the dose is reduced by approximately 9%. Further, Toth et al. (2007) reported that automatic tube modulation was expected to reduce patient effective doses in chest CT examinations by approximately 10%. The authors noted that longitudinal modulation would account for most (two-thirds) of the dose reduction, and angular modulation accounts for the remaining one-third (ibid).

Patient Positioning

When a patient is not centered in the CT gantry isocenter, which means the patient is not centered in the scan field-of-view, image noise and patient dose increase because of poor bowtie filter performance. Studies on phantoms have shown that *miscentering* the patient by as little as 3 cm increased surface dose by 18%, and miscentering by 6 cm increased surface dose by as much as 41% (Toth et al., 2007).

Iterative Image Reconstruction

The goal of *image reconstruction* in CT is to create an image of the X-ray transmission (attenuation measurements) through the patient. There are several defined sets of rules (algorithms) to perform this task, and the pioneering work of Sir Godfrey

Hounsfield involved the use of the algebraic reconstruction technique, a class of iterative algorithms (Verona et al., 2011). These initial iterative algorithms later were replaced by analytic reconstruction algorithms of which the filtered back projection algorithm became the workhorse of CT image reconstruction. One of the major problems with the filtered back projection algorithm is noise; another is streak artifacts. Today, the *iterative reconstruction* (IR) algorithm has resurfaced because of the availability of high-speed computing (ibid). The primary advantages of iterative image reconstruction algorithms are to reduce image noise and minimize the higher radiation dose inherent in the filtered back projection algorithm. All major CT manufacturers offer IR algorithms as of 2014. For example, GE Healthcare offers the Adaptive Statistical IR (ASIR) and Model-Based IR (MBIR) algorithms; Siemens Healthineers offers the Sonogram-Affirmed Image Reconstruction (SAFIRE) and the Advanced Modeled Iterative Reconstruction (ADMIRE); and Canon Medical Systems offer the Adaptive Iterative Dose Reduction (AIDR) and the Adaptive Iterative Dose Reduction 3-Dimensional (AIDR 3D)

The iterative image reconstruction process generally uses the filtered back projection CT image data, referred to as the *measured projections*, to create *simulated projections*. The simulated projections are compared with the initial measured projections to determine differences in image noise. Once this difference is determined, it is applied to the simulated projection to correct for inconsistencies.

The system reconstructs a new CT image, and the process repeats until the difference between the measured and simulated projections is minor enough to be acceptable. This iterative process results in images that are true representations of the subject being scanned with reduced noise and artifacts. Several studies have demonstrated reductions in radiation dose using IR that vary from 30% to 50%. (McCollough et al., 2009; Verona et al., 2011. These studies have included dose reductions in pediatric studies, CT abdominal studies, and CT angiography.

DOSE OPTIMIZATION IN CT

When discussing how to closely follow the ALARA principle and balance the need for patient radiation protection with the need for acquiring high-quality diagnostic images. In short, the previously discussed principle of optimization based on the ICRP radiation protection framework refers to optimization as keeping radiation doses ALARA so as not to compromise the diagnostic quality of the image. Optimization therefore deals with both radiation dose and image quality. Dose reduction strategies relate to adjusting and controlling the technical factors affecting the dose to decrease patient dose. The effect of these factors (e.g., mAs, kV, pitch, scan field-of-view, beam collimation, AEC, overbeaming and overranging, and iterative image reconstruction) on patient dose has been researched by multiple authors. CT dose metrics also have been reviewed. Several articles specifically addressing CT dose reduction are included throughout this text.

A checklist for dose optimization is provided by Goo (2012) and includes body size-adapted, CT protocols, tube current modulation, optimal tube voltage at equivalent radiation dose, longitudinal scan range, repeated scans, scan modes, and noise-reducing IR algorithms.

Research on Dose Optimization and Image Quality

Dose optimization seeks to find a balance in being able to provide optimum image quality by understanding a combination of CT dose and image quality parameters. CT image quality has been described in terms of high-contrast spatial resolution, low-contrast resolution, temporal resolution, CT number accuracy and uniformity, image noise, and image artifacts. Research has continued to determine the best methods for lowering radiation dose in CT examinations without compromising the diagnostic quality of images. These studies often are complex so they can follow precise scientific methods, including identifying the problem, performing a literature review, stating the goals regarding the investigation of the problem, and designing a methodology to find a solution to the problem. Scientific methods also include data collection, analysis, and interpretation of the data and dissemination of the study findings. In general, research on optimizing dose and image quality involves various methodologies to demonstrate dose reduction without a loss of image quality. To determine optimal image quality, McCollough et al. (2006) stressed that studies must involve quantitative metrics such as image noise and observer performance.

In a special issue of the journal *Radiation Protection Dosimetry* dedicated to optimization strategies in medical imaging for fluoroscopy, radiography, mammography, and CT, several studies identified at least four important requirements for dose and image-quality optimization research:

- Ensure *patient safety*.
- Determine the *level of image quality* required for a particular diagnostic task.
- Acquire *images at various exposure levels from high to low* and in such a manner that accurate diagnosis can still be made.
- Use *reliable and valid methodologies* for the dosimetry, image acquisition, and evaluation of image quality using human observers, keeping in mind the nature of the detection task.

To accomplish these requirements, CT dose and image-quality optimization studies must ensure that the following minimum essential elements are considered:

- The CT imaging system is calibrated to ensure consistent and reliable performance.
- The dosimeters used to capture dose levels are calibrated.
- Researchers use appropriate phantoms (anthropomorphic phantoms and phantoms for determining objective image-quality parameters) and acceptable dose measurement methodology for acquiring scans at different exposure levels.
- Images are assessed in two phases:

    1. Expert observers evaluate image quality based on a defined and specific criterion (such as the appearance of image noise) to establish an optimized dose level.

2. The same set of observers is used to assess images obtained at various dose levels, including an optimized dose level, using established, valid, and reliable observer performance methods. *Observer performance methods* include receiver operating characteristics and visual grading analysis methods. The task of pathology detection requires a different observer performance test than that of detecting normal anatomical structures.

Receiving operator characteristic is the more common observer performance method. Under this method, a study's observers determine whether an image contains a lesion or pathology. The observer assigns a grade on a scale (e.g., 1–5) that rates the observer's level of confidence in the decision.

A *visual grading analysis* assigns a grade to the image's quality based on a comparison with a reference image. Visual grading analysis is based on the assumption that an observer's ability to see and evaluate normal anatomy correlates to the ability to evaluate pathology or abnormal findings.

Findings from CT Dose Optimization Studies

Some studies that reduce patient dose markedly by reducing kilovolt, changing pitch, adjusting beam width or collimation, or by using iterative image reconstruction do not address the important consideration of optimizing image quality while reducing dose. For the most part, the studies did not include observer performance methods to evaluate image quality at these reduced exposures. One of the fundamental problems with this approach to dose management is that the dose may be so low that the diagnostic quality of the image is compromised, thus endangering the integrity of the clinical diagnosis and necessitating repeat examinations.

Other research in CT, however, has included methods of dose and image-quality optimization, which include valid and reliable dosimetry, observer image-quality assessment, and statistical analysis of results. Examples include the following:

- Sohaib et al. (2001) examined the effect of reducing milliampere seconds on image quality and patient dose in sinus CT examinations. The authors reported a dose reduction from 13.5 mGy at 200 mAs to 3.1 mGy at 50 mAs ($p < 0.05$) without loss of image quality. The study used an observer performance method that involved visual grading analysis.
- Russell et al. (2008) examined dose-image quality in neck volume CT and showed that automatic tube current modulation reduced the CTDI by 20% with the noise index set at 11.4 and by 34% with the noise index set at 20.2. The dose reductions were made without compromising image quality significantly.

THE ROLE OF THE RADIOGRAPHER IN DOSE OPTIMIZATION

The increasing use of CT as a clinical tool in medicine coupled with the fact that the modality has recently been cited as the largest and most rapidly growing source of medical ionizing radiation exposure has provided an increasingly important rationale for dose reduction and image-quality optimization in CT. All professionals who work in CT should follow ALARA principles. Radiographers play an important role in lowering the CT dose without compromising image quality.

The radiology community has responded to concerns regarding dose and image-quality optimization. One approach has been to examine closely the role of all individuals who have responsibility in optimizing dose in CT. Strauss et al. (2010) and Matthews and Brennan (2009) identified radiologists, physicians, medical physicists, radiographers, and CT manufacturers in this regard. Strauss et al. have described ten steps to optimize image quality and reduce radiation dose in CT. The first of these steps is to increase awareness and understanding of CT radiation dose issues among radiographers.

Strauss et al. (2010) described the need for education in CT physics and CT equipment and registration with the American Registry of Radiologic Radiographers. The authors also noted that radiographers should explore the Image Gently Web site at www.imagegently.org and should "take the pledge" provided on the site to demonstrate their commitment to patient care and safety.

The radiographer is central to CT image acquisition and generally is responsible for equipment start-up procedures and patient care and communications throughout the entire examination, along with patient positioning, communications with the radiologist regarding all clinical aspects of the examination, and overall radiation protection of the patient and other staff present during the examination. As a result, the radiographer plays a significant role in patient dose and image-quality optimization in CT through a thorough understanding of the following factors:

- The risks of radiation and CT dose.
- Current technical advances in CT.
- CT dose metrics, particularly $CTDI_{vol}$, the DLP and effective dose, and associated units.
- CT image-quality metrics such as spatial resolution, contrast resolution, noise, and artifacts.
- The technical factors affecting patient dose in CT, including exposure technique factors (kV and mAs), AEC, pitch, effective milliampere seconds, slice thickness, scan field-of-view, beam collimation, noise-reducing algorithms (IR algorithms), anatomical coverage, overbeaming and overranging, patient centering, and noise index.
- Scan protocols and reviewing the protocols with the radiologist on an ongoing basis to optimize dose and image quality.
- The prescan and postscan display of CT dose reports shows the $CTDI_{vol}$, the DLP, and effective dose.
- How to get involved with the development or implementation of a CT dose-monitoring or dose-tracking system for the radiographer's CT department. Monitoring and tracking should include items such as dose capture, conversion of absorbed dose to effective dose, patient-specific storage, dose analytics, dose communication, and data export.

- How to participate in research on CT patient dose and image-quality optimization. This requires a fundamental knowledge of CT equipment and dosimeter calibration, image acquisition details, observer performance measures, and appropriate statistical tools.
- How to ensure continuous professional development through relevant continuing education activities.

CONCLUSION

The increasing use of CT in medical imaging and the relatively large doses delivered by CT scanning compared with other diagnostic imaging modalities necessitate an emphasis by all radiology professionals to optimize image quality and minimize patient dose from CT examinations. In addition, concerns about the stochastic risk of radiation from within the profession and from the public and media emphasize education of all parties involved in ordering and providing CT examinations or in the design, manufacture, and quality control of CT equipment.

When conducting CT examinations, radiologic radiographers should understand the basic concepts of CT dosimetry with respect to the CTDI and its variants, the DLP, and effective dose. In particular, radiographers should understand how the selection of technical factors, including the recently implemented IR algorithms, affects patient dose in CT. Finally, radiologic radiographers must understand the distinction between CT dose reduction and CT dose optimization and the application of ALARA and remain active participants in optimizing patient dose and image quality.

REFERENCES

Berrington de Gonzalez A, Mahesh M, Kim KP, et al. Projected cancer risks from computed tomographic scans performed in the United States in 2007. *Arch Intern Med.* 2009;169(22):2071–2077. doi:10.1001/archintern med.2009.440.

Brenner DJ, Hall EJ. Computed tomography: An increasing source of radiation exposure. *N Engl J Med.* 2007;357(22):2277–2284.

Bushberg JT, Seibert JA, Leidholdt EM, Boone JM. *The Essential Physics of Medical Imaging.* 3rd ed. Philadelphia, PA: Lippincott Williams & Wilkins; 2012.

Christner JA, Zavaletta VA, Eusemann CD, Walz-Flannigan AL, McCollough CH. Dose reduction in helical CT: Dynamically adjustable z-axis x-ray beam collimation. *AJR Am J Roentgenol.* 2010;194(1):W49–W55. doi:10.2214/AJR.09.2878.

Coakley, FV, Gould R, Yeh BM, Arenson RL. CT radiation dose: What can you do right now in your practice? *AJR Am J Roentgenol.* 2011;196(3):619–625. doi:10.2214/AJR.10.5043.

Cody D, McNitt-Gray M. CT image quality and patient dose, definite, methods and trade offs. In: Frush DP, Huda W, eds. *RSNA Categorical Course in Diagnostic Radiology Physics: From Invisible to Visible – The Science and Practice of X ray Imaging and Dose Optimization.* 2006, 141–155.

Dauer LT, Brooks AL, Hoel DG, Morgan WF, Stram D, Tran P. Review and evaluation of updated research on health effects associated with low-dose ionizing radiation. *Radiat Protect Dosimetry.* 2010;140(2):103–136. doi:10.1093/rpd/ncq141.

Goo HW. CT radiation dose optimization and estimation: An update for radiologists. *Korean J Radiol.* 2012;13(1):1–11. doi:10.3348/kjr.2012.13.1.1.
Hendee WR, O'Connor MK. Radiation risks in medical imaging: Separating fact from fantasy. *Radiology.* 2013;264(2), 312–320. doi:10.1148/radiol.12112678.
Hricak H, Brenner DJ, Adelstein SJ, Frush DP, et al. Managing radiation use in medical imaging: A multifaceted challenge. *Radiology.* 2011;258(3):889–905. doi:10.1148/radiol.10101157.
Kanal KM, Stewart BK, Kolokythas O, Shuman WP. Impact of operator-selected image noise index and reconstruction slice thickness on patient radiation dose in 64-MDCT. *AJR Am J Roentgenol.* 2007;189(1):219–225.
Kaza RK, Platt JF, Goodsitt MM, et al. Emerging techniques for dose optimization in abdominal CT. *Radiographics.* 2014;34(1):4–17. doi:10.1148/rg.341135038.
Mahesh M. *MDCT Physics: The Basics: Technology, Image Quality and Radiation Dose.* Philadelphia, PA: Lippincott Williams & Wilkins; 2009.
Mathews JD, Forsythe AV, Brady Z, et al. Cancer risk in 680,000 people exposed to computed tomography scans in childhood or adolescence: Data linkage study of 11 million Australians. *BMJ.* 2013;346:1–18. doi:10.1136/bmj.f2360.
Matthews K, Brennan P. Optimization of x-ray examinations: General principles and an Irish perspective. *Radiography.* 2009;15:262–268.
McCollough C, Bruesewitz MR, Kofler JM Jr. CT dose reduction and dose management tools: Overview of available options. *Radiographics.* 2006;26(2):503–512.
McCollough CH, Primak AN, Braun N, Kofler J, Yu L, Christner J. Strategies for reducing radiation dose in CT. *Radiol Clin North Am.* 2009;47(1):27–40. doi:10.1016/j.rcl.2008.10.006.
McNitt-Gray MF. AAPM/RSNA physics tutorial for residents: Topics in CT: Radiation dose in CT. *Radiographics.* 2002;22(6):1541–1553.
National Research Council. *Health Risks from Exposure to Low Levels of Ionizing Radiation: BEIR VII Phase 2.* Washington, DC: National Academic Press; 2006.
Pearce MS, Salotti JA, Little MP, et al. Radiation exposure from CT scans in childhood and subsequent risk of leukemia and brain tumors: A retrospective cohort study. *Lancet.* 2012;80(9840):499–505. doi:10.1016/S0140-6736(12) 60815-0.
Russell MT, Fink JR, Rebeles F, Kanal K, Ramos M, Anzal Y. Balancing radiation dose and image quality: Clinical applications of neck volume CT. *Am J Neuoradiol.* 2008;29(4):727–731. doi:10.3174/ajnr.A0891.
Seeram E. *Computed Tomography: Physical Principles, Clinical Applications, and Quality Control.* Philadelphia, PA: Saunders Elsevier; 2009.
Sohaib SA, Peppercorn PD, Horrocks JA, Keene MH, Kenyon GS, Reznek RH. The effect of decreasing mAs on image quality and patient dose in sinus CT. *Br J Radiol.* 2001;74(878):157–161.
Strauss KJ, Goske MJ, Kaste SC, et al. Image gently: Ten steps you can take to optimize image quality and lower CT dose for pediatric patients. *AJR Am J Roentgenol.* 2010;194(4):868–873. doi:10.2214/AJR.09.4091.
The 2007 recommendations of the International Commission on Radiological Protection. ICRP Publication 103. *Ann ICRP.* 2007;37(2–4):1–332.
Tian X, Li X, Segars WP, Paulson EK, Frush DP, Samei E. Pediatric chest and abdominopelvic CT: Organ dose estimation based on 42 patient models. *Radiology.* 2014;270(2):535–547. doi:10.1148/radiol.13122617.
Toth T, Ge Z, Daly MP. The influence of patient centering on CT dose and image noise. *Med Phys.* 2007;34(7):3091–3101.

U.S. Food and Drug Administration. Radiation-emitting products: Pediatric x-ray imaging. http://www.fda.gov/Radiation-EmittingProducts/RadiationEmitting ProductsandProcedures/MedicalImaging/ucm298899.htm. Updated March 20, 2014. Accessed April 10, 2014.

Verona GA, Ceschiu RC, Clayton BL, Sutcavage T, Tadross SS, Panigrahy A. Reducing abdominal CT radiation dose with the adaptive statistical iterative reconstruction technique in children. *Pediatr Radiol.* 2011;41(9):1174–1182. doi:10.1007/s00247-011-2063-x.

Wallace AB, Goergen SK, Schick D, Soblusky T, Jolley D. Multidetector CT dose: Clinical practice improvement strategies from a successful optimization program. *J Am Coll Radiol.* 2010;7(8):614–624. doi:10.1016/j.jacr.2010.03.015.

Winklehner A, Karlo C, Puippe G, et al. Raw data-based iterative reconstruction in body CTA: Evaluation of radiation dose saving potential. *Eur Radiol.* 2011;21(12):2521–2526. doi:10.1007/s00330-011-2227-y.

Section 3

Patient Care

5 Patient Care in Computed Tomography

Tarni Nelson
Charles Sturt University

Christopher M Hayre
University of Exeter

CONTENTS

INTRODUCTION

This chapter explores how patient care in the Computed Tomography (CT). Department is multi-faceted with a shift from a technical focus to a more patient-centred approach. Coincided with this, however, we assert a requirement of technical skill and aptitude. CT radiographers must have a strong understanding and correlation between high levels of communication skill with their patients, their families and other healthcare workers within the interdisciplinary team. It is the role of radiographers to acquire and produce high-quality images whilst also simultaneously facilitating patient care. Radiographers must undertake rigorous training in this modality to understand imaging parameters, contrast enhancement and phasing, recognition of pathology and contraindications to CT scanning. In a fast-paced CT environment,

DOI: 10.1201/9781003132554-8

radiographers must be agile in technique modification whilst maintaining patient care and recognising that every patient experience can vary from one to the next.

The authors reflect on the importance of being a holistic radiographer, which encompasses strong interpersonal skill alongside a high level of technical prowess. CT radiographers need to provide best patient care, whilst performing their task often under highly robust and an emotionally charged healthcare environments. This must be managed whilst autonomous integration of Workplace Health and Safety policies and procedures is being adhered to in order to maintain holistic care of the patient. With a background of CT exposure in an array of public hospitals, including major trauma centres and large teaching hospitals, this chapter offers the perspective fundamentally working primarily within the Public Health sector both within Australian settings and internationally.

PATIENT COMMUNICATION AND PATIENT PREPARATION

Medical imaging, as a speciality, is a diagnostic tool for many diseases and plays an integral role in the patient's pathway. It is used for acute diagnosis, monitoring of disease, progression and predicting outcomes (European Society of Radiology, 2010). As healthcare professionals, it is our role to provide specific services to requiring individuals. Effective communication is an integral requirement within the healthcare sphere and its importance is demonstrated by regulatory body capabilities. The Australian Health Practitioner Regulation Agency (AHPRA) values the importance of communication and thus a requirement of a practising healthcare worker. A high level of communication skill is not only essential in establishing and maintaining effective patient–practitioner relationships but also cemented within the healthcare team. These skills transfer across all medical imaging modalities; however, they remain crucial in CT in order to maintain a high level of patient care.

Many studies support the importance of effective communication in healthcare. When compared with other healthcare professionals, the period of communication between patient and radiographer is considerably shorter and more focused (Pollard et al., 2019). This means that Medical Radiation Practitioners have less time to build trust and rapport whilst delivering an explanation of the procedure or examination. CT is a fast-paced, robust, medical imaging environment in which there can be barriers to optimal patient care. These barriers could be radiographer, patient or environmental dependent. For example, often junior radiographers can be overwhelmed with learning CT in the environment as they fail to have the interpersonal skills and strong communication for patients. With such CT scanning technology, there is more dependency on a high level of radiographer ability, particularly in the acute setting to have a thorough understanding between anatomy, pathology, best scan phasing and parameters to provide optimal imaging for the pathology in question. Often used in the acute setting, CT requires close liaison with trauma teams, physicians and surgeons, thus collaboration with a number of professionals, with limited room for error (Blocker et al., 2013). Due to the speed of CT scans, time is often not a luxury and the decision to perform urgent reviews or add complimentary imaging should be performed quickly, recognising the importance of higher-level thinking skills held by the scanning radiographer. With high dependency patients and a team of trained experts, a strong awareness of the deteriorating patient and scanning parameters must be understood at a competent level by the CT radiographer. Altered states of patient consciousness pose another barrier to communication in CT. For example, hemodynamically unstable patients can present to CT; therefore, alongside other healthcare professionals, the CT clinician must understand vital signs and be able to produce optimal images whilst allowing for the nursing team to keep the patient stable. This could be through effective communication with fellow staff, allowing the treating team to attend to the patient in between planning and acquisition during CT examinations.

The use of diagnostic imaging as a tool within medicine has increased dramatically over the past few decades (Smith-Bindman, 2008). With developments in cross-sectional medical imaging and improvements in technology resulting in decreases in radiation dose, CT has cemented itself as a service used within many patient pathways. The vast majority of patients entering a hospital will undergo some form of imaging pathway, whether in the acute A&E setting, for pre-operative planning or for investigation of disease progression. Radiographers have a strong technical focus and awareness around radiation safety; however, interpersonal skills extend beyond simply obtaining diagnostic images. CT radiographers will observe patients at their most vulnerable; thus, it is imperative that they alleviate patient distress and anxiety around patient visits. Often patients are fearful of findings of the scan, contributing to much anxiety ahead of the procedure–for example, CT interventional cases whereby nodules or masses are biopsied for pathological study and diagnosis. There can be an array of characteristics that can influence the radiographer–patient interaction, including the personality and experience of the radiographer, the patient's cognitive state, patient injury or ailment, the age of the patient and behavioural traits of the patient (Booth, 2008). Additionally, on top of these intrinsic factors, extrinsic factors can intrude on the radiographer–patient relationship, such as time constraints, overflowing department and equipment malfunctioning.

There are factors that limit or act as a barrier to effective communication, which can ultimately lead to suboptimal patient care, patient dissatisfaction and increased anxiety and compromise patient safety (Almutairi, 2015). Such barriers can include low literacy levels, language and cultural differences between practitioner and patient. When delivering holistic health, it is imperative that the healthcare worker possesses a myriad of professional attributes to enable for a high level of healthcare delivery. Cultural competency and humility, intellectual humility, the ability to actively listen, one's awareness around paralinguistic cues and non-verbal communication are all important interpersonal skills of the radiographer to accommodate diversity and achieve better healthcare outcomes, therefore limiting the likelihood of adverse events. With such skills, the patient can be more informed and empowered over their health, and subsequently, aid in reducing anxiety levels.

CT radiographers must hold a high level of interpersonal skills alongside being credible and have an extensive knowledge base within the profession, allowing them to display empathy and use active and effective listening strategies whilst developing a respectful rapport with the patient (Dauer et al., 2011). Effective communication in the CT department with patients allows for assessment of their cognitive state and mental capacity around informed consent. At the very centre of periprocedural care is patient identification, and then furthermore, confirmation of the correct examination or procedure.

Patient awareness around radiation risk is still a common theme globally. Informed consent concerning medical imaging and ionising radiation fosters a shared decision-making process around the patient's own health. As the World Health Organisation has recognised ionising radiation as a carcinogen at low doses, supported within the current radiobiological paradigm, there is an increased importance around informed consent and improving patient knowledge about the risks of ionising radiation when undergoing CT. As a basis for informed consent, patients should be made aware of the risks associated with having a CT examination, as well as the risks associated from intravenous administration of contrast agents (Sanelli et al., 2004). Information exchange is integral to empowering the patient with knowledge, utilising two-way communication, and therefore, culminating in informed consent. Radiographers must ensure that the patient has a full understanding of the procedure and has had explanation and time to ask questions. This is not only for interventional CT procedures such as injections, drainages or biopsies, but for contrast-enhanced CT and non-contrast-enhanced CT, where patients do not lack mental capacity.

Dietary Restrictions

In many clinical centres, it is common for patients to withhold the consumption of food or liquid ahead of the administration of intravenous (IV) contrast medium for CT scanning. Prior to the introduction of contrast of non-ionic, low osmolarity, the IV contrast previously used within CT scanning was ionic in nature with a high osmolar composition. This medium saw higher rates of emetic complications, which rationalised the preparative fasting for most CT contrast-enhanced examinations. This historical concern was centred on pulmonary aspiration of gastric contents, and therefore, preparative fasting was utilised ahead of a contrast-enhanced CT scans in order to minimise the risk of aspirational pneumonitis (Lee et al., 2012). Fasting of patients is not always possible, particularly when the consideration of patients in the accident and emergency environment or urgent inpatients for investigation of any source of internal bleeding.

As global trends in the utilisation of CT are increasing from its first introduction in the 1970s, including those requiring the administration of contrast medium, the need of pre-procedural fasting has come under review. In procedures that fasting could specifically aid in the optimal imaging to the region of interest, of course it should be utilised in the pre-procedural workup. These procedures include CT virtual colonography studies, where it is crucial that the bowel wall is free from any food obstruction or artefact, therefore enabling accurate intraluminal visualisation. Similarly, any procedure requiring general anaesthesia or sedation should involve preparative fasting (Barbosa et al., 2018). However, there is no evidence to suggest that nutrition or hydration needs to be withheld from patients any longer; often pre-hydration is more beneficial to reduce likelihood of nephrotoxicity or possibility of decline in glomerular filtration rate (GFR) after contrast media exposure (Bader et al., 2004). Along with this pre-procedural measure, part of the preparation when undertaking contrast-enhanced examination is recent biochemistry, laboratory results of the patient must be checked by the scanning clinician, specifically the GFR and creatinine levels. This ascertains that the renal function of the patient can tolerate and properly excrete the ionic contrast agent, without causing contrast-induced acute kidney injury (CI-AKI).

Sedation

Sedation of patients in the imaging suite is not uncommon. In the event of a patient undergoing a CT interventional procedure or for paediatric imaging, sedation may be required. Liaisons with all parties are needed to achieve optimal diagnostic images, whilst adhering to ALARA and not otherwise compromising the patient's health and safety any further, especially if at greater anaesthetic or sedation risk. With modern CT scanners and the rapidity of scan time, patients may need little to no sedation in some cases. For example, with the introduction of CT in the 1980s, the first head scan took 5 minutes; whereas for modern scanners, a diagnostic series can be obtained as quickly as 2 seconds. Each patient must have an individualised scan plan to enable cross-sectional imaging to occur optimally and safely. In the context of paediatric imaging, there are alternate methods of non-pharmacological sedation to allow for radiological imaging to occur, such as sleep deprivation, parental involvement, distraction and play therapy (Arlachov and Ganatra, 2012).

CONTRAST AGENTS: CONTRAST SPECIFICATIONS

CT is generally a non-invasive tool that allows for three-dimensional visualisation and differentiation of internal structures. Where it is difficult in some studies to differentiate between adjacent structures, to assess vessel occlusion or stenosis, or to see perfusion of organs, the use of contrast imaging agents allows for better visualisation and differentiation of tissues. As indicated above, non-ionic contrast mediums are typically used, replacing previously used ionic agents (Ho et al., 2012). Contrast that contains a high level of viscosity must be kept warm to allow for speedy administration. The viscosity of contrast agents needs to be considered as it can affect the rate at which the medium can be delivered, therefore subsequently compromising optimal image quality, by either missing the bolus at its optimal enhancement or not injecting at a high enough flow rate to ensure adequate opacification and Hounsfield Units are reached. The quantity of contrast to be administered depends on the weight of the patient. Currently, 1–1.5 ml/kg is employed when administering IV contrast. Various factors lead to a reduction in contrast dose administration, including acquisition speed, injection rate and the use of Dual Energy CT (Bhalla et al., 2019). Recent advancements in multi-detector CT have resulted in a reduction of contrast dose and radiation dose to the patient.

Injection of IV contrast parameters varies depending on the anatomy being imaged, the phasing of the scan, the pathology under investigation, cardiac output and length of the scan. Furthermore, the IV cannula size can act as a further barrier to injection rates. Patients with poor peripheral IV access and smaller cannula size make it difficult to achieve a desired injection flow rate. For example, when performing a CT scan of the pulmonary arteries, commonly known as a 'CTPA', a high level of pulmonary arterial enhancement may be affected by the flow rate restriction due to cannula size obtainable (Uysal et al., 2010). The level of vascular enhancement is, therefore, dependent on the flow rate by the radiographer and is determined by the number of iodine molecules administered to the patient per second. Therefore, the radiographer must carefully select a vessel that tolerates high-pressure injection and produces optimal enhancement of the desired region of interest, whilst minimising pain or discomfort to the patient.

The optimal goal when imaging CT is achieving maximum enhancement using minimal contrast medium. The preferable route of administration of IV iodinated contrast is through a peripheral IV cannula. The peripheral IV access in conjunction with the use of a power injector allows for a reliable, consistent delivery of contrast at the selected flow rate according to the desired scan. By undertaking a bolus-tracked contrast scan, using low levels of radiation, the radiographer can actively observe contrast filling the region of interest and begin the scan, ensuring optimal contrast enhancement. For patients with poor peripheral access, or patients undergoing chemotherapy or dialysis, a central venous catheter (CVC) may be in situ. These are typically observed in patients from high dependency units. There are various types of CVCs that may be used in the clinical setting: most frequently, tunnelled and non-tunnelled CVC's, ports and peripherally inserted catheters (Buijis et al., 2017). Because CT examinations require a high injection rate to obtain optimal contrast opacification of intrinsic structures, and this is generally not achievable through the use of CVCs, where a slower flow rate is required to avoid damage to the device subsequently resulting in less concentration of contrast agent. There are discrepancies between clinical sites and clinicians around the appropriateness of utilising CVC for contrast injection in CT via a power injector. Radiologists and clinical guidelines are hesitant to use CVC for the injection of contrast medium due to the associated risks of complications including catheter rupture, vessel injury, mediastinal haematoma, contrast extravasation, cardiac arrhythmia and latter complications of infection (Sanelli et al., 2004). It is also difficult to have a standardised protocol around the use of CVCs due to variances in manufacturing them. Limitations around varied manufacturers include materials, lengths used and luminal diameters (Sanelli et al., 2004).

Phasing of contrast enhancement is difficult to obtain when a hand injection is undertaken. Hand injections are used rather than power injections in a few cases. They can be used when imaging paediatric patients, or in instances where the speed of injection does not need to be high or constant – for example, undertaking a post contrast-enhanced brain imaging to assess hypervascular metastases. Contrast enhancement can also be affected by other external factors, including patient body habitus and cardiac output, tissue characteristics, contrast agent type, volume, injection time, scan timing and saline solution flushing (Buijis et al., 2017; Caruso et al., 2018). There are many factors that contribute to suboptimal contrast enhancement to the region of interest, thus imperative that radiographers can recognise and adjust parameters to avoid this. To minimise the amount of iodinated contrast required for some angiogram studies, a saline bolus may be used by the clinician to ensure that the contrast is pushed through rapidly. There are many other advantages of utilising saline to encompass iodine injection. It enables any residual contrast to be 'pushed through' intravenously thus limiting venous artefact and omitting the peripheral site from the injection. With the IV administration of contrast medium, the likelihood of a vascular air embolism is also present. These emboli are typically reported as non-fatal events, whereby for most produces producing no symptoms in patients (Sodhi et al., 2015). When an air embolus is present within the IV injection, post administration there may be manifestation of clinical symptoms including acute dyspnoea, chest pain, seizures, gasping, cyanosis or hypotension (Sodhi et al., 2015).

Accidental venous injection of air has been reported in 11%–23% of patients, and it has the potential to be fatal with consequences culminating in cardiac or respiratory arrest, seizures and cognitive decline (Authority, 2020). Upon using a pressure injector, there is a potential for an air embolus, either via cannula insertion, microbubbles in the contrast itself or the power injector line, failing to be primed ahead of administration. Therefore, it is imperative that radiographers check for any free air within the cannula when inserting, whilst ensuring no bubbles are present when loading contrast or injector tubing. The most frequently used devices in hospitals and within imaging departments are peripheral venous catheters. These are used frequently in the CT suite, as they are an in-dwelling lumen allowing for continual IV access. However, these can be associated with a high risk of bloodstream infection (Zhang et al., 2016). The use of peripheral IV cannulation is to facilitate the administration of iodinated medium to the patient for a contrast-enhanced CT examination. Figure 5.1 depicts the multitude of factors that contribute to the optimal enhancement of internal structures using contrast media.

There is much importance around hand hygiene among healthcare workers to reduce the rate of infection from the introduction of peripherally inserted cannulas. Hand hygiene is considered one of the most important steps in preventing the transmission of infection (Chan et al., 2012). Globally, sufficient hand hygiene is recognised as minimising the spread of infection. Hand hygiene is washing the hands with plain or microbial soap and water, or the use of an alcohol-based skin rub. Similarly, utilising aseptic techniques in relation to cannulation can prevent the spread of infection.

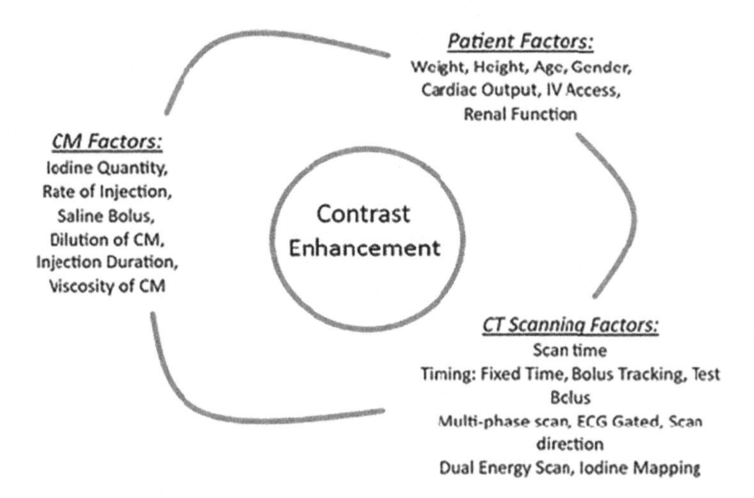

FIGURE 5.1 Multitude of factors contributing to optimal enhancement of internal structures via contrast media.

Interventional procedures are increasingly performed in the CT suite, heightening the importance of aseptic technique and sterile field protocols. These practices include proper hand hygiene, gowning, gloving, preparing the region of interest, draping, maintaining a sterile field and cleanliness of the CT environment and equipment (Chan et al., 2012). Ensuring stock that is utilised ahead of expiry dates is another important safety measure to implement ahead of usage. The role of the CT radiographer not only surrounds optimal imaging and communication with interventional radiologists but it also focuses around cleaning and disinfecting the CT scanner and patient devices in order to eliminate any risk of cross-contamination between patients.

Contrast Complications and Adverse Effect

To ensure the correct pathway of IV contrast media via a peripheral cannula, the radiographer first must ensure that the cannula is correctly within the venous system. This involves hand injected saline, in order to 'flush' the line, and secondly, the aspiration of blood with backflow from the peripheral line (Indrajit et al., 2015). This needs to occur ahead of the injection to ensure that no extravasation of the contrast agent is likely to occur. Some clinical centres perform test injections with the power injector ahead of the scan to ensure that the vein and IV cannula can withstand the pressure of the injection ahead of the scan. Extravasation occurs when the contrast agent escapes the IV lumen and accumulates within the surrounding soft tissue during the injection. Patients should be educated ahead of the use of their IV access to immediately report pain or discomfort caused by the IV contrast or initial saline flush. When extravasation has occurred, most patients experience burning at the injection site, swelling and tenderness. Cessation of the injection must occur immediately to limit the extent of damage to the surrounding structures and further pain to the patient. Many patients recover without further injury; however, in extreme cases, it can lead to skin ulceration at and around the site, tissue necrosis, or in extreme situations, compartment syndrome.

Sites more prone to extravasation injury are where there is less soft tissue protection for underlying structures, such as the dorsum of the hand or foot (Al-Benna et al., 2013). Much literature is mixed in the review of extravasation of iodinated contrast. Application of cold packs help with symptom relief and reduce heat felt by the patient at the site. Hot packs, however, increase localised vasodilation, thereby diluting the extravasated iodine (Al-Benna et al., 2013). Elevation of the affected limb is also recommended to promote resorption of the contrast medium. In addition to extravasation, hypersensitivity reactions can occur from iodinated contrast mediums. Although rarer now with the use of non-ionic contrast media, with the dramatic increase in CT examinations over the last decade, reactions can occur. These reactions range from resulting in urticaria and pruritus to severe reactions such as cardiopulmonary arrest (Briguori, 2003). Acute reactions can be further categorised into mild, moderate and severe. Mild contrast reactions generally resolve without any specific treatment. Patients may experience vomiting, headache or flushing. Moderate reactions can be a heightened effect of the mild symptoms, alongside mild hypotension and bronchospasm (Thomsen and Morcos, 2002). Of the most severity, patients may experience severe bronchospasm, deterioration of their level of consciousness, laryngeal oedema, cardiac arrest as well as potentially pulmonary collapse (Thomsen and Morcos, 2002). Adverse reactions to IV contrast agents in CT are rare, with moderate and severe being very uncommon. The prompt recognition and associated treatment of adverse side effects from the contrast agent by the CT radiographer is integral in preventing the patient's condition from deteriorating further. Imaging guidelines state that an outpatient must be retained for a time period of 30 minutes, with their cannula in situ after their examination involving contrast media to ensure that no delayed hypersensitivity reaction has occurred (RANZCR, 2018).

Contrast media nephrotoxicity is another associated risk when performing a contrast-enhanced CT scan. CI-AKI is a decline in renal function following the administration intravenously or intra-arterially of an iodinated contrast agent. Contrast agents can lead to acute renal failure that begins soon after the administration of the medium, and renal decline occurring within days. In some cases, acute renal failure is irreparable, contributing to an increase in patient mortality and morbidity. The best treatment for contrast-induced renal failure is prevention rather than cure. The gold standard in the prevention of contrast-induced nephrotoxicity remains uncertain; however, some recommendations include pre- and post-procedural hydration, reduction in the quantity of contrast agent used and the use of a contrast agent of low osmolarity (Briguori, 2003). The Royal Australian and New Zealand College of Radiologists (RANZCR) guidelines around the administration of IV contrast in CT in regards to CI-AKI indicate that patients with estimated glomerular filtration rates of

- >45 mL/min likely to be non-existent;
- <45 mL/min likely to be low or non-existent;
- <30 mL/min severe renal impairment is noted, and the risk vs benefit must be considered. Periprocedural hydration should be considered. This should be discussed in conjunction with renal physicians.

As well as these guidelines are important to ensure that the patient has no history of kidney disease coupled with no recent renal surgery or dialysis. Ahead of the administration of an IV contrast media in CT, some further clinical questions must be asked to the patient in order to minimise the risk of hypersensitivity to contrast media:

- Ask if the patient has had an injection of contrast before and as to whether a prior reaction has occurred, their likelihood of another subsequent allergic reaction is increased by tenfold (Callahan et al., 2014). The prior reaction must be recorded and discussed with a radiologist and the referring team.
- Patients should be screened for asthma, as patients who have a clinical history of asthma have a sixfold increased risk of hypersensitivity reaction to contrast medium.
- Multiple allergies can increase the likelihood of an acute reaction to iodinated contrast agents also. According to the RANZCR, one allergic reaction that does not increase a patient's likelihood of reaction to iodinated IV contrast medium is an allergy to topical iodine solutions.
- It is important to ascertain whether the patient has Diabetes Mellitus or has been prescribed Metformin due to the increased risk of lactic acidosis.

Oral & Rectal Contrast

When investigating the gastrointestinal tract, alternate contrast agents may be utilised including oral and rectal contrasts. Within this, the CT radiographer can use positive or negative oral contrast alongside the use of IV contrast if required. The indications for administering oral contrast for a certain time period ahead of the CT examination include the investigation of bowel leaks, gastrointestinal fistulae, fluid collections or in the event of bowel tagging, ahead of a CT colonography. The CT radiographer must be mindful that, whilst many patients will orally intake the contrast, some may have the only access points through an oro- or naso-gastric tube or stoma, and must consider the timing of its movement through the GI tract to best assess the region of interest. Furthermore, contrast can be retrogradely administered through the rectum.

The utilisation of positive oral contrast in abdominopelvic CT allows for visualisation of bowel wall and allows for delineation of the bowel from its surrounding anatomical structures (Pollentine, Ngan-Soo and McCoubrie, 2013). The use of water-soluble iodinated oral contrast is preferred in many instances, as well as being reported as more palatable of the patient when compared to alternatives and also used in therapeutic instances, such as resolution of post-operative small bowel obstruction (Pollentine, Ngan-Soo and McCoubrie, 2013). Complications may arise with the administration of some oral or rectal contrast agents, for instance, the contrast agent leaking into the mediastinal or peritoneal cavity. In the investigation of an oesophageal or gastrointestinal perforation, water-soluble iodinated contrast is the preferred positive agent to reduce the likelihood of potential complications around peritonitis if a bowel leak is apparent. Its alternative, barium sulphate solution is contraindicated in the investigation of a bowel leak due to it being an insoluble substance (Ghahremani and Gore, 2021). Should there be the presence of a perforation of the bowel and barium spills into the peritoneal cavity alongside bowel contents and faecal matter, bacteria can lead to peritonitis (Ghahremani and Gore, 2021). Therefore, it is important that CT radiographers avoid the use of barium sulphate as a rectal or oral contrast when a bowel leak is of clinical suspicion. The CT radiographer's understanding of contrast agents is integral to eliminating harm to the patient. It must be understood that the use of water-soluble iodinated contrast should not be used in the event when a trachea-oesophageal fistula is suspected because if this pathology is confirmed the use of it can lead to pneumonitis (Hegde et al., 2013).

An alternative to rectal liquid contrast is the inflation of the bowel to assess the wall lumen in the event of a CT colonography. Optimal inflation of the bowel by the CT radiographer or radiologist is critical for the assessment of the wall to avoid lowering the sensitivity of detecting any intraluminal polyps or masses (Shinners et al., 2006). Unfortunately, often the patient is rather uncomfortable throughout this examination to ensure diagnostic distension of the colon. The commonly used options to inflate the colon during a CT colonography include room air and carbon dioxide (CO_2). These are currently the two best approaches, however, evidence suggests that CO_2 may be better tolerated by the patient due to its ability to be reabsorbed by the bowel wall much more rapidly than room air (Shinners et al., 2006). Being one hundred and fifty times faster in reabsorption, CO_2 also shows signs of improved bowel distention, allowing for technical success in the procedure, minimising patient discomfort and the need for more complex investigations, such as a colonoscopy (Shinners et al., 2006).

CONSIDERATIONS FOR HIGH-RISK PATIENTS

Pregnant Women

Patients who are pregnant may experience non-obstetrical acute health emergencies during the course of their pregnancy, which need diagnosis and subsequent treatment. With modern CT increasing in its sphere of diagnosis of diseases, this trend has to be increased with pregnant women. Due to CT utilising ionising radiation, this can be detrimental to an unborn foetus. Iodinated contrast may be used during pregnancy; as the literature supports, there is little of the agent that crosses the placenta to the foetus (Sadro and Dubinsky, 2013). Unquestionably, the patient must be informed and consented to the administration of the contrast agent, and is aware of the risks of ionising radiation ahead of consenting to the ionising examination. Appendicitis, pulmonary embolism, acute trauma and renal colic are among some of the non-obstetrical emergencies commonly seen clinically. Various clinical tests must be undertaken to diagnose and treat the pregnant patient alongside foetal monitoring. Ultimately, foetal survival is linked to maternal survival, and therefore, all efforts must be made to save the pregnant patient (Sadro and Dubinsky, 2013).

Paediatrics

Like a fetus, children are more sensitive to radiation-induced carcinogenesis as they have more years remaining in life for a potential cancer to develop. With that said, paediatric CT has increased over the last decade. The fundamentals of radiation in medicine stem from justification and optimisation, and the benefit of the CT scan for the paediatric patient must be outweighed by the paediatric radiologist and treating team. In turn, dose optimisation strategies must be implemented by the CT radiographer. With modern CT scanners and dose reduction strategies, CT has become further utilised due to its enhanced sensitivity and specificity over alternate non ionising methods where CT is the gold standard for the pathology in question.

When performing CT imaging on children, the preparation prior to the examination varies from the pre-planning of an adult examination. The way children process information is different from adults due to varying cognitive abilities and communication skills (Desai and Pandya, 2013). It is not uncommon to see paediatric healthcare workers greet young patients through the concept of play – by offering toys or asking about their hobbies and generating small, lighthearted conversation. It is important when dealing with children that a supportive and trusted environment is created, with rapport built with the child as well as their caregiver. Parents and caregivers play an integral role in the facilitation of effective communication between practitioner and the juvenile patient. The parents must be included in the healthcare examination process, as they can be helpful in reducing the child's anxiety levels.

Furthermore, the carer of the child can help nurse the paediatric patient through a *feed and wrap* technique, with the plan to avoid sedation or anaesthesia – scanning the infant whilst they sleep (Antonov et al., 2017). This can mean settling the child in a familiar environment and then dimming lights and reducing noise in the scan room as they enter to avoid disturbing the sleeping child. Sitting and getting down to the patients eye level is helpful in fostering a connection with the child. At times, anaesthesia may be required to sedate the child to ensure the examination is optimal whilst adhering to ALARA principles. In this environment, communication between the healthcare worker and the parent/caregiver is vital.

Dialysis Patients

Patients who are undergoing dialysis for renal failure or decreased renal function, whether it be haemodialysis or peritoneal dialysis, have an increased likelihood of decreased renal function following exposure to an agent that is nephrotoxic (Davenport et al., 2020). Should contrast administration be required in the event of a life-threatening diagnosis, the agent should not be withheld due to renal insufficiency. Should the presentation not be life threatening, consultation must be made between the treating team, the radiologist and the renal physician.

Diabetic Patients & Metformin

Metformin is a pharmaceutical used as an anti-diabetic drug in non-insulin-dependent diabetes mellitus. Metformin controls blood glucose levels and decreases the amounts of blood sugar produced by the liver (Nasri and Rafieian-Kopaei, 2014). Whilst metformin is not nephrotoxic, the administration of iodinated contrast intravenously is a potential concern for further renal damage in patients with AKI or chronic kidney injury. Iodine administration may precipitate lactic acidosis in the diabetic patient who is prescribed metformin. Lactic acidosis in diabetic patients is widely understood. Lactic acid within the body is metabolised and eliminated by the renal system. Lactic acidosis is a rare complication, whereby it occurs when the iodinated contrast causes renal failure and the patient continues to take Metformin (Rasuli and Hammond, 1998). To avoid the complication of contrast-induced lactic acidosis, Metformin is withheld for a 48-hour time period, post injection of iodine, during which time any CI-AKI will be clinically apparent (Figure 5.2). If renal function is then normal, Metformin can be resumed.

Iodine Allergy

It is not uncommon for patients to have hypersensitivities to iodine, and therefore, this must be identified in the pre-procedural checks and correct course of action implemented to ensure patient safety. Reactions from contrast agents remain unpredictable and occur sporadically. Premedication may be considered in patients that have a risk of mild or moderate reactions, but there is limited evidence to support that premedication prevents acute, severe reactions. Premedication can be in the form of steroid cover or antihistamines ahead of the administration of contrast media (RANZCR, 2018).

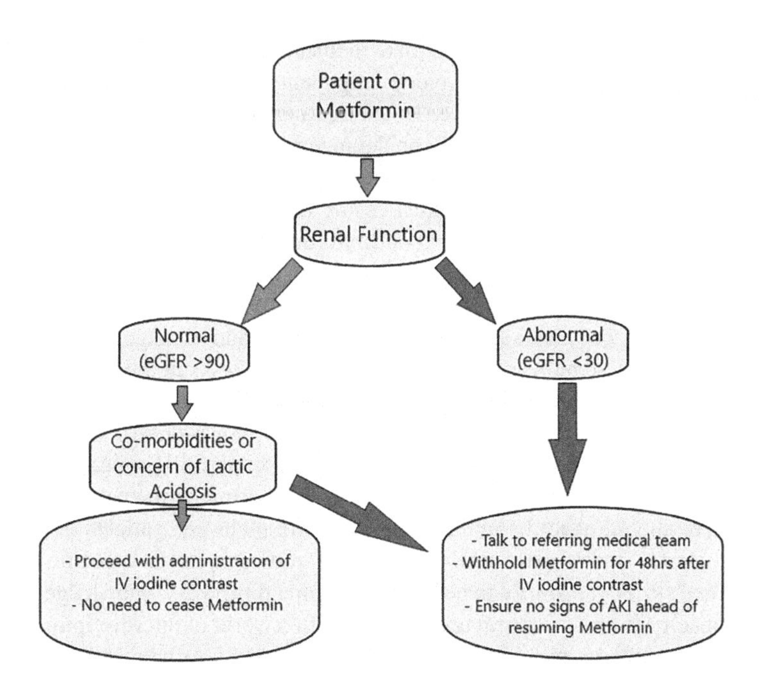

FIGURE 5.2 Flow chart indicating when to withhold Metformin and when to allow it to be continued – based on RANZCR, 2018 guidelines. (Adapted from McCartney et al. (1999).)

Hyperthyroidism

Iodinated intravascular contrast media is one of the highest volume medical drugs in use, compared with any other pharmaceutical; however, with no known therapeutic effects, it only must be used for optimal diagnostic information, without causing any adverse effects to the patient (Katzberg and Haller, 2006). With the increased use of CT as a diagnostic tool, IV contrast media has increasingly become a common source of excess iodine uptake within examined patients (Lee et al., 2015). Following the use of contrast within a CT examination, iodine stores can remain within the system of a healthy thyroid for 4–6 weeks (RANZCR, 2018). Patients with no prior thyroid dysfunction can suffer from thyroid complications post administration; however, patients with known thyroid dysfunction are more likely to suffer post CT examination (Lee et al., 2015). In patients with thyroid dysfunction, radiological iodinated contrast, used in the CT suite, can attribute to and cause excess iodine intake by the thyroid gland. In extreme cases, patients may experience a 'thyroid storm' or thyrotoxicosis. This clinically manifests as tissues exposed to higher than normal levels of thyroid hormone and can affect all major organs within the body (Carroll and Matfin, 2010).

Thyroid storms are more commonly seen in patients with underlying Graves' disease, particularly when untreated; therefore, the CT radiographer must be aware of this ahead of administering large amounts of IV iodinated contrast. In patients where thyrotoxicosis is known, it is preferred that iodinated contrast medium is withheld, unless there is a strong indication to administer it, and this should be done in consultation with an endocrinologist (RANZCR, 2018). Without prior treatment, a thyroid storm could occur and can be fatal requiring immediate medical attention. We never want to compromise patient safety if it can be avoided. In patients with known thyroid issues, thyroid function tests should be conducted by the treating physician in the weeks following iodinated contrast media use to ensure no derangements in values (RANZCR, 2018).

Ultimately, the CT suite is an agile department that requires problem solving and critical thinking. The radiographer must ensure that patient safety is never compromised, patient comfort is achieved and optimal imaging is performed to allow for an accurate and rapid diagnosis. Hybrid approaches in the CT suite are shaping modern medicine; however, the professional fundamentals around patient safety in regard to communication, contrast agents and complications and management of high-risk patients collectively remain as some of the most crucial tasks of the CT radiographer. The technical prowess required to be a competent CT radiographer is increasing with these innovations in modern medical technology; however, this should not overshadow the importance of the patient and interpersonal skills around achieving a well-rounded imaging examination. In a busy CT department, the value of humanity in healthcare should never be undervalued. CT clinicians see patients in their most vulnerable states and to be a well-rounded CT radiographer is a recipe of strong interpersonal skills, the ability to be human, technical prowess, knowledge, attitudes and the capacity to be an integral team member. In a world of interdisciplinary teams and various healthcare providers, CT radiographers need to be mindful that at the crux of healthcare is wiping tears, providing patients with warm blankets and holding patients' or parents' hands as we alleviate their anxieties. This diverse skillset is the epitome of a trusted healthcare professional.

REFERENCES

2018. *Iodinated Contrast Media Guideline.* [ebook] Sydney: The Royal Australian and New Zealand College of Radiologists (RANZCR). Available at: <https://www.ranzcr.com/search/ranzcr-iodinated-contrast-guidelines> [Accessed 30 June 2021].

Al-Benna, S., O'Boyle, C. and Holley, J., 2013. Extravasation Injuries in Adults. ISRN Dermatology, 2013, pp. 1–8.

Almutairi, K., 2015. Culture and language differences as a barrier to provision of quality care by the health workforce in Saudi Arabia. *Saudi Medical Journal*, 36(4), pp. 425–431.

Antonov, N., Ruzal-Shapiro, C., Morel, K., Millar, W., Kashyap, S., Lauren, C. and Garzon, M., 2016. Feed and wrap MRI technique in infants. *Clinical Pediatrics*, 56(12), pp. 1095–1103.

Arlachov, Y. and Ganatra, R., 2012. Sedation/anaesthesia in paediatric radiology. *The British Journal of Radiology*, 85(1019), pp. e1018–e1031.

Authority, P., 2004. *Venous Air Emboli and Automatic Contrast Media Injectors.* [online] Pennsylvania Patient Safety Authority. Available at: <http://patientsafety.pa.gov/ADVISORIES/Pages/200412_13.aspx>

Bader, B., Berger, E., Heede, M., Silberbaur, I., Duda, S., Risler, T. and Erley, C., 2004. What is the best hydration regimen to prevent contrast media-induced nephrotoxicity? *Clinical Nephrology*, [online] 62(07), pp. 1–7. Available at: <https://pubmed.ncbi.nlm.nih.gov/15267006/> [Accessed 30 June 2021].

Bae, K., 2010. Intravenous contrast medium administration and scan timing at CT: Considerations and approaches. *Radiology*, 256(1), pp. 32–61.

Barbosa, P., Bitencourt, A., Tyng, C., Cunha, R., Travesso, D., Almeida, M. and Chojniak, R., 2018. JOURNAL CLUB: Preparative fasting for contrast-enhanced CT in a cancer center: A new approach. *American Journal of Roentgenology*, 210(5), pp. 941–947.

Bhalla, A., Das, A., Naranje, P., Irodi, A., Raj, V. and Goyal, A., 2019. Imaging protocols for CT chest: A recommendation. *Indian Journal of Radiology and Imaging*, 29(3), p. 236.

Blocker, R., Shouhed, D., Gangi, A., Ley, E., Blaha, J., Gewertz, B., Wiegmann, D. and Catchpole, K., 2013. Barriers to trauma patient care associated with CT scanning. *Journal of the American College of Surgeons*, 217(1), pp. 135–141.

Booth, L., 2008. The radiographer-patient relationship: Enhancing understanding using a transactional analysis approach. *Radiography*, 14(4), pp. 323–331.

Briguori, C., Tavano, D. and Colombo, A., 2003. Contrast agent-associated nephrotoxicity. *Progress in Cardiovascular Diseases*, 45(6), pp. 493–503.

Buijs, S., Barentsz, M., Smits, M., Gratama, J. and Spronk, P., 2017. Systematic review of the safety and efficacy of contrast injection via venous catheters for contrast-enhanced computed tomography. *European Journal of Radiology Open*, 4, pp. 118–122.

Callahan, M., Servaes, S., Lee, E., Towbin, A., Westra, S. and Frush, D., 2014. Practice patterns for the use of iodinated IV contrast media for pediatric CT studies: A survey of the society for pediatric radiology. *American Journal of Roentgenology*, 202(4), pp. 872–879.

Carroll, R. and Matfin, G., 2010. Review: Endocrine and metabolic emergencies: Thyroid storm. *Therapeutic Advances in Endocrinology and Metabolism*, 1(3), pp. 139–145.

Caruso, D., De Santis, D., Rivosecchi, F., Zerunian, M., Panvini, N., Montesano, M., Biondi, T., Bellini, D., Rengo, M. and Laghi, A., 2018. Lean body weight-tailored iodinated contrast injection in obese patient: Boer versus James Formula. *BioMed Research International*, 2018, pp. 1–6.

Chan, D., Downing, D., Keough, C., Saad, W., Annamalai, G., d'Othee, B., Ganguli, S., Itkin, M., Kalva, S., Khan, A., Krishnamurthy, V., Nikolic, B., Owens, C., Postoak, D., Roberts, A., Rose, S., Sacks, D., Siddiqi, N., Swan, T., Thornton, R., Towbin, R., Wallace, M., Walker, T., Wojak, J., Wardrope, R. and Cardella, J., 2012. Joint practice guideline for sterile technique during vascular and interventional radiology procedures: From the society of interventional radiology, association of perioperative registered nurses, and association for radiologic and imaging nursing, for the society of interventional radiology (Wael Saad, MD, Chair), Standards of Practice Committee, and Endorsed by the Cardiovascular Interventional Radiological Society of Europe and the Canadian Interventional Radiology Association. *Journal of Vascular and Interventional Radiology*, 23(12), pp. 1603–1612.

Dauer, L., Thornton, R., Hay, J., Balter, R., Williamson, M. and St. Germain, J., 2011. Fears, feelings, and facts: interactively communicating benefits and risks of medical radiation with patients. *American Journal of Roentgenology*, 196(4), pp. 756–761.

Davenport, M., Perazella, M., Yee, J., Dillman, J., Fine, D., McDonald, R., Rodby, R., Wang, C. and Weinreb, J., 2020. Use of intravenous iodinated contrast media in patients with kidney disease: Consensus statements from the American College of Radiology and the National Kidney Foundation. *Radiology*, 294(3), pp. 660–668.

Desai, P. and Pandya, S., 2013. Communicating with children in healthcare settings. *The Indian Journal of Pediatrics*, 80(12), pp. 1028–1033.

Ghahremani, G. and Gore, R., 2021. Intraperitoneal barium from gastrointestinal perforations: Reassessment of the prognosis and long-term effects. *American Journal of Roentgenology*, [online] 217(1), pp. 117–123. Available at: <https://www-ajronline-org.ezproxy.csu.edu.au/doi/pdf/10.2214/AJR.20.23526>.

Hegde, R., Kalekar, T., Gajbhiye, M., Bandgar, A., Pawar, S. and Khadse, G., 2013. Esophagobronchial fistulae: Diagnosis by MDCT with oral contrast swallow examination of a benign and a malignant cause. *Indian Journal of Radiology and Imaging*, 23(2), p. 168.

Ho, J., Kingston, R., Young, N., Katelaris, C. and Sindhusake, D., 2012. Immediate hypersensitivity reactions to IV non-ionic iodinated contrast in computed tomography. *Asia Pacific Allergy*, 2(4), p. 242.

Indrajit, I., Sivasankar, R., D'Souza, J., Pant, R., Negi, R., Sahu, S. and PI, H., 2015. Pressure injectors for radiologists: A review and what is new. *Indian Journal of Radiology and Imaging*, 25(1), p. 2.

Insights into Imaging, 2010. The future role of radiology in healthcare. 1(1), pp. 2–11.

Katzberg, R. and Haller, C., 2006. Contrast-induced nephrotoxicity: Clinical landscape. *Kidney International*, [online] 69, pp. S3–S7. Available at: <https://www.kidney-international.org/article/S0085-2538(15)51385-9/fulltext> [Accessed 16 August 2021].

Lee, B., Ok, J., Abdelaziz Elsayed, A., Kim, Y. and Han, D., 2012. Preparative fasting for contrast-enhanced CT: Reconsideration. *Radiology*, 263(2), pp. 444–450.

Lee, S., Rhee, C., Leung, A., Braverman, L., Brent, G. and Pearce, E., 2015. A review: Radiographic iodinated contrast media-induced thyroid dysfunction. *The Journal of Clinical Endocrinology & Metabolism*, 100(2), pp. 376–383.

McCartney, M., Gilbert, F., Murchison, L., Pearson, D., McHardy, K. and Murray, A., 1999. Metformin and contrast media — A dangerous combination? *Clinical Radiology*, 54(1), pp. 29–33.

Nasri, H. and Rafieian-Kopaei, M., 2014. Metformin: Current knowledge. *Journal of Research in Medical Sciences*, [online] 19(7), pp. 658–664. Available at: <https://www.ncbi.nlm.nih.gov/pmc/articles/PMC4214027/> [Accessed 16 August 2021].

Pollard, N., Lincoln, M., Nisbet, G. and Penman, M., 2019. Patient perceptions of communication with diagnostic radiographers. *Radiography*, 25(4), pp. 333–338.

Pollentine, A., Ngan-Soo, E. and McCoubrie, P., 2013. Acceptability of oral iodinated contrast media: a head-to-head comparison of four media. *The British Journal of Radiology*, 86(1025), p. 20120636.

Rasuli, P. and Hammond, I. 1998, Metformin and contrast media: Where is the conflict? *Canadian Association of Radiologists Journal*, 49(3), pp. 161–166.

Sadro, C. and Dubinsky, T., 2013. *Article - CT in pregnancy: Risks and benefits.* [online] Appliedradiology.com. Available at: <https://www.appliedradiology.com/communities/Pediatric-Imaging/ct-in-pregnancy-risks-and-benefits>.

Sanelli, P., Deshmukh, M., Ougorets, I., Caiati, R. and Heier, L., 2004. Safety and feasibility of using a central venous catheter for rapid contrast injection rates. *American Journal of Roentgenology*, 183(6), pp. 1829–1834.

Shinners, T., Pickhardt, P., Taylor, A., Jones, D. and Olsen, C., 2006. Patient-controlled room air insufflation versus automated carbon dioxide delivery for CT colonography. *American Journal of Roentgenology*, [online] 186(6), pp. 1491–1496. Available at: <https://www.ajronline.org/doi/10.2214/AJR.05.0416>.

Smith-Bindman, R., Miglioretti, D. and Larson, E., 2008. Rising use of diagnostic medical imaging in a large integrated health system. *Health Affairs*, 27(6), pp. 1491–1502.

Sodhi, K., Saxena, A., Chandrashekhar, G., Bhatia, A., Singhi, S., Khandelwal, N. and Agarwal, R., 2015. Vascular air embolism after contrast administration on 64 row multiple detector computed tomography: A prospective analysis. *Lung India*, 32(3), p. 216.

Thomsen, H. and Morcos, S., 2002. Radiographic contrast media. *BJU International*, 86, pp. 1–10.

Uysal Ramadan, S., Kosar, P., Sonmez, I., Karahan, S. and Kosar, U., 2010. Optimisation of contrast medium volume and injection-related factors in CT pulmonary angiography: 64-slice CT study. *European Radiology*, 20(9), pp. 2100–2107.

Wang, C., Cohan, R., Ellis, J., Caoili, E., Wang, G. and Francis, I., 2008. Frequency, outcome, and appropriateness of treatment of nonionic iodinated contrast media reactions. *American Journal of Roentgenology*, 191(2), pp. 409–415.

Zhang, L., Cao, S., Marsh, N., Ray-Barruel, G., Flynn, J., Larsen, E. and Rickard, C., 2016. Infection risks associated with peripheral vascular catheters. *Journal of Infection Prevention*, 17(5), pp. 207–213.

Section 4

Cross-Sectional Anatomy

6 Cross-Sectional Anatomy of the Head

Arjun Burlakoti, Harsha Wechalekar, and Nicola Massy-Westropp
University of South Australia

Lars Kruse
Dr Jones and Partners

Shayne Chau
University of Canberra

CONTENTS

DOI: 10.1201/9781003132554-10

AXIAL CT – AT THE LEVEL OF THE CEPHALIC END OF FALX CEREBRI

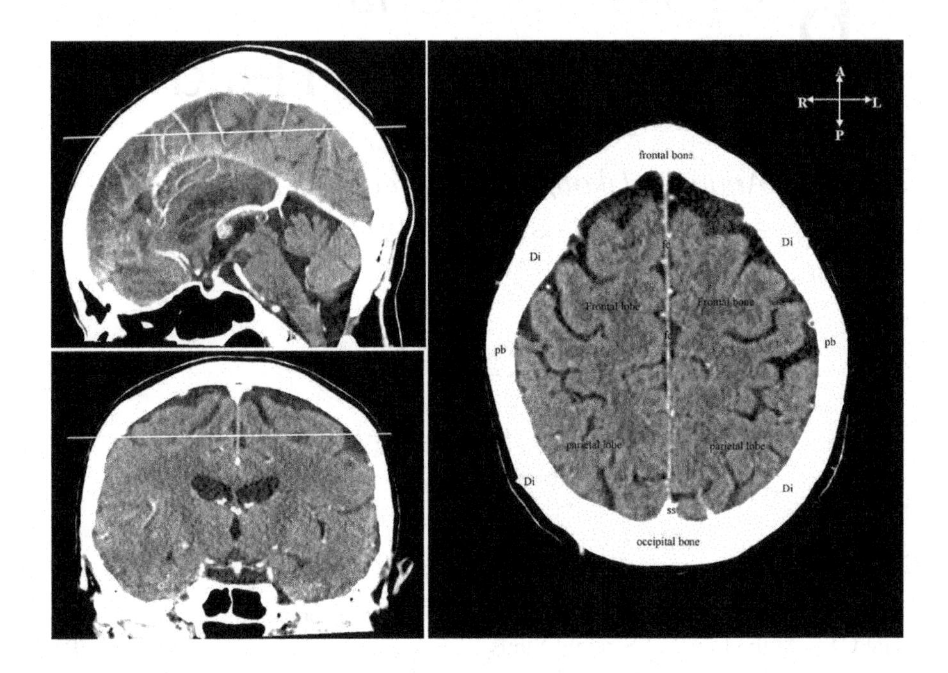

Di – diploë	pb – parietal bone
fc – falx cerebri	ss – superior sagittal sinus

AXIAL CT – AT THE LEVEL OF STRAIGHT SINUS

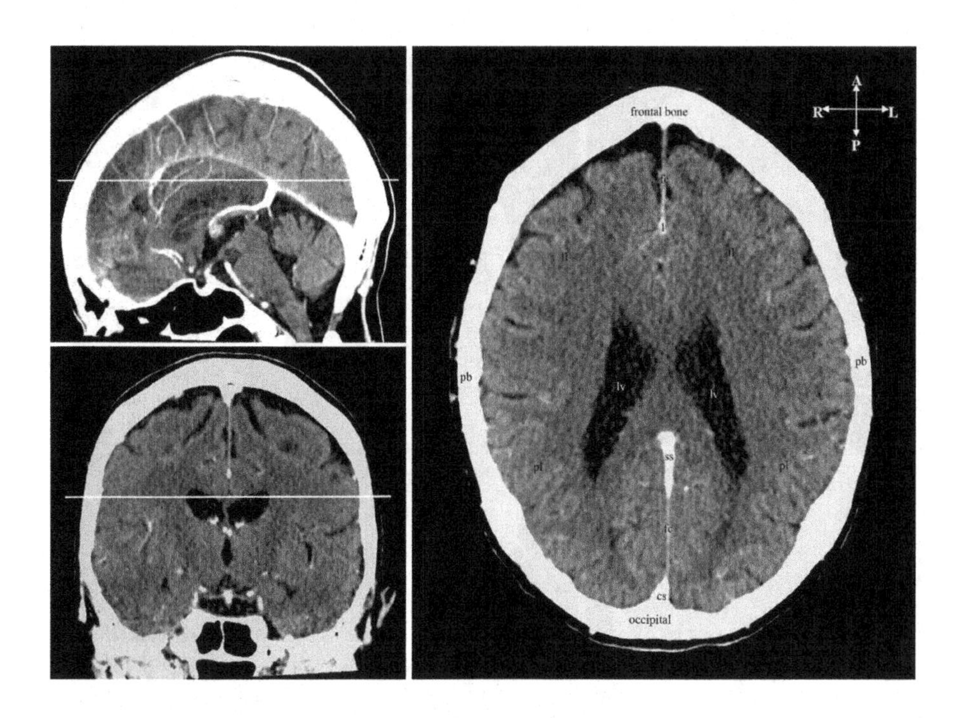

1 – anterior cerebral artery	lv – lateral ventricle	cs – superior sagittal sinus
fl – frontal lobe	pl – parietal lobe	pb – parietal bone
fc – falx cerebri	ss – straight sinus	

AXIAL CT – AT THE LEVEL OF PINEAL GLAND

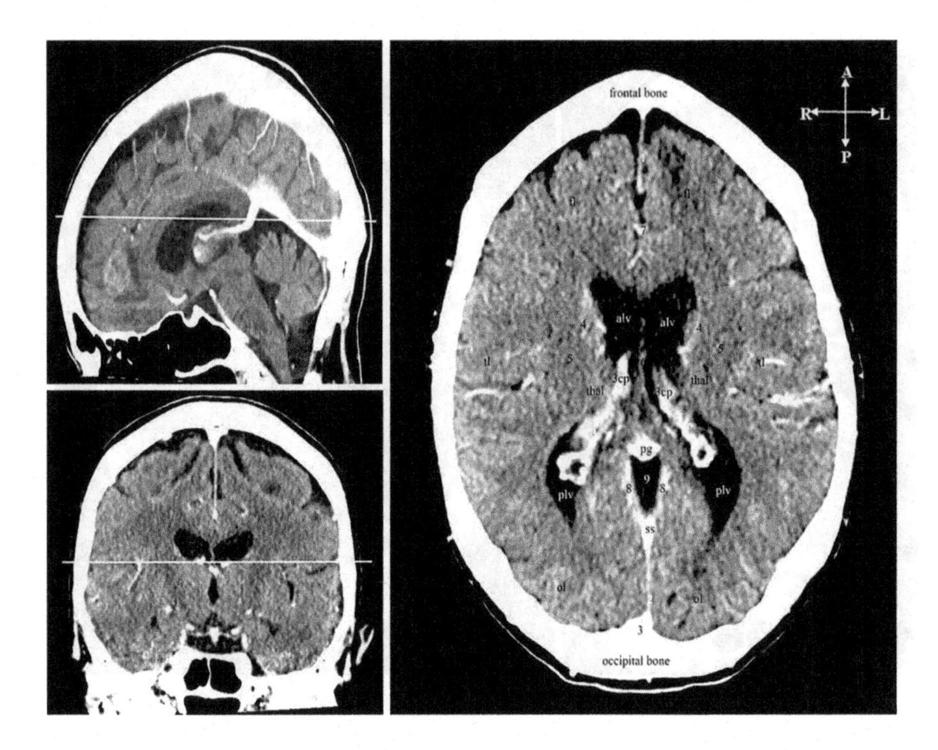

1 and 2 – falx cerebri	plv – posterior horn of the lateral ventricle
3 – confluence of sinuses	thal – thalamus
4 – head of the caudate nuclei	pg – pineal gland
5 – lentiform nuclei	fl – frontal lobe
6 – interventricular septum	tl – temporal lobe
7 – anterior cerebral artery	ol – occipital lobe
8 – tentorium cerebelli	3cp – third ventricle choroid plexus
9 – superior cerebellar cistern	alv – anterior horn of the lateral ventricle
	ss = straight sinus

AXIAL CT – AT THE LEVEL OF GREAT CEREBRAL VEIN

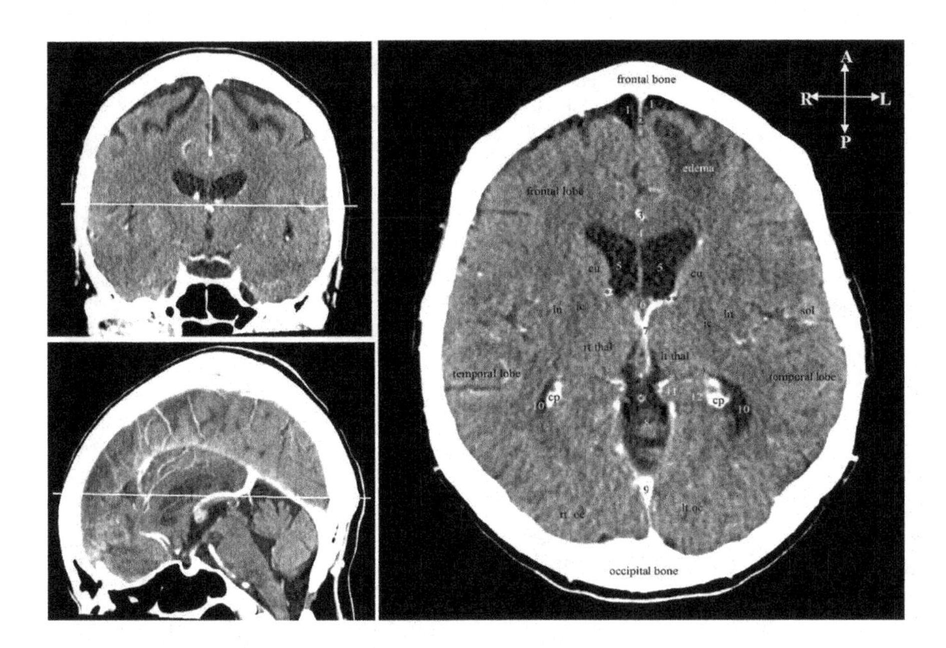

1 – anterior paramedian cistern
2 – falx cerebri
3 – anterior cerebral artery
4 – genu of corpus callosum
5 – anterior horn lateral ventricle
6 – fornix
7 – internal cerebral vein
8 – superior cerebellar cistern
9 – straight sinus
10 – posterior horn lateral ventricle
11 – parahippocampal gyrus
12 – hippocampus
cu – head of caudate nucleus
ln – lentiform nucleus
ic – internal capsule
cp – choroid plexus
rt/lt oc – right and left occipital lobes
rt/lt thal – right and left thalami
* – great cerebral vein
** – basal vein
Sol – space occupying lesion

AXIAL CT – AT THE LEVEL OF THE CONFLUENCE OF SINUSES

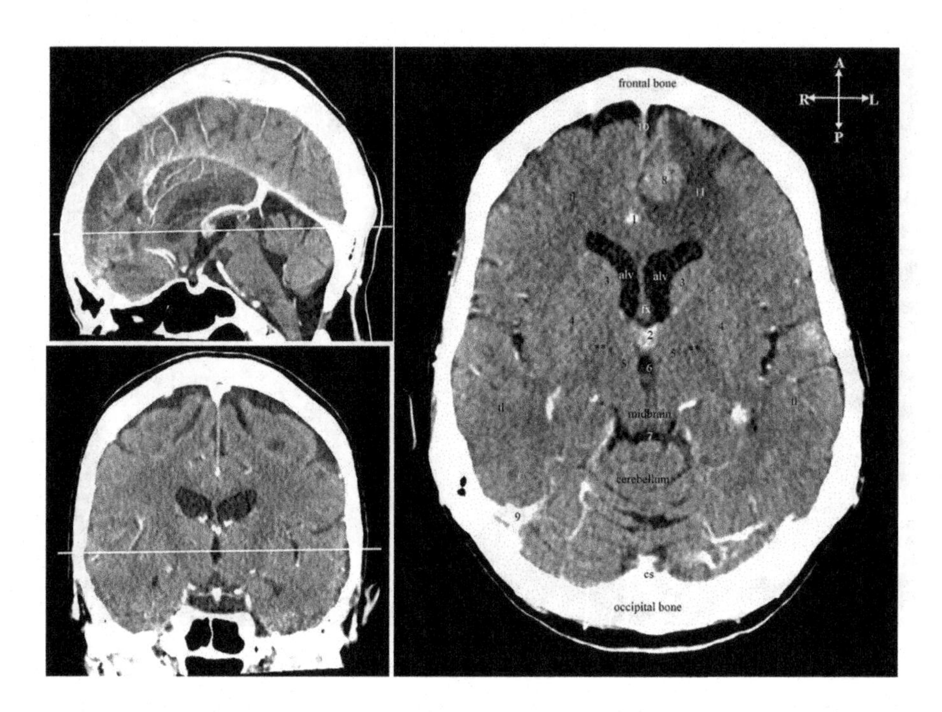

1 – anterior cerebral artery	7 – quadrigeminal cistern	fx – fornix
2 – choroid plexus of the third ventricle	8 – sol (space-occupying lesion)	cs – confluence of sinus
3 – head of caudate nucleus	9 – petrosal sinus	alv – anterior horn of the lateral horn
4 – lentiform nucleus	10 – falx cerebri	tl – temporal lobe
5 – thalamus	11 – oedema	** – internal capsule
6 – interpeduncular cistern	fl – frontal lobe	

AXIAL CT – AT THE LEVEL OF THE GENU OF CORPUS CALLOSUM

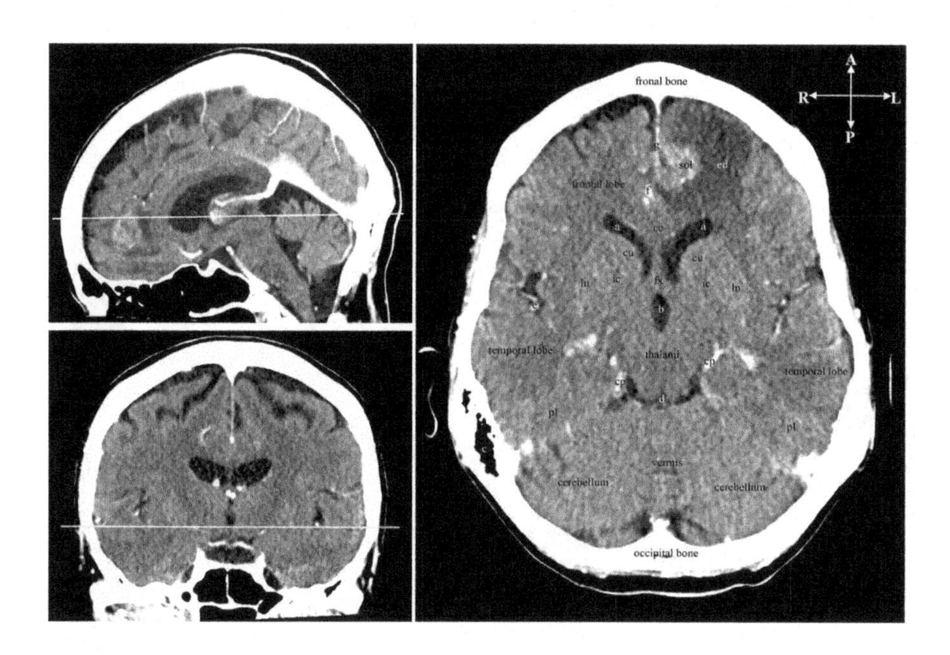

---

sol – space-occupying lesion (secondary metastatic lesions)	ln – lentiform nucleus	c – mastoid air cells
ed – oedema in the frontal lobe	fx – fornix	d – quadrigeminal cistern
co – corpus callosum	cp – choroid plexus	e – branch of middle cerebral artery
cu – caudate nuclei	a – lateral ventricle	f – anterior cerebral artery
ic – internal capsule	b – third ventricle	g – falx cerebri

AXIAL CT – AT THE LEVEL OF THE TERMINAL PART OF BASILAR ARTERY IN PREPONTINE CISTERN

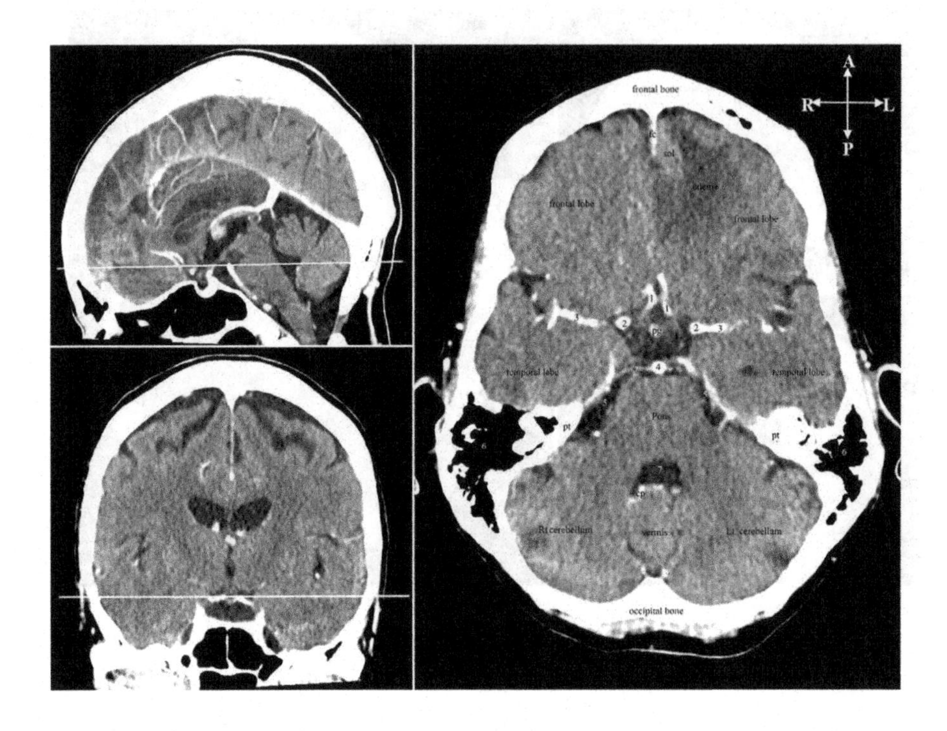

1 – anterior cerebral artery
2 – internal carotid artery
3 – middle cerebral artery
4 – basilar artery
5 – prepontine cistern
6 – tympanic cavity
7 – fourth ventricle

fc – falx cerebri
sol – space-occupying metastatic lesion
cp – choroid plexus
pt – petrous part of the temporal bone
* – posterior cerebral artery
.. – occipital sinus

AXIAL CT – AT THE LEVEL OF EXTERNAL OCCIPITAL PROTUBERANCE

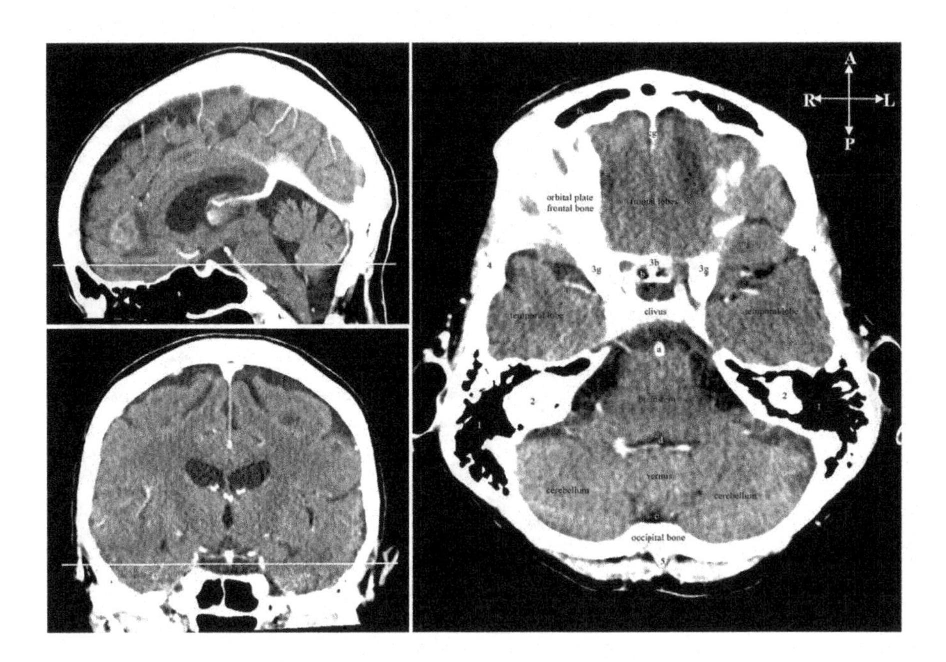

a – basilar artery	3b – body of sphenoid bone
b – sphenoidal air sinus	3g – greater wing of the sphenoid
c – occipital sinus	4 – squamous part of the temporal bone
d – fourth ventricle	5 – external occipital protuberance
1 – tympanic cavity	fs – frontal sinus
2 – petrous part of the temporal bone	cg – crista galli

AXIAL CT – AT THE LEVEL OF ETHMOIDAL AIR CELLS

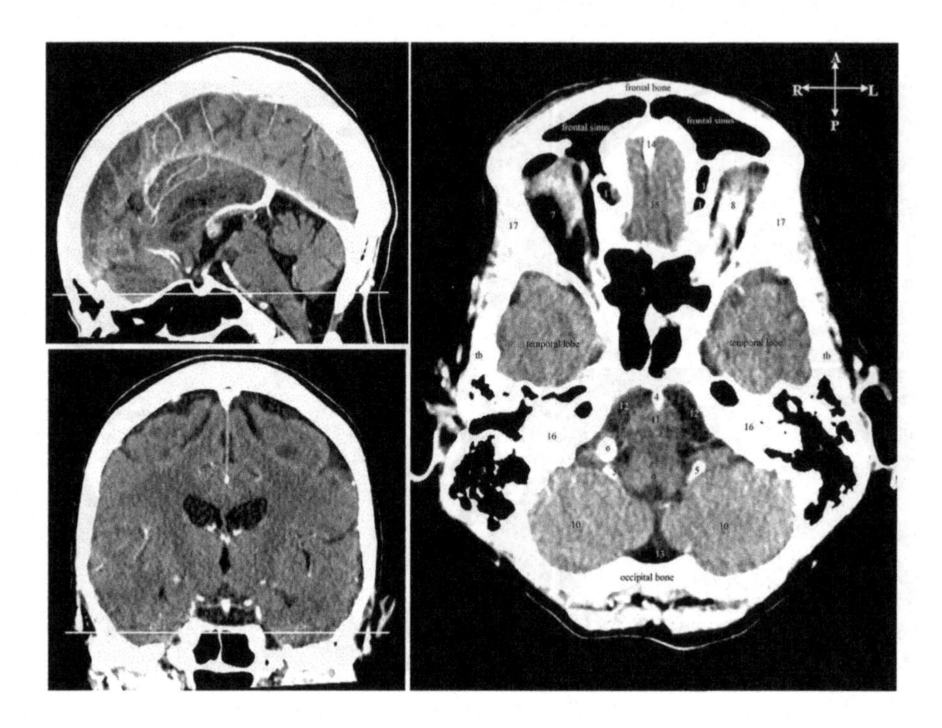

- 1 – ethmoidal air sinuses
- 2 – sphenoidal air sinus
- 3 – mastoid air cells
- 4 – basilar artery
- 5 – posterior inferior cerebellar artery
- 6 – vertebral artery
- 7 and 8 – orbital cavity with contents
- 9 – vermis
- 10 – right and left cerebellar hemispheres
- 11 – lower end of the pons
- 12 – prepontine cistern
- 13 – occipital sinus
- 14 – crista galli
- 15 – frontal lobe
- 16 – pterous part of the temporal bone
- 17 – greater wing of the sphenoid bone
- tb – temporal bone

AXIAL CT – AT THE LEVEL OF POSTERIOR NASAL CHOANAE

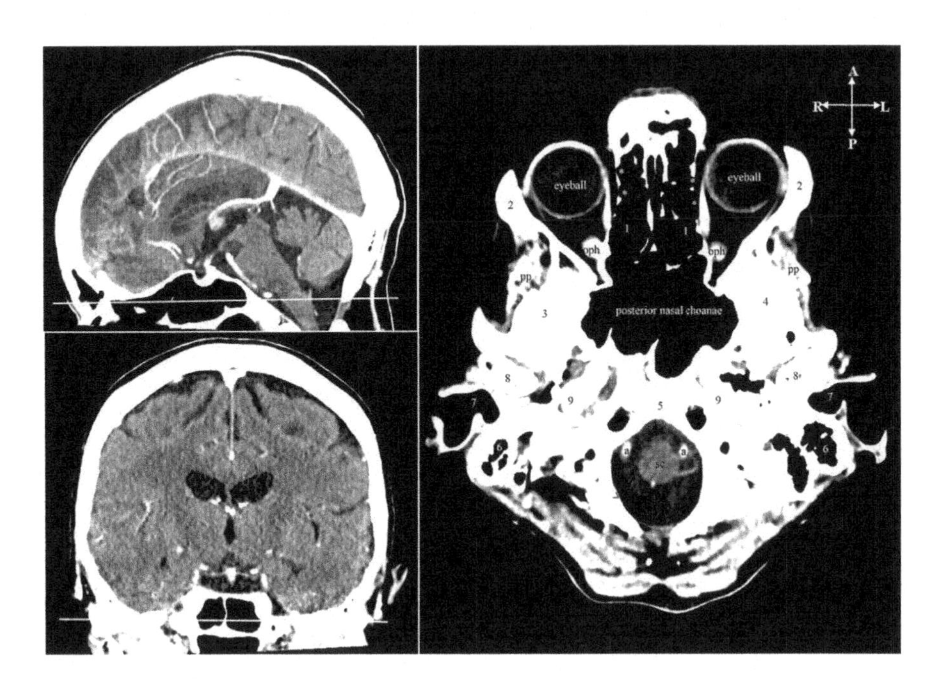

1 – nasal cavity	9 – petrous part of the temporal bone
2 – zygomatic bone	a – vertebral arteries
3 and 4 – temporal bone	sc – spinal cord
5 – basilar part of the occipital bone	oph – ophthalmic artery
6 – mastoid air cells	** – ethmoidal sinuses
7 – external acoustic meatus	^ – foramen magnum
8 – head of the mandible	pp – pterygoid plexus of veins

7 Cross-Sectional Anatomy of the Neck

Arjun Burlakoti, Harsha Wechalekar, and Nicola Massy-Westropp
University of South Australia

Lars Kruse
Dr Jones and Partners
Medical Imaging

Shayne Chau
University of Canberra

CONTENTS

DOI: 10.1201/9781003132554-11

AXIAL CT – AT THE LEVEL OF THE CONDYLE OF THE MANDIBLE

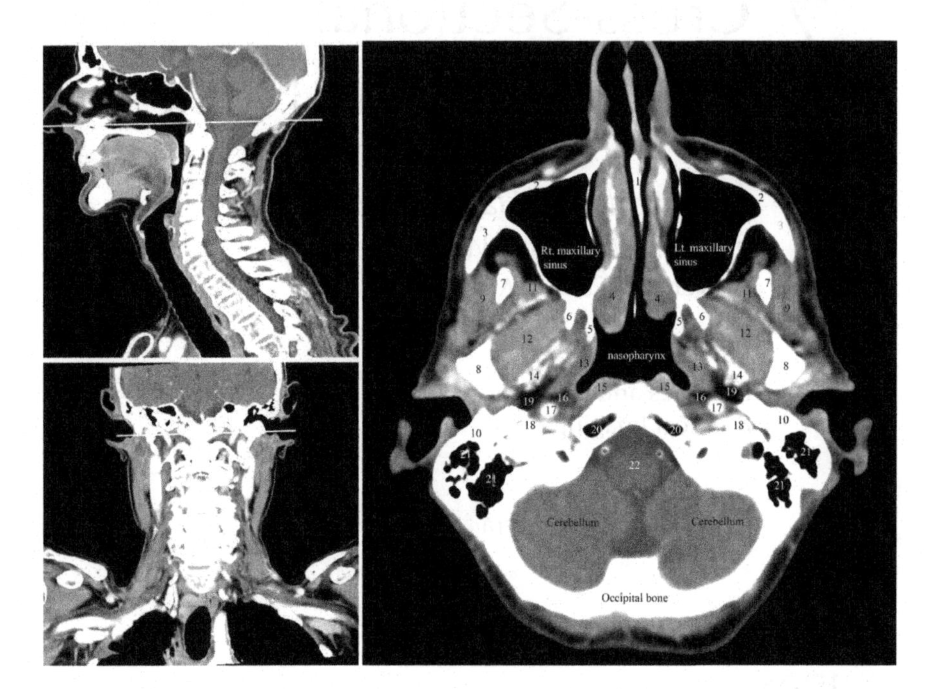

1 – vomer
2 – maxillary process of the zygomatic bone
3 – temporal process of the zygomatic bone
4 – inferior conchae
5 – medial pterygoid plate
6 – lateral pterygoid plate
7 – coronoid process of the mandible
8 – condyle of the mandible
9 – masseter
10 – mastoid process
11 – temporalis
12 – lateral pterygoid muscle
13 – medial pterygoid muscle
14 – pterygoid venous plexus
15 – prevertebral muscles
16 – auditory tube
17 – internal carotid artery
18 – internal jugular vein
19 – auditory canal
20 – condylar canals
21 – mastoid air cells
22 – medulla oblongata
** – vertebral arteries
rt – right
lt – left

AXIAL CT – AT THE LEVEL OF INFERIOR NASAL CONCHA

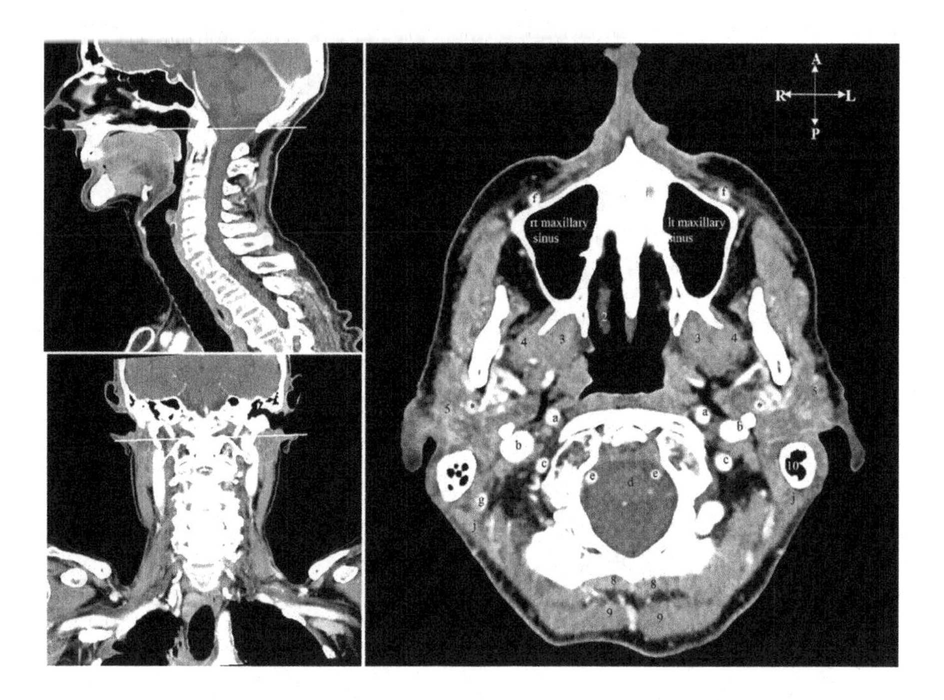

2 – inferior nasal concha	a – internal carotid artery
3 – medial pterygoid muscles	b – internal jugular vein
4 – lateral pterygoid muscles	c – suboccipital plexus of veins
5 – parotid gland	d – medulla
6 – prevertebral muscles	e – vertebral arteries
7 – masseter	f – facial veins
8 – rectus capitis posterior minor	g – suboccipital veins
9 – semispinalis capitis	h – salpingopharyngeus muscle
10 – mastoid air cells	i – levator veli palatini
11 – temporalis	j – splenius capitis
** – retromandibular veins	

AXIAL CT – AT THE LEVEL OF C1

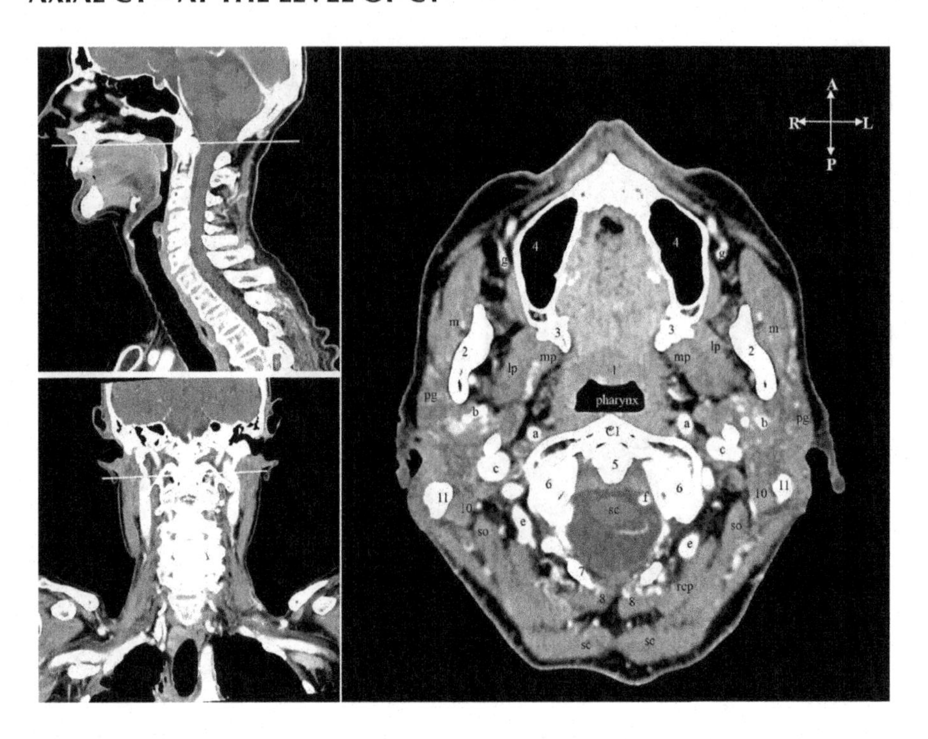

1 – musculus uvulae
2 – ramus of the mandible
3 – pterygoid process
4 – maxillary sinus
5 – dens (or odontoid process)
6 – lateral atlantoaxial joints
7 – posterior arch of C1
8 – rectus capitis posterior minor
9 – sternocleidomastoid
10 – posterior belly of digastric
11 – mastoid process
a – internal carotid artery
b – retromandibular vein
c – internal jugular vein
d – vertebral vein
e – suboccipital venous plexus
f – vertebral artery
g – facial vein
m – masseter
lp – lateral pterygoid
mp – medial pterygoid
rcp – rectus capitis posterior major
pg – parotid gland
so – superior obliquus capitis
sc – semispinalis capitis
sc – spinal cord

AXIAL CT – AT THE LEVEL OF THE DENS

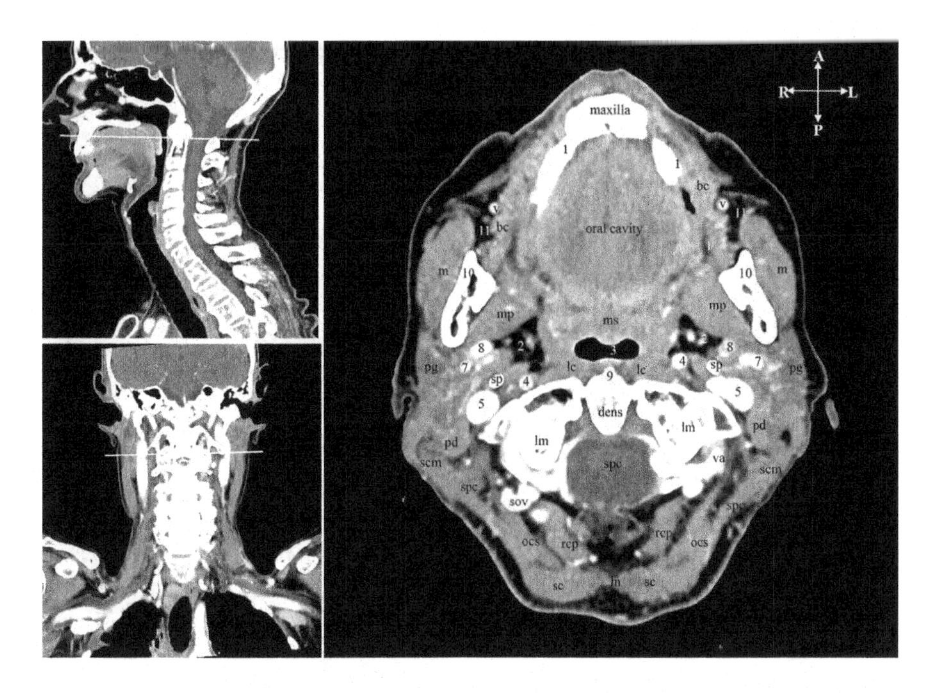

1 – alveolar spaces in the maxilla
2 – para-pharyngeal spaces
3 – oropharynx
4 – internal carotid artery
5 – internal jugular vein
7 – retromandibular vein
8 – external carotid artery
9 – anterior tubercle of the atlas
10 – mandible (ramus)
11 – retromaxillozygomatic space
v – facial vein
ms – muscles of the soft palate
pg – parotid gland
lm – lateral mass of atlas
Va – vertebral artery
m – masseter
mp – medial pterygoid muscle
sov – suboccipital venous plexus
scm – sternocleidomastoid muscle
pd – posterior belly of digastric
spc – cervial part of the spinal cord
rcp – rectus capitis posterior major
ocs – obliquus capitis superior
spc – splenius capitis
ln – ligamentum nuchae
bc – buccinator
sp – styloid process
sc – semispinalis capitis
lc – longus colli

AXIAL CT – AT THE LEVEL OF POSTERIOR ARCH OF C2

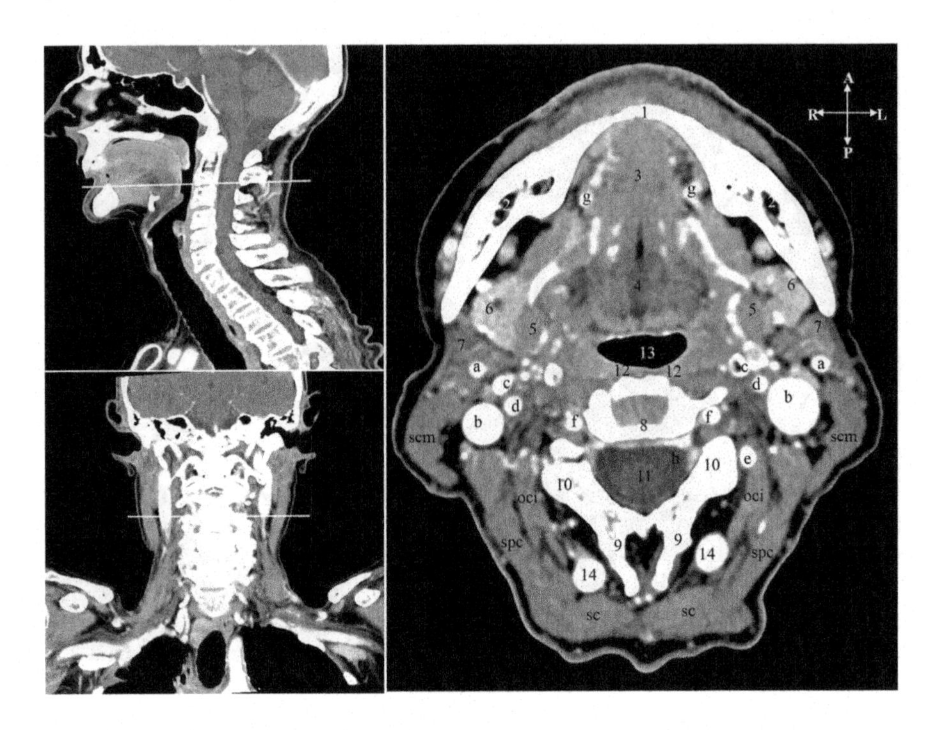

1 – body of the mandible
2 – alveolar spaces
3 – tongue muscles
4 – root of the tongue
5 – posterior belly of digastric
6 – submandibular gland
7 – parotid gland
8 – vertebral body-C2
9 – spinous process-C2
10 – superior articular process
11 – spinal cord
12 – prevertebral muscles (longus colli)
13 – oropharynx
14 – suboccipital venous plexus
scm – sternocleidomastoid muscle
oci – obliquus capitis inferior
spc – splenius capitis
sc – semispinalis capitis
a – retromandibular vein
b – internal jugular vein
c – external carotid artery
d – internal carotid artery
e – vertebral vein
f – vertebral artery
g – lingual artery
h – vertebral canal

AXIAL CT – AT THE LEVEL OF C3

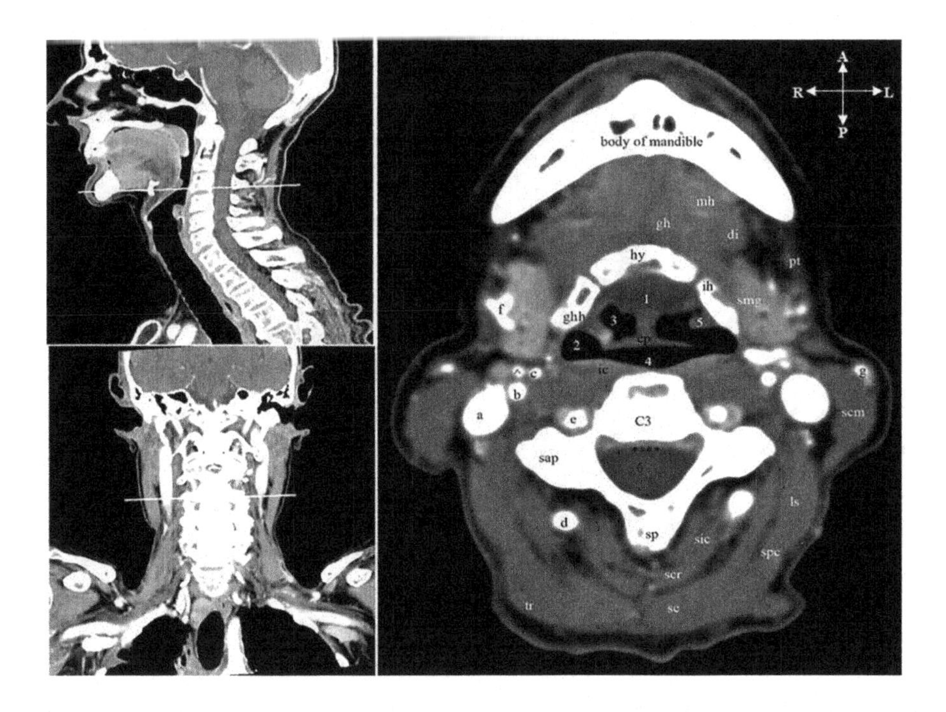

1 – median hyoepiglottic fold
2 – pyriform fossa
3 – epiglottic valleculae
4 – laryngopharynx
5 – lateral glossoepiglottic fold
6 – spinal cord
a – internal jugular vein
b – internal carotid artery
c – external carotid artery
d – suboccipital venous plexus
scm – sternocleidomastoid

e – vertebral artery
f – facial vein
g – external jugular vein
^ – occipital artery
**** – Internal vertebral venous plexus
gh – geniohyoid
mh – mylohyoid
di – anterior belly digastric
pt – platysma
smg – submandibular gland
ls – lesser horn of the hyoid bone

ghh – greater horn of the hyoid bone
sc – semispinalis capitis
scr/sic – semispinalis cervicis
spc – splenius capitis
ls – levator scapulae
sap – superior articular process
sp – spinous process
ic – inferior pharyngeal constrictor
hy – body of hyoid bone

AXIAL CT – AT THE LEVEL OF C4

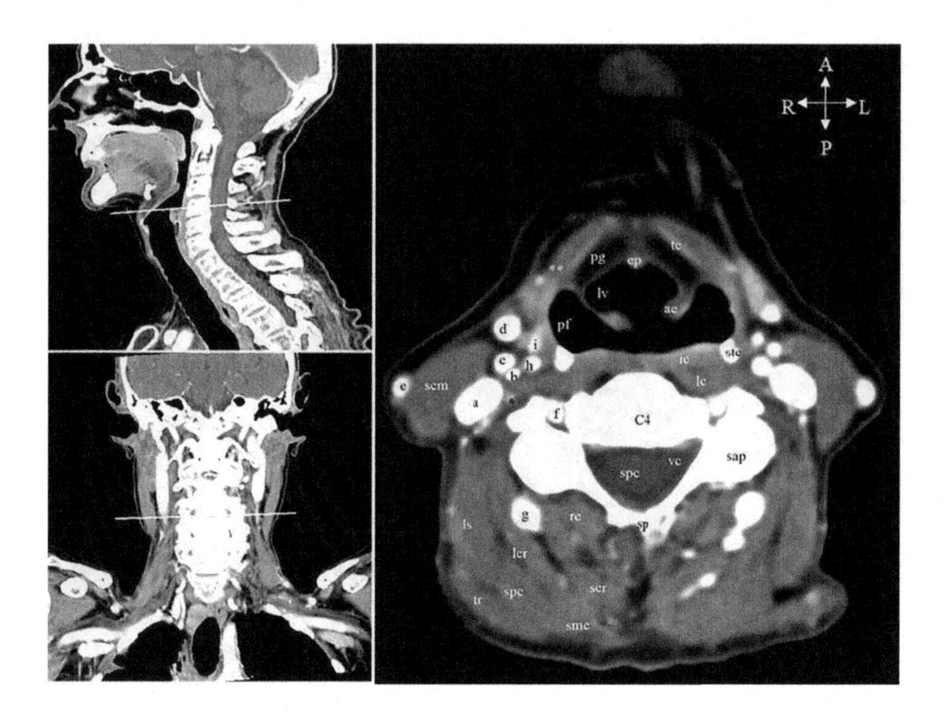

tc – thyroid cartilage
ae – aryepiglottic fold
ep – epiglottis
pg – paraepiglottic fat
lv – laryngeal vestibule
pf – piriform fossa
stc – superior horn of the thyroid cartilage
ic – inferior constrictor
lc – longus colli
scm – sternocleidomastoid
spc – spinal cord
vc – vertebral canal
sp – spinous process of C4 vertebra
rc – rotatores cervicis
lcr – longissimus cervicis
ls – levator scapulae
spc – splenius capitis
smc – semispinalis capitis
scr – semispinalis cervicis
tr – trapezius
a – internal jugular vein
b – internal carotid artery
c – external carotid artery
d – common facial vein
e – external jugular vein
f – vertebral artery
g – suboccipital vein
h – superior thyroid vein
i – superior thyroid artery
* – vagus nerve
*** – infrahyoid muscles

AXIAL CT – AT THE LEVEL OF C5

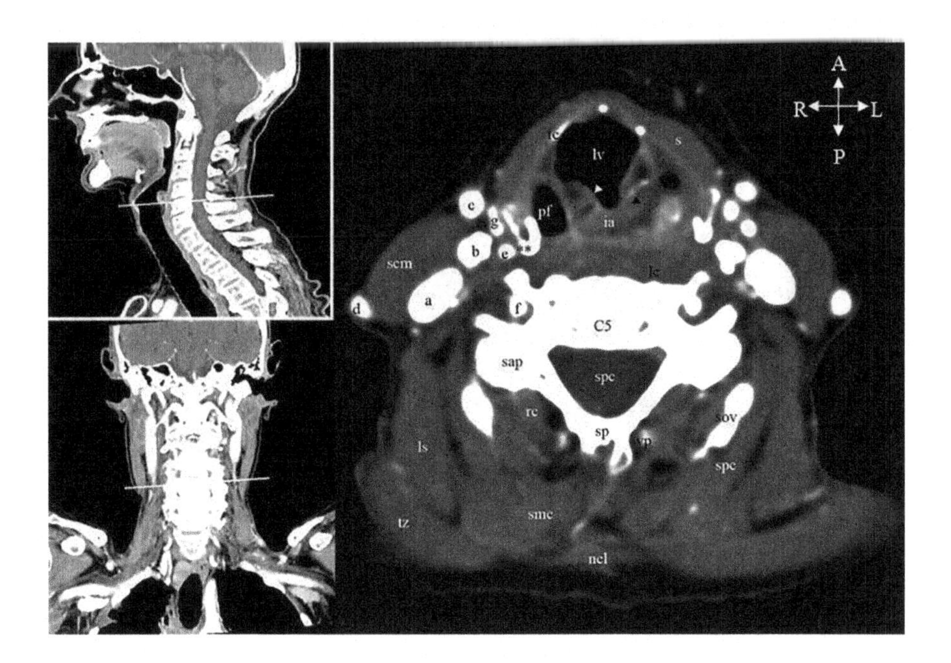

tc – lamina of the thyroid cartilage
s – strap muscles
lv – laryngeal vestibule

white arrowhead – aryepiglottic fold
black arrowhead – corniculate and cuneiforms cartilage
ia – interarytenoid muscle
pf – piriform fossa
lc – longus colli
sap – superior articular process
spc – spinal cord

sp – spinous process
sov – suboccipital plexus of veins
vp – external vertebral venous plexus
rc – rotator cervicis
spc – splenius capitis

smc – semispinalis capitis
ncl – nuchal ligament
ls – levator scapulae
t – trapezius

scm – sternocleidomastoid
a – internal jugular vein
b – bifurcation of common carotid artery
c – facial vein
d – external jugular vein

e – superior thyroid vein
f – vertebral artery
g – superior thyroid artery
** – thyroid cartilage horn

AXIAL CT – AT THE LEVEL OF C6

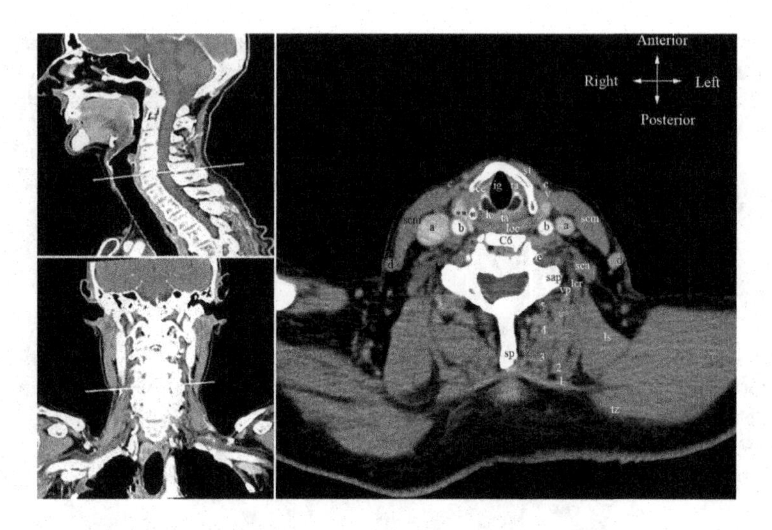

1-splenius capitis
2-spenius cervicis
3- semispinalis capitis
4-semispinalis capitis
5-cervical component of multifidus muscle
lcr-longissimus cervicis
ls-levator scapulae
sca-scalene muscles
tz-trapezius
vp-external vertebral venous plexus

sap-superior articular process
sp-spinous process
scm-sternocleidomastoid
ig-infraglottic cavity
ct-thyroarytenoid muscle
st-sternothyroid
*-inferior horn of the thyroid cartilage
**-right lobe of the thyroid gland
ce-upper margin of conus elasticus
lc-lamina of cricoid cartilage

a-internal jugular vein
b-common carotid artery
c-anterior jugular vein
d-external jugular vein
e-vertebral artery
v-veins of the neck
ta-transverse arytenoid muscle
loc-longus colli

8 Cross-Sectional Anatomy of the Thoracic System

Arjun Burlakoti, Harsha Wechalekar, and Nicola Massy-Westropp
University of South Australia

Lars Kruse
Dr Jones and Partners
Medical Imaging

Shayne Chau
University of Canberra

CONTENTS

DOI: 10.1201/9781003132554-12

C7/T1 VERTEBRAL LEVEL

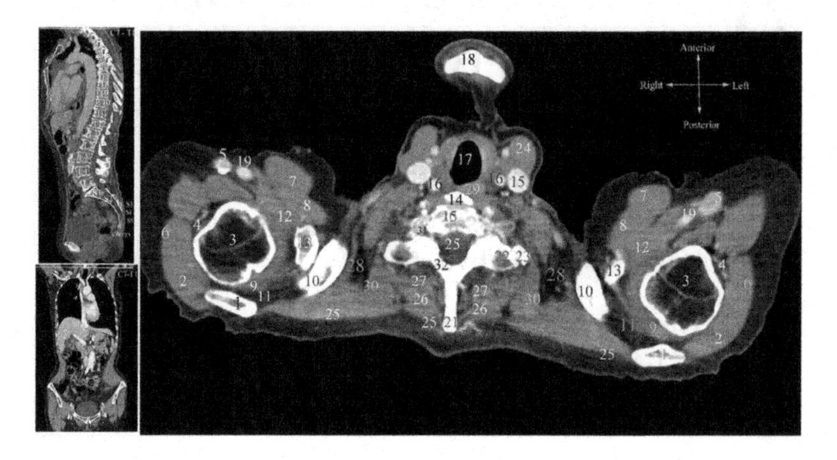

FIGURE 8.1 Axial computed tomography (CT) scan: cervicothoracic junction and C7/T1 vertebral level.

1 – acromion process
2 – posterior deltoid
3 – bone marrow in the medullary cavity, proximal end of humerus
4 – subdeltoid synovial bursa
5 – cephalic vein drains into the axillary vein
6 – lateral deltoid
7 – pectoralis major muscle sternocostal part
8 – pectoralis major muscle clavicular part
9 – supraspinatus muscle
10 – lateral end of clavicle
11 – subacromial bursa positioned superior to the supraspinatus muscle
12 – coracobrachialis and the short head of biceps brachii muscle
13 – coracoid process
14 – C7 vertebral body
15 – internal jugular vein
16 – common carotid artery
17 – trachea
18 – mental region of mandible
19 – axillary artery continues as brachial artery in the arm
20 – intervertebral disc between C7 and T1 vertebrae
21 – spinous process of T1
22 – transverse process of T1
23 – articular tubercle of the first rib
24 – sternocleidomastoid muscle
25 – trapezius muscle
26 – erector spinae group of muscles
27 – semispinalis group of muscles
28 – cervicoaxillary canal
29 – oesophagus
30 – levator scapulae muscle
31 – intervertebral foramen between C7 and T1
32 – lamina

T2/T3 THORACIC VERTEBRAL LEVEL

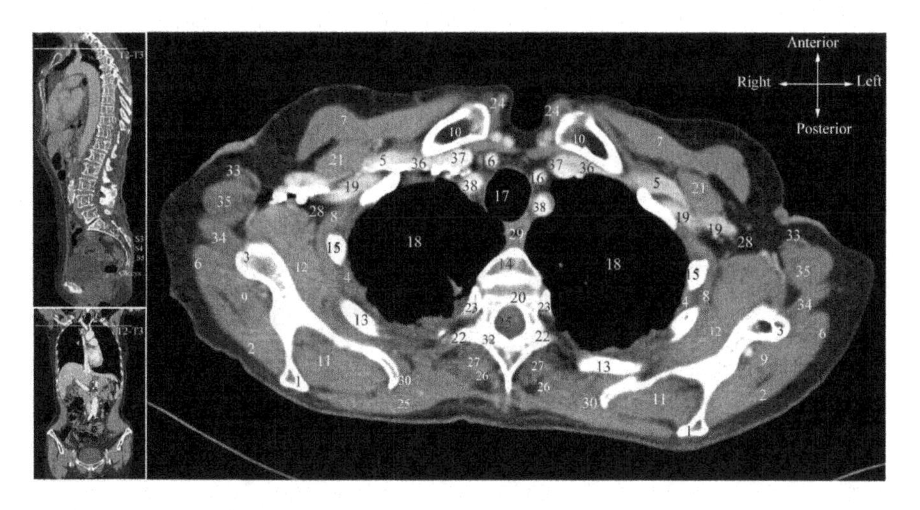

FIGURE 8.2 Axial computed tomography (CT) scan: T2/T3 vertebral level.

1 – spine of scapula
2 – posterior deltoid muscle
3 – superior lateral border of scapula
4 – intercostal muscles
5 – axillary vein drains into the subclavian vein
6 – lateral deltoid muscle
7 – pectoralis major muscle
8 – serratus anterior (superior) muscle
9 – infraspinatus muscle
10 – medial end of clavicle
11 – supraspinatus muscle
12 – subscapularis muscle in the subscapular fossa
13 – angle of the third rib
14 – intervertebral disc between T2 and T3
15 – body of the second rib
16 – common carotid arteries
17 – trachea
18 – apices of the lungs
19 – axillary arteries
20 – T3 vertebral body
21 – pectoralis minor muscle
22 – transverse process of T3 vertebra
23 – head of the third rib
24 – sternocleidomastoid muscle
25 – trapezius muscle (intermediate)
26 – erector spinae group of muscles
27 – semispinalis group of muscles
28 – cervicoaxillary canal
29 – oesophagus
30 – levator scapulae muscle
31 – vertebral foramen with spinal cord
32 – lamina
33 – latissimus dorsi muscle
34 – teres minor muscle
35 – teres major muscle
36 – subclavian veins
37 – brachiocephalic veins
38 – subclavian arteries

T3/T4 THORACIC VERTEBRAL LEVEL

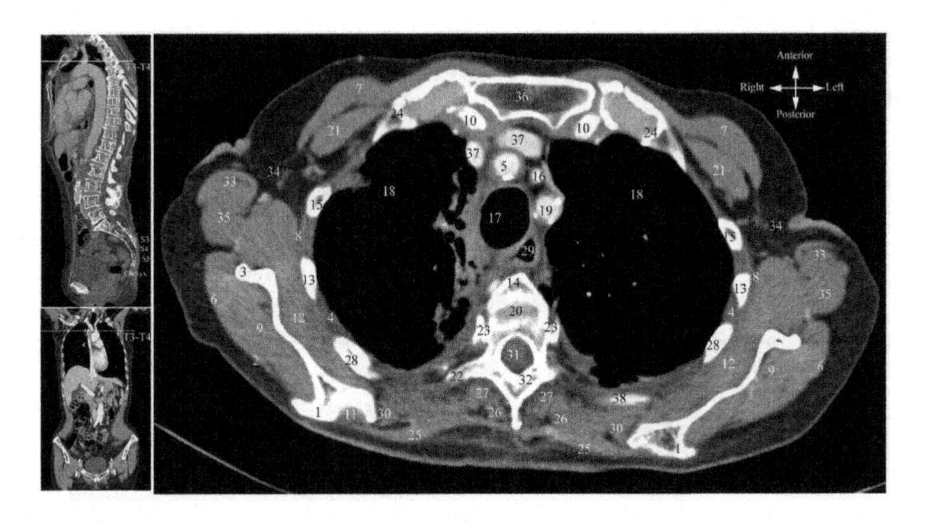

FIGURE 8.3 Axial computed tomography (CT) scan: T3/T4 level.

1 – root of spine of scapula
2 – posterior deltoid muscle
3 – lateral border of scapula
4 – intercostal muscles
5 – brachiocephalic trunk (artery)
6 – lateral deltoid muscle
7 – pectoralis major muscle
8 – scapulothoracic joints
9 – infraspinatus muscle
10 – medial end of clavicle
11 – right supraspinatus muscle
12 – subscapularis muscle in the subscapular fossa
13 – costotransverse joint third rib articulating with the fourth rib
14 – inferior portion of T3 vertebral body
15 – second rib
16 – left common carotid arteries
17 – trachea
18 – superior lobes of the lungs
19 – left subclavian artery
20 – T3/T4 intervertebral disc
21 – pectoralis minor muscle
22 – transverse process of T4 vertebra
23 – head of the fourth rib articulating forming the fourth costovertebral joint
24 – anterior end of the first rib
25 – trapezius muscle (intermediate)
26 – erector spinae group of muscles
27 – semispinalis group of muscles
28 – angle of the fourth rib
29 – oesophagus
30 – rhomboid minor muscle
31 – vertebral foramen with spinal cord
32 – lamina
33 – latissimus dorsi muscle
34 – axilla
35 – teres major muscle
36 – manubrium
37 – brachiocephalic veins
38 – angle of left fifth rib

T5 THORACIC VERTEBRAL LEVEL

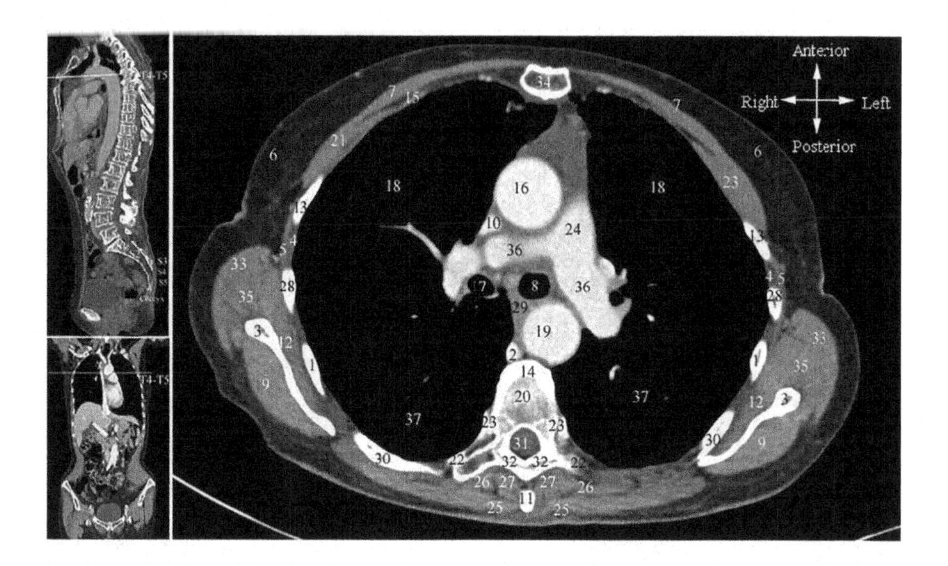

FIGURE 8.4 Axial computed tomography (CT) scan: T4/T5 vertebral level.

---

1 – fifth rib
2 – azygos vein
3 – lateral border of scapula
4 – intercostal muscles
5 – serratus anterior (inferior) muscles
6 – subcutaneous adipose tissue
7 – pectoralis major muscle
8 – left primary bronchus
9 – infraspinatus muscle
10 – superior vena cava
11 – spinous process of T5
12 – subscapularis muscle in the subscapular fossa
13 – body of the third rib
14 – vertebral body T5
15 – right second rib (anterior end)
16 – ascending aorta
17 – right primary bronchus
18 – superior lobes of the lungs
19 – descending thoracic aorta
20 – intervertebral disc T5/T6
21 – pectoralis minor muscle
22 – transverse process of T6 vertebra articulating with the articular tubercle of the sixth rib forming the costotransverse joint
23 – head of the sixth rib articulating forming the sixth costovertebral joint
24 – pulmonary trunk
25 – trapezius muscle (intermediate)
26 – erector spinae group of muscles
27 – semispinalis group of muscles
28 – fourth rib
29 – oesophagus
30 – angle of the sixth rib
31 – vertebral foramen with spinal cord
32 – vertebral laminae
33 – latissimus dorsi muscle
34 – sternum (just inferior to the sternal angle
35 – teres major muscle
36 – right and left pulmonary arteries
37 – inferior lobes of the lungs

T9 THORACIC VERTEBRAL LEVEL

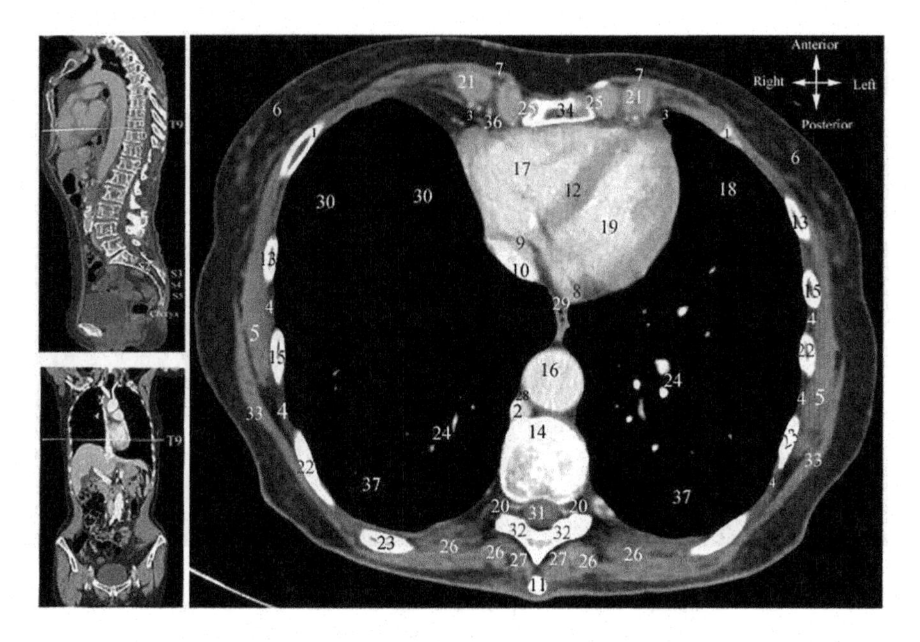

FIGURE 8.5 Axial computed tomography (CT) scan: T9 vertebral level.

---

1 – fifth rib
2 – azygos vein
3 – costomediastinal recesses
4 – intercostal muscles
5 – serratus anterior (inferior) muscles
6 – subcutaneous adipose tissue
7 – rectus abdominis muscles
8 – left atrium (posterior inferior aspect)
9 – right atrium (inferior most aspect)
10 – inferior vena cava
11 – spinous process of T8
12 – interventricular septum
13 – body of the sixth rib
14 – vertebral body T9
15 – body of the seventh rib
16 – descending thoracic aorta
17 – right ventricle
18 – superior lobe of the left lung
19 – left ventricle
20 – intervertebral foramina
21 – costal cartilages
22 – angle of the eighth rib
23 – angle of the ninth rib
24 – pulmonary veins
25 – sternochondral joint
26 – erector spinae group of muscles
27 – semispinalis thoracis muscles
28 – thoracic duct
29 – oesophagus
30 – middle lobe of the right lung
31 – vertebral foramen with spinal cord

---

9 Cross-Sectional Anatomy of the Abdominopelvic System

Arjun Burlakoti, Harsha Wechalekar, and Nicola Massy-Westropp
University of South Australia

Lars Kruse
Dr Jones and Partners
Medical Imaging

Shayne Chau
University of Canberra

CONTENTS

INTRODUCTION

Visualization of the upper quadrants of the abdomen involves viewing as high as the seventh thoracic vertebra in the axial plane, hence imaging the lower lobes of both lungs and the ventricles of the heart. At this level, the upper portion of the right lobe

DOI: 10.1201/9781003132554-13

of the liver can be seen. The abdominopelvic cavity can then be followed inferiorly to a level below the pubic symphysis.

Key digestive, urinary and reproductive systems may be identified as well as blood vessels, connective tissues and potential spaces. After viewing this section, readers will be familiar with the liver, portal vein, pancreas, spleen, ascending, transverse, descending and sigmoid colon, cecum, jejunum, ileum and rectum. Blood vessels including the abdominal aorta, celiac trunk, renal veins, superior and inferior mesenteric arteries and the common, internal and external iliac vessels, and inferior vena cava can be viewed. The kidneys, bladder and reproductive organs will also become familiar. Readers may become familiar with the intraperitoneal and retroperitoneal spaces and structures occupying these spaces.

Structures within the abdomen are often divided into intraperitoneal and retroperitoneal. Structures are not enclosed by peritoneal membrane and do not receive their blood supply from the vessels within the mesentery. These posterior abdominal structures include the oesophagus, most of the duodenum and pancreas; the inferior vena cava and aorta; adrenal glands, kidneys and ureters; the ascending and descending colon and rectum.

T11 IMAGES FROM LOWER THORACIC VERTEBRAL LEVELS SHOW BOTH THE THORAX AND ABDOMEN

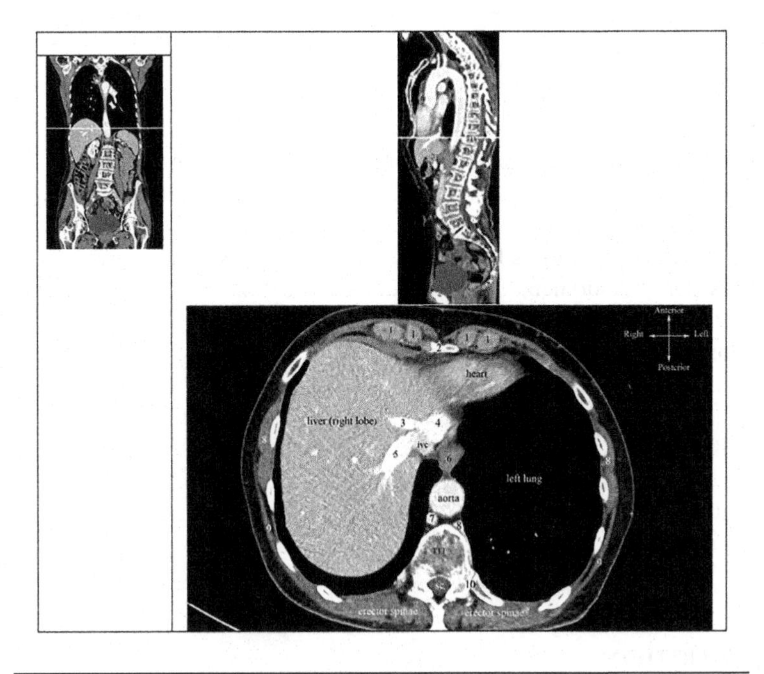

1 – costal cartilages	5 – right hepatic vein	9 – latissimus dorsi
2 – sternum	6 – oesophagus	10 – costotransverse joint
3 – middle hepatic vein	7 – azygous vein	ivc – inferior vena cava
4 – left hepatic vein	8 – hemiazygos vein	sc – spinal cord

T12 UPPER

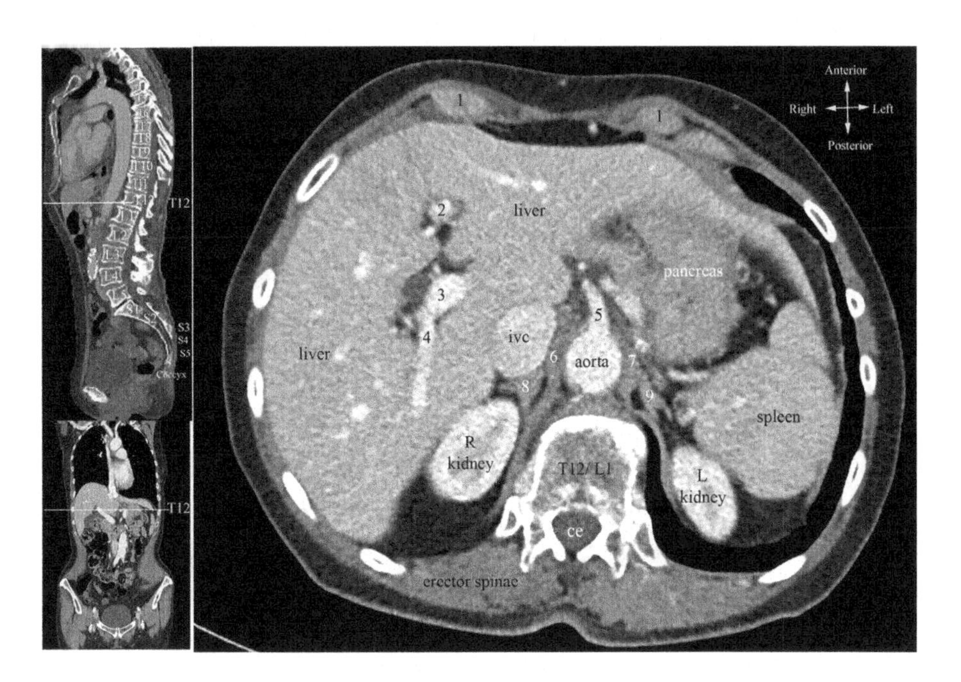

1	costal cartilage	5	celiac trunk	9	left adrenal gland
2	left portal vein	6	right crus of the diaphragm	10	spinal cord
3	portal vein (main)	7	left crus of the diaphragm	ivc	inferior vena cava
4	right portal vein	8	right adrenal gland	ce	cauda equina

T12 LOWER – SPLENIC ARTERIES PANCREAS

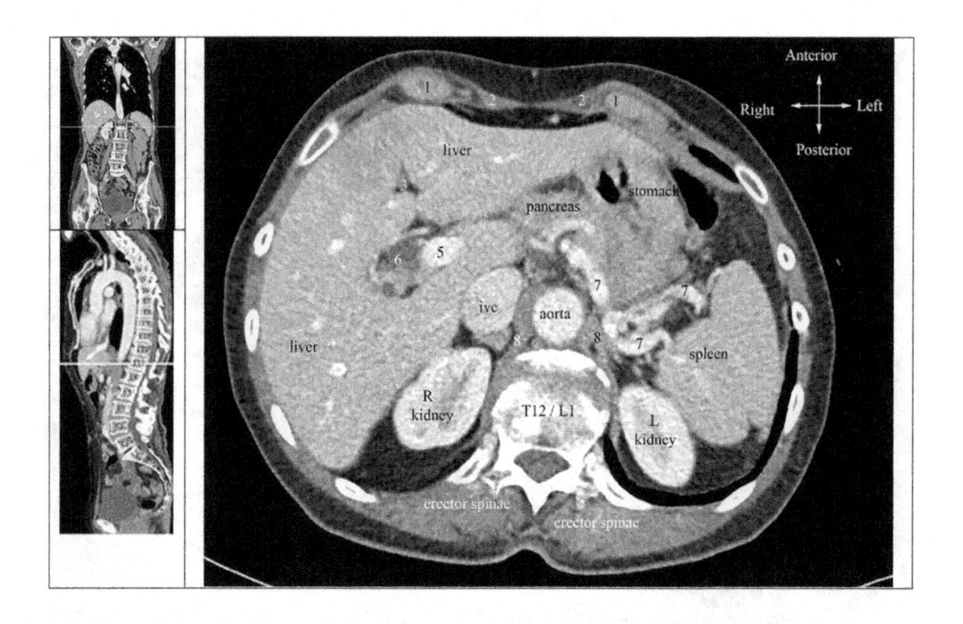

1 – costal cartilage
2 – rectus abdominis
3 – falciform ligament
4 – stomach
5 – main portal vein
6 – gall bladder
7 – splenic vessels
8 – diaphragm
ivc – inferior vena cava
sc – spinal cord

CORONAL POSTERIOR ABDOMEN

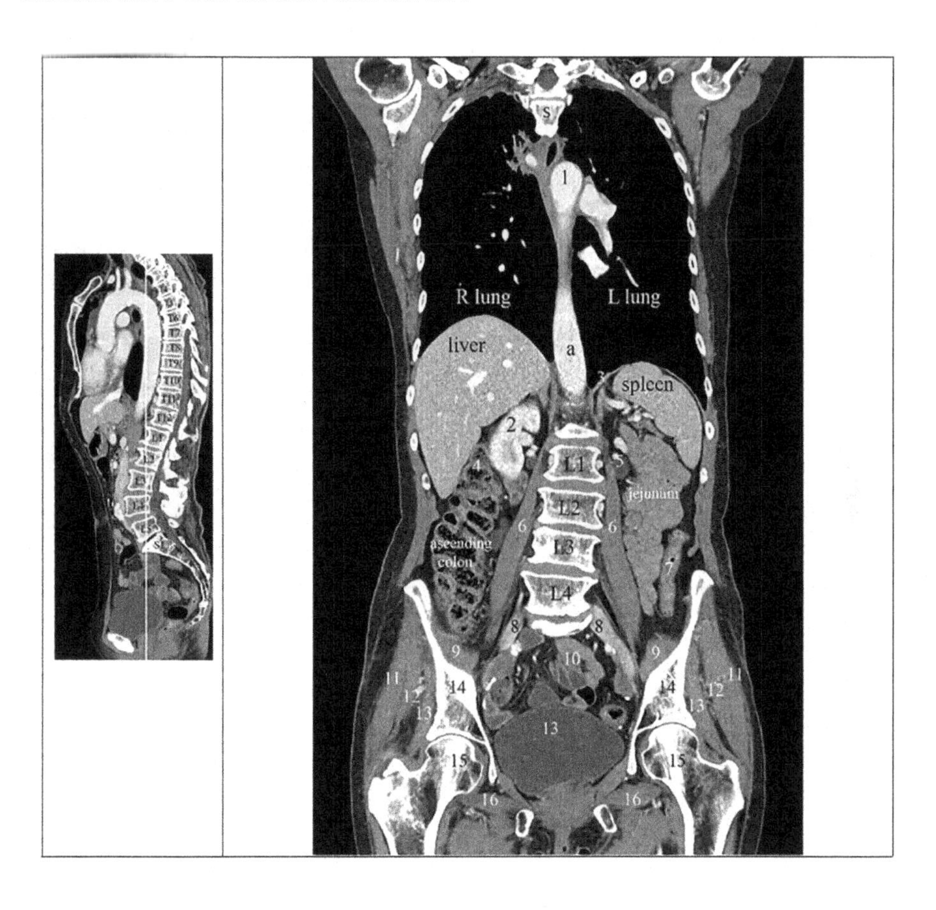

a – aorta	5 – left renal pelvis	11 – gluteus maximus
s – sternum	6 – psoas major	12 – gluteus medius
1 – aorta (thoracic)	7 – descending colon	13 – pelvic cavity – urinary bladder
2 – right kidney	8 – common iliac arteries	14 – ilium
3 – diaphragm	9 – iliacus	15 – head of femur
4 – hepatic flexure	10 – ileum	16 – obturator externus

L1 LOWER

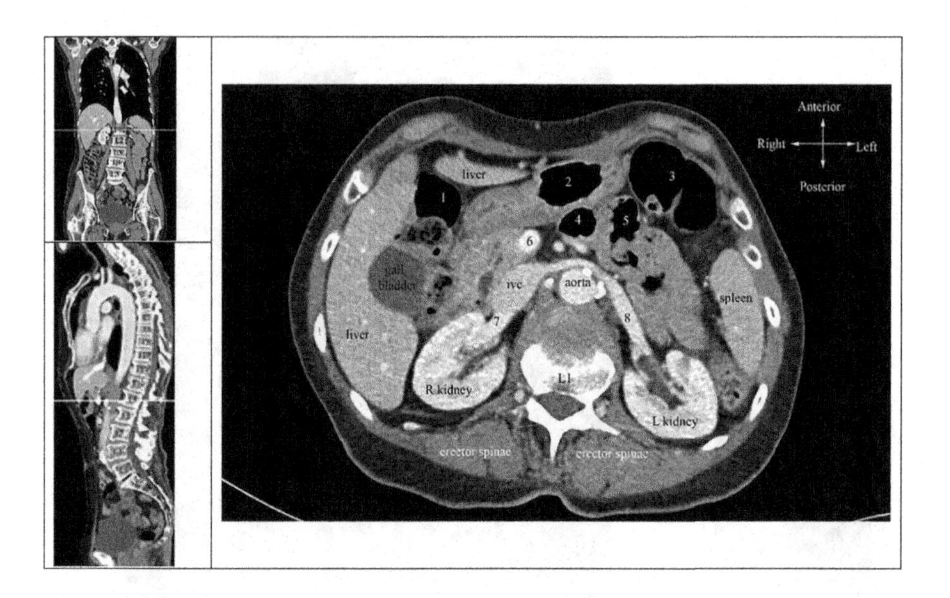

1 – hepatic flexure of colon
2 – stomach
3 – splenic flexure of colon
4 – duodenum (third part)
5 – duodenum (fourth part)
6 – portal vein
7 – right renal vein
8 – left renal vein
ivc – inferior vena cava

L2 – TRANSVERSE COLON HEAD OF PANCREAS

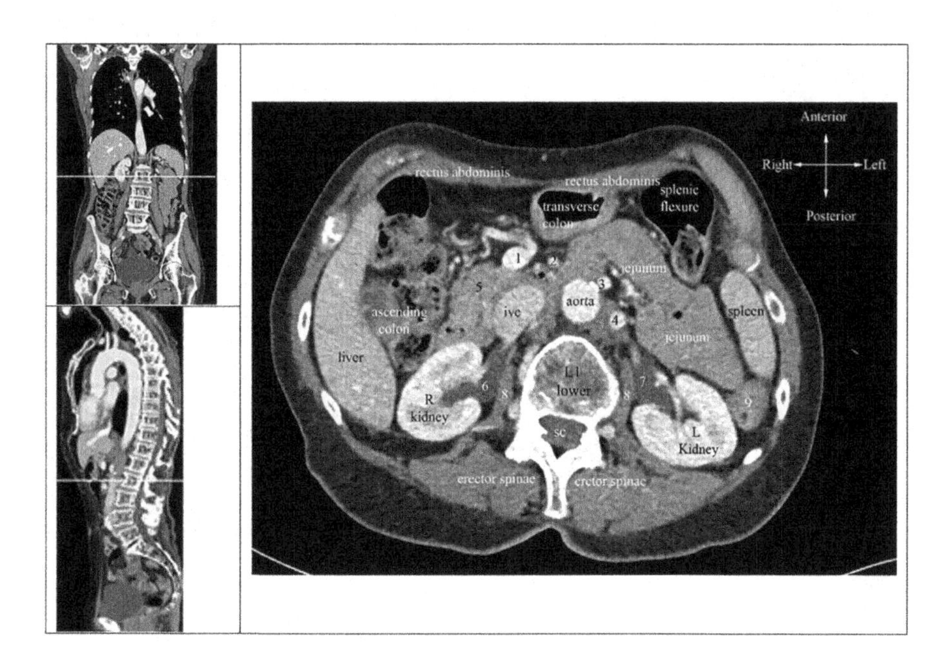

1 – superior mesenteric vein (or confluence of portal vein)	5 – head of pancreas	9 – descending colon
2 – superior mesenteric artery	6 – right renal pelvis	ivc – inferior vena cava
3 – inferior mesenteric vein	7 – left renal pelvis	sc – spinal cord
4 – left gonadial vein	8 – right and left crus of diaphragm	

L3

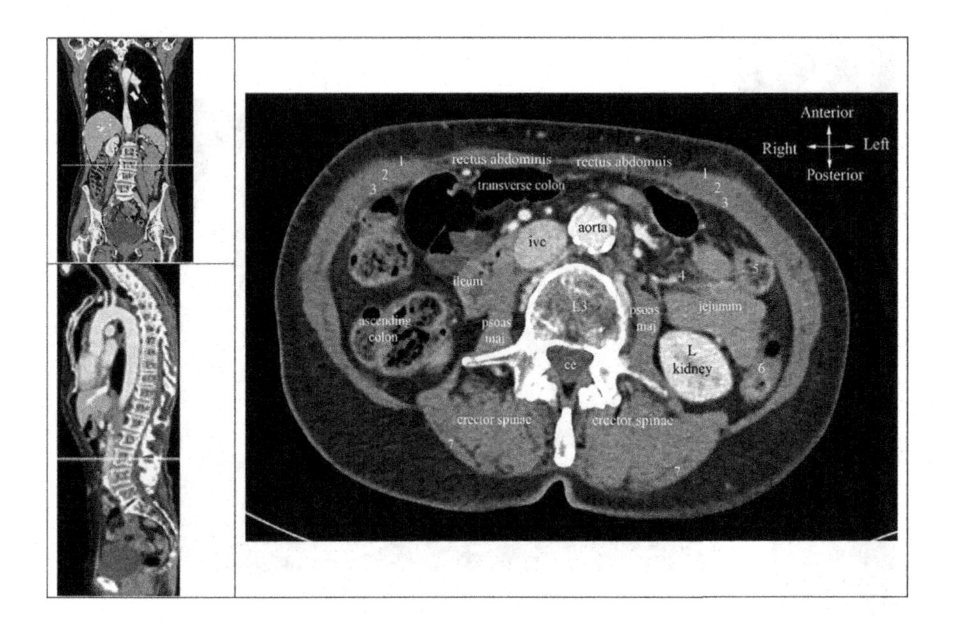

1 – external oblique	4 – mesentery	7 – latissimus dorsi
2 – internal oblique	5 – descending colon	ce – cauda equina of spinal cord
3 – transversus abdominus	6 – descending colon	ivc – inferior vena cava

L4

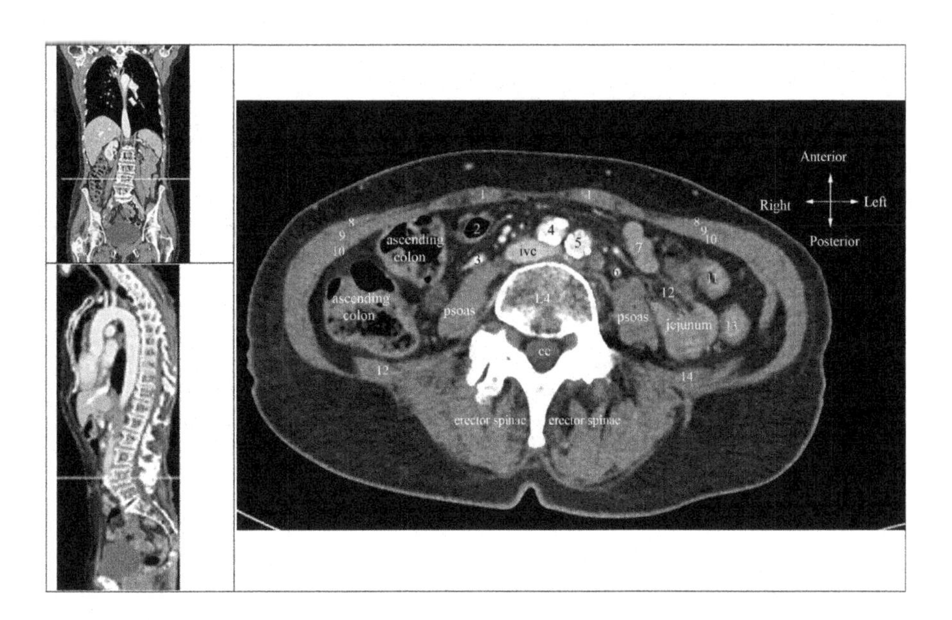

1. rectus abdominis
2. ileum
3. right ureter
4. right common iliac artery
5. left common iliac artery
6. left ureter
7. jejunum
8. external oblique
9. internal oblique
10. transversus abdominis
11. jejunum
12. mesentery
13. descending colon
14. quadratus lumborum

ce cauda equina
ivc inferior vena cava

L5/S1 – ILIAC VESSELS

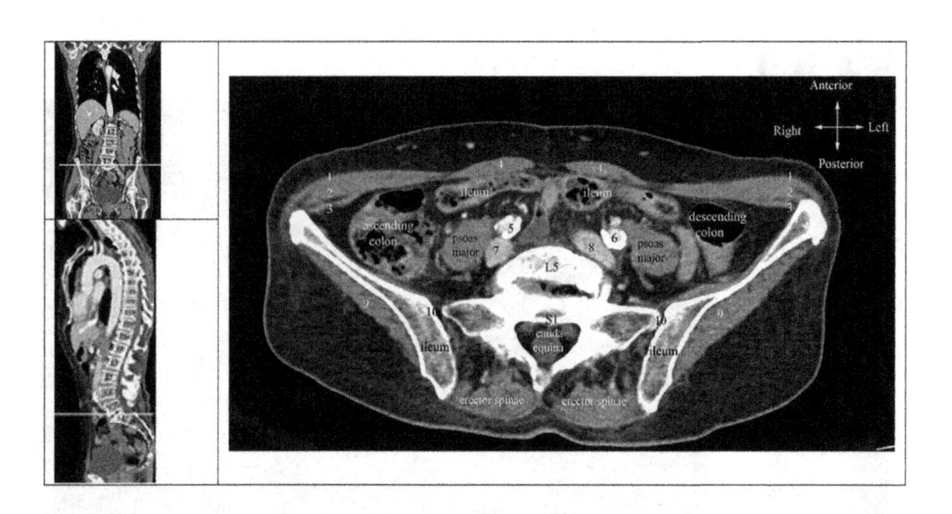

1 – external oblique
2 – internal oblique
3 – transversus abdominis
4 – rectus abdominis
5 – Right common Iliac artery
6 – left common iliac artery
7 – right common iliac vein
8 – left common iliac vein
9 – gluteus medius
10 – sacroiliac joints

S3

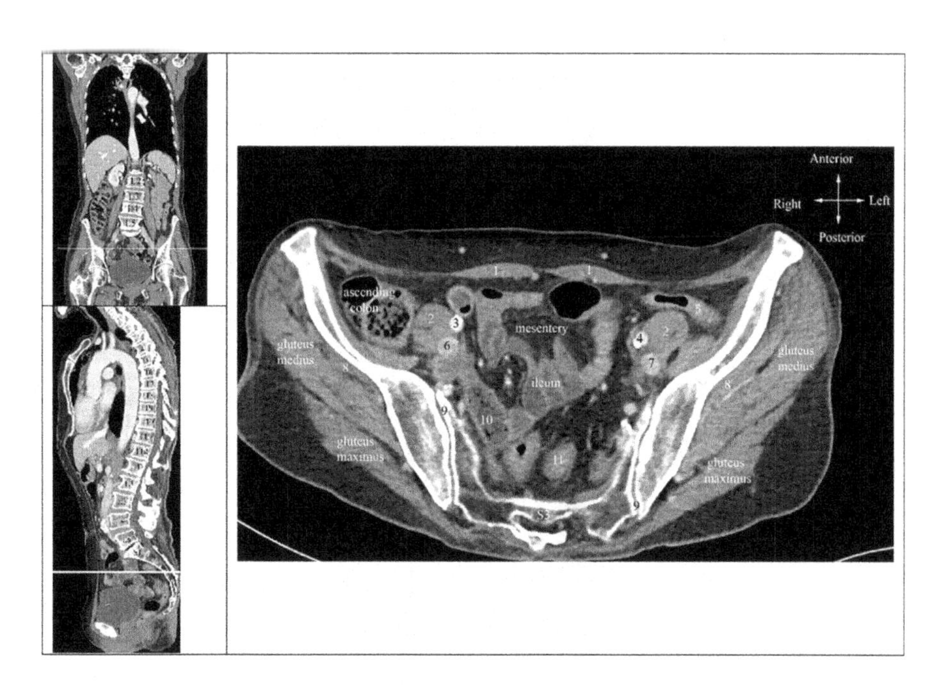

1 – rectus abdominis
2 – psoas major
3 – right external iliac artery
4 – left external iliac artery
5 – sigmoid colon
6 – right internal iliac vein
7 – left internal iliac vein
8 – gluteus minimus
9 – sacroiliac joints
10 – rectosigmoid junction
11 – ileum

MID-SAGITTAL – MALE

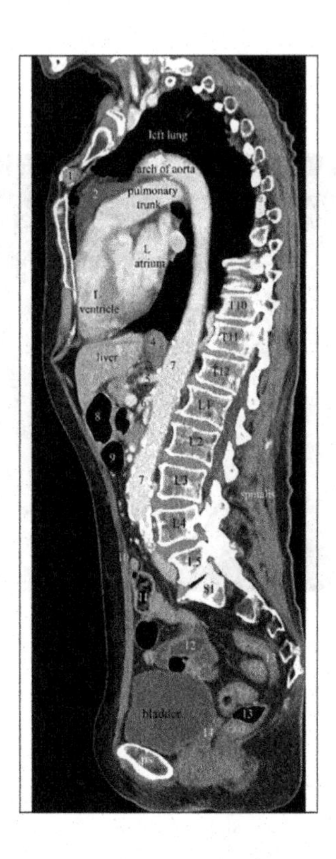

1 – sternal angle
2 – left brachiocephalic vein (or the first part of superior vena cava)
3 – costal cartilage
4 – abdominal part of oesophagus
5 – celiac trunk
6 – superior mesenteric artery
7 – aorta (abdominal)
8 – stomach
9 – transverse colon
10 – rectus abdominis
11 – ileum
12 – sigmoid colon
13 – rectum
14 – seminal vesicle
ps – pubic symphysis

COCCYX – MALE

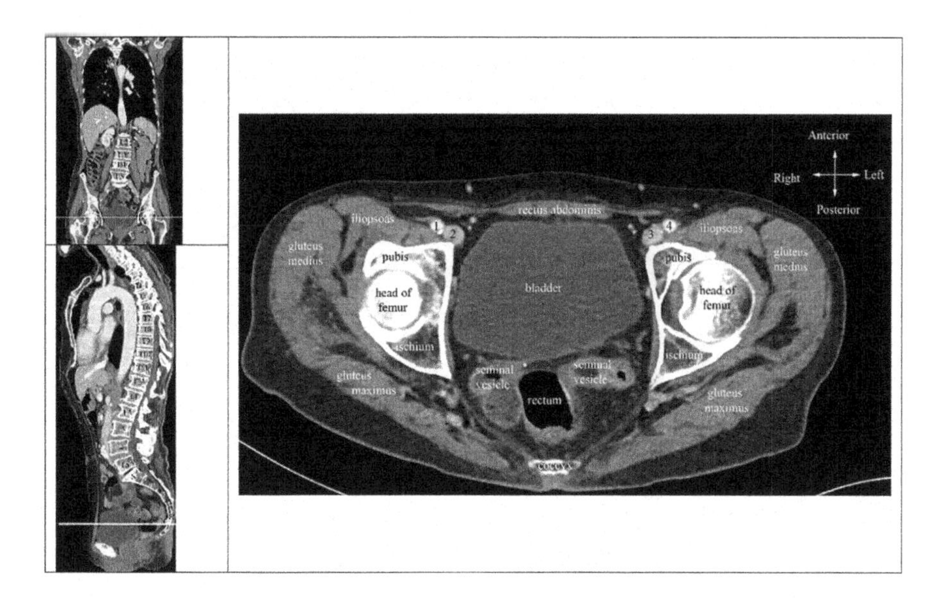

1 – right femoral artery	3 – left femoral vein
2 – right femoral vein	4 – left femoral artery

COCCYX – FEMALE

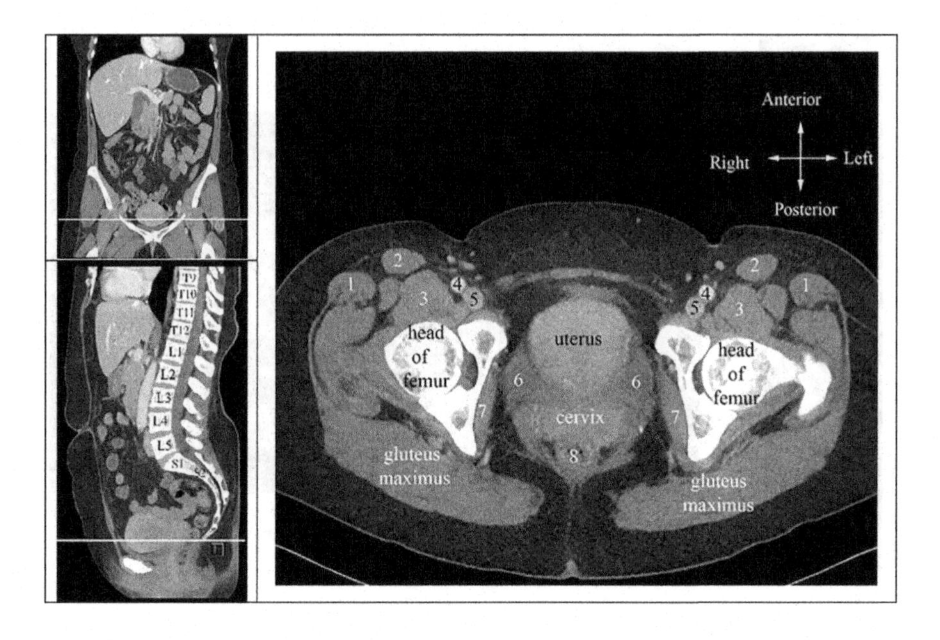

1 – tensor fascia latae	5 – left and right external iliac veins
2 – sartorius	6 – partial volume of the urinary bladder
3 – iliopsoas	7 – obturator internus
4 – left and right external iliac arteries	8 – rectum

10 Cross-Sectional Anatomy of the Upper Limb

Arjun Burlakoti, Harsha Wechalekar, and Nicola Massy-Westropp
University of South Australia

Lars Kruse
Dr Jones and Partners
Medical Imaging

Shayne Chau
University of Canberra

CONTENTS

DOI: 10.1201/9781003132554-14

T1 VERTEBRAL LEVEL

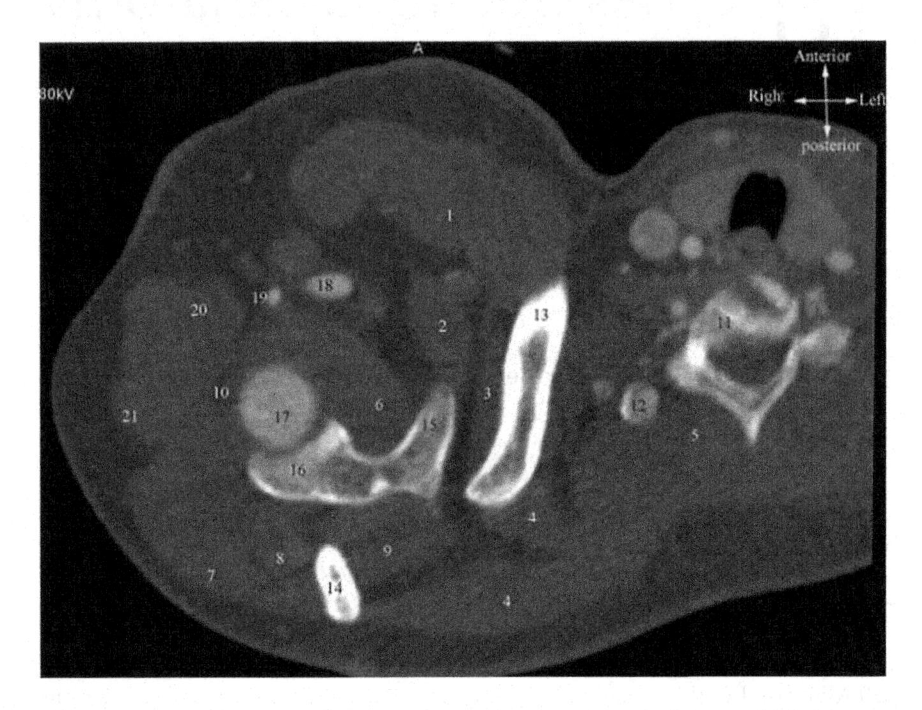

FIGURE 10.1 Axial computed tomography (CT) scan – right glenohumeral joint, T1 vertebral level.

1 – pectoralis major muscle
2 – pectoralis minor muscle
3 – subclavius muscle
4 – trapezius attached to the lateral clavicle and acromion process
5 – semispinalis cervicis muscle
6 – subscapularis muscle
7 – deltoid muscle (posterior)
8 – infraspinatus muscle
9 – supraspinatus muscle
10 – subdeltoid-subacromial bursa
11 – body of first thoracic (T1) vertebra
12 – transverse process of T1
13 – clavicle bone
14 – acromion process
15 – coracoid process of scapula
16 – glenoid fossa
17 – head of humerus
18 – axillary artery
19 – subscapular artery
20 – deltoid muscle (anterior)
21 – deltoid muscle (lateral)

LEFT MID ARM LEVEL

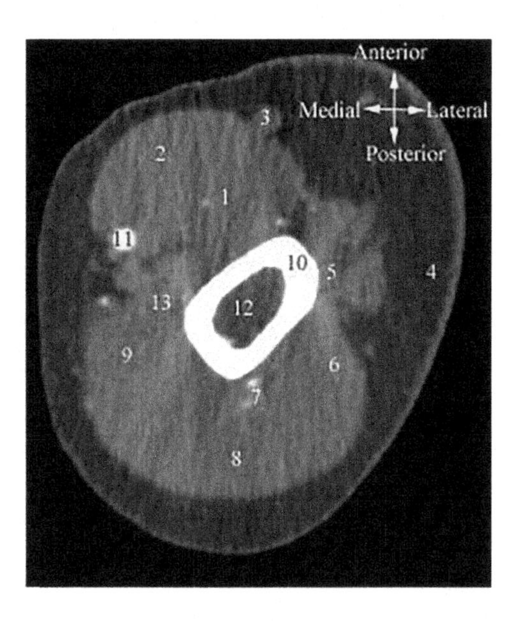

FIGURE 10.2 Axial computed tomography (CT) scan – left mid-arm level.

1 – brachialis muscles
2 – biceps brachii muscle
3 – cephalic vein (superficial vein)
4 – subcutaneous tissue
5 – deltoid muscle and tendon
6 – lateral head of triceps brachii muscle
7 – deep artery of arm (profunda brachii artery)
8 – long head of triceps brachii muscle
9 – medial head of triceps brachii muscle
10 – humerus (compact bone)
11 – brachial artery in the arm
12 – bone marrow in the medullary cavity–mid humerus
13 – coracobrachialis muscle

LEFT DISTAL ARM LEVEL

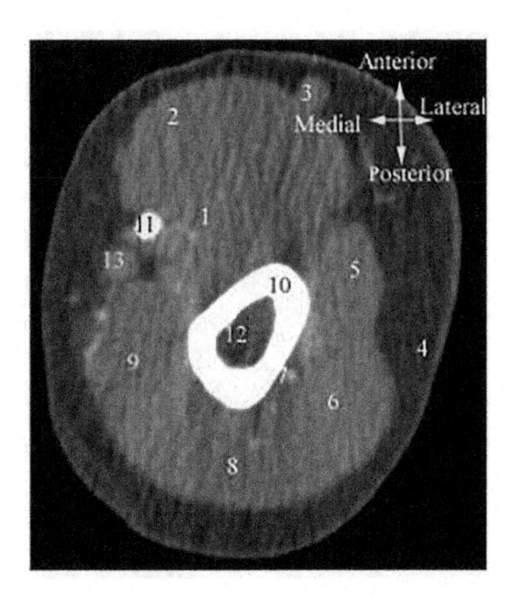

FIGURE 10.3 Axial computed tomography (CT) scan – left distal arm level.

1 – brachialis muscles
2 – biceps brachii muscle
3 – cephalic vein (superficial vein)
4 – subcutaneous tissue
5 – brachioradialis muscle
6 – lateral head of triceps brachii muscle
7 – deep artery of arm (profunda brachii artery)
8 – long head of triceps brachii muscle
9 – medial head of triceps brachii muscle
10 – humerus (compact bone)
11 – brachial artery in the arm
12 – bone marrow in the medullary cavity–mid humerus
13 – brachial vein

LEFT CUBITAL FOSSA LEVEL

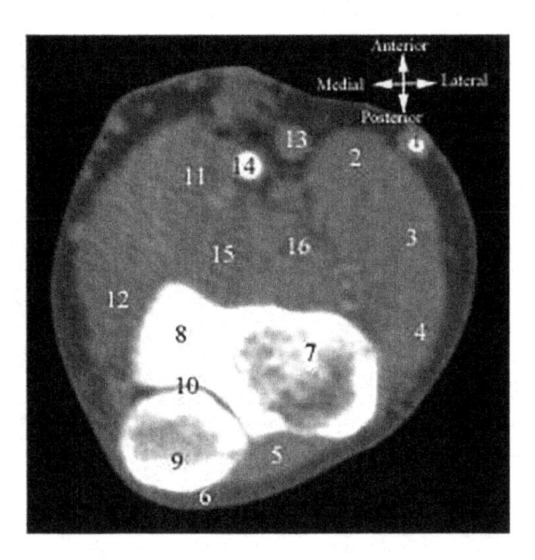

FIGURE 10.4 Axial computed tomography (CT) scan – left cubital fossa level.

---

1 – intravenous needle into the cephalic vein (superficial vein)
2 – brachioradialis muscle
3 – extensor carpi radialis longus muscle
4 – extensor carpi radialis brevis muscle
5 – anconeus muscle
6 – triceps brachii muscle tendon
7 – capitulum of distal humerus
8 – trochlea of distal humerus
9 – olecranon process of ulna
10 – olecranon process of ulna in the olecranon fossa on humerus
11 – pronator teres muscle
12 – flexor carpi ulnaris muscle
13 – median cubital vein
14 – brachial artery in the cubital fossa

LEFT PROXIMAL RADIOULNAR JOINT LEVEL

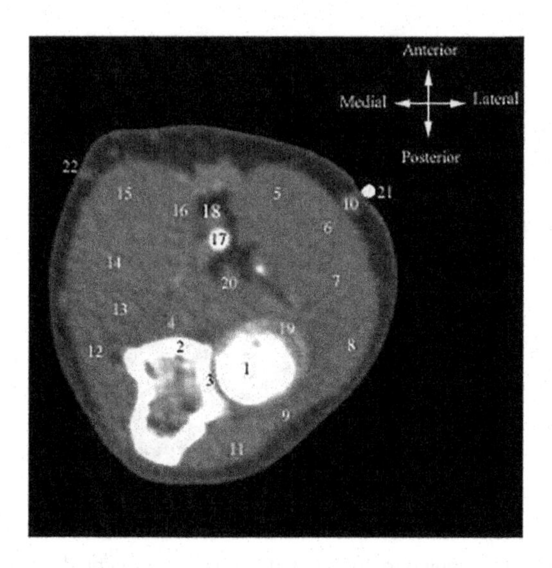

FIGURE 10.5 Axial computed tomography (CT) scan – left proximal radioulnar joint level.

- 1 – head of radius
- 2 – ulnar tuberosity
- 3 – radial notch of ulna
- 4 – brachialis muscle
- 5 – brachioradialis muscle
- 6 – extensor carpi radialis longus muscle
- 7 – extensor carpi radialis brevis muscle
- 8 – extensor digitorum muscle
- 9 – anconeus muscle
- 10 – cephalic vein
- 11 – extensor carpi ulnaris
- 12 – flexor carpi ulnaris muscle
- 13 – flexor digitorum profundus muscle
- 14 – flexor digitorum superficialis muscle
- 15 – flexor carpi radialis
- 16 – pronator teres muscle
- 17 – brachial artery in the cubital fossa
- 18 – brachial vein
- 19 – supinator muscle
- 20 – biceps brachii tendon
- 21 – intravenous needle next to the cephalic vein (superficial vein)
- 22 – basilic vein (superficial vein)

LEFT MID FOREARM LEVEL

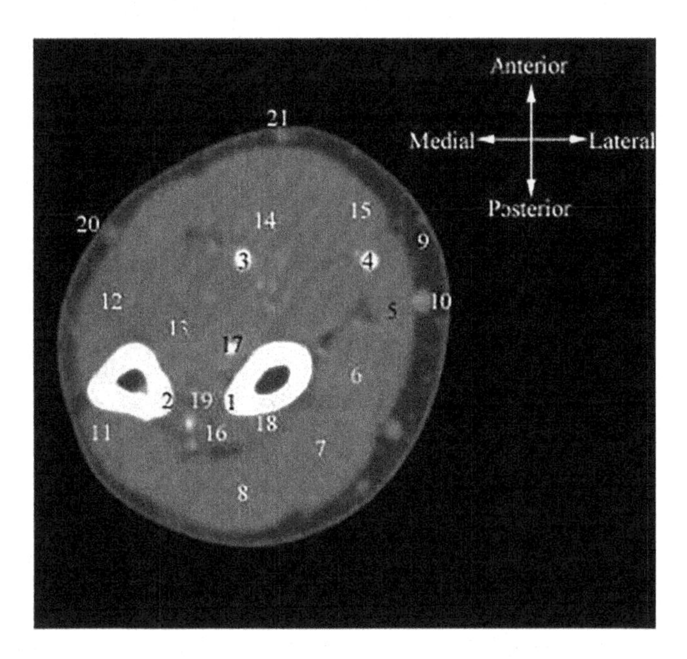

FIGURE 10.6 Axial computed tomography (CT) scan – left mid forearm level.

1 – interosseous border of radius	8 – extensor digitorum muscle	15 – flexor carpi radialis
2 – interosseous border of ulnar	9 – subcutaneous tissue	16 – extensor pollicis longus (deep extensor group)
3 – ulnar artery	10 – cephalic vein	17 – common interosseous artery of forearm
4 – radial artery	11 – extensor carpi ulnaris	18 – abductor pollicis longus (deep extensor group)
5 – brachioradialis muscle	12 – flexor carpi ulnaris muscle	19 – interosseous membrane
6 – extensor carpi radialis longus muscle	13 – flexor digitorum profundus muscle	20 – basilic vein (superficial vein)
7 – extensor carpi radialis brevis muscle	14 – flexor digitorum superficialis muscle	21 – median antebrachial vein (superficial vein)

LEFT DISTAL FOREARM/PROXIMAL WRIST LEVEL

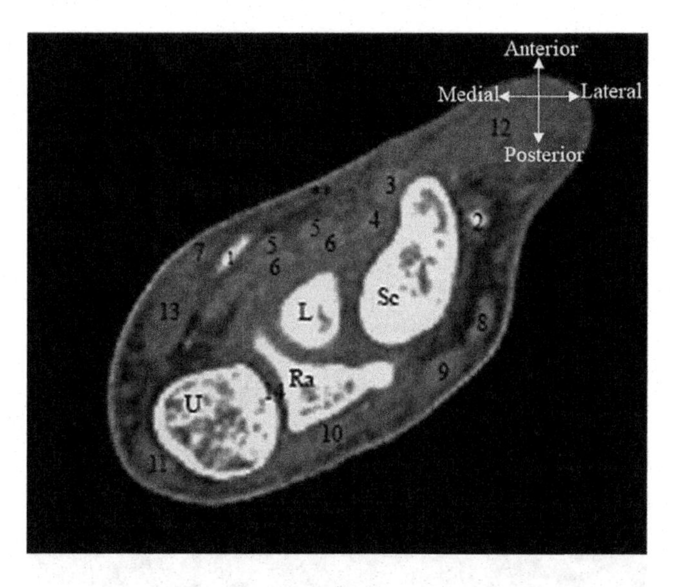

FIGURE 10.7 Axial computed tomography (CT) scan – left distal forearm or proximal wrist.

Ra – distal radius
U – head of the ulna
L – lunate bone
Sc – scaphoid bone
** – palmar aponeurosis
1 – ulnar artery
2 – radial artery
3 – flexor carpi radialis
4 – flexor pollicis longus
5 – flexor digitorum superficialis
6 – flexor digitorum profundus
7 – flexor carpi ulnaris
8 – abductor pollicis longus
9 – extensor pollicis longus
10 – extensor digitorum
11 – extensor carpi ulnaris
12 – thenar eminence
13 – hypothenar eminence
14 – distal radioulnar joint

LEFT MID CARPAL LEVEL

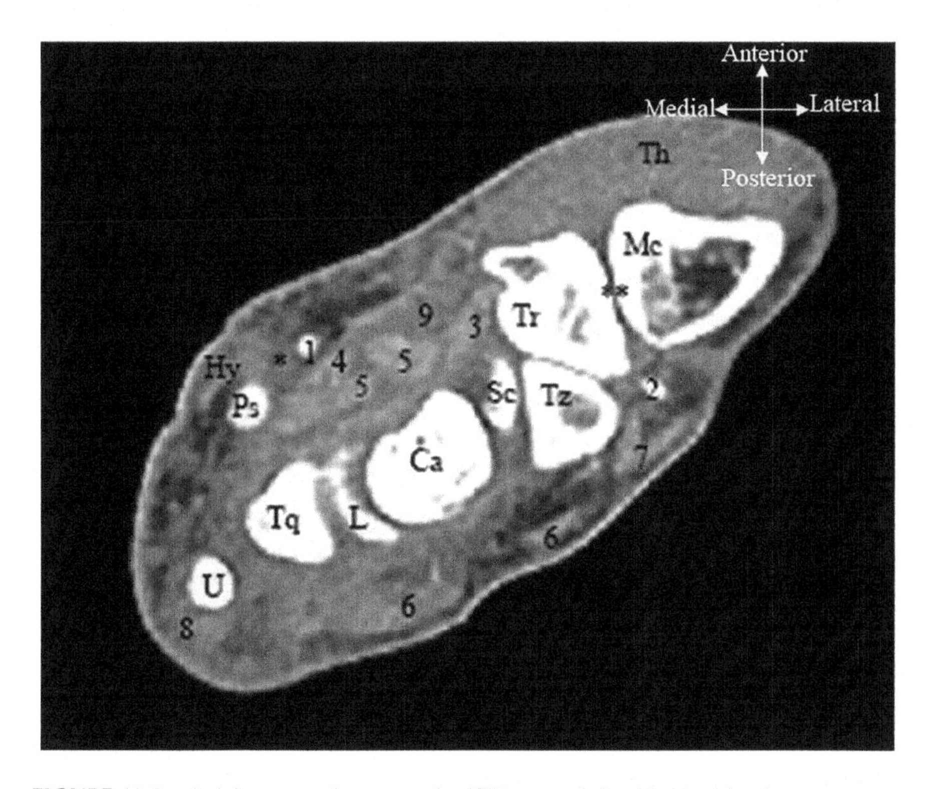

FIGURE 10.8 Axial computed tomography (CT) scan – left mid carpal level.

Mc – base of the first metacarpal	* – ulnar nerve
Tr – trapezium	** – first carpometacarpal joint
Tz – trapezoid	1 – ulnar artery
Sc – scaphoid	2 – radial artery
Ca – capitate	3 – flexor pollicis longus
L – lunate	4 – flexor digitorum superficialis tendon
Tq – triquetral	5 – flexor digitorum profundus tendon
U – ulnar styloid	6 – extensor digitorum tendon
Ps – pisiform	7 – extensor pollicis longus
Th – thenar eminence	8 – extensor carpi ulnaris
Hy – hypothenar eminence	9 – median nerve

LEFT DISTAL CARPAL LEVEL

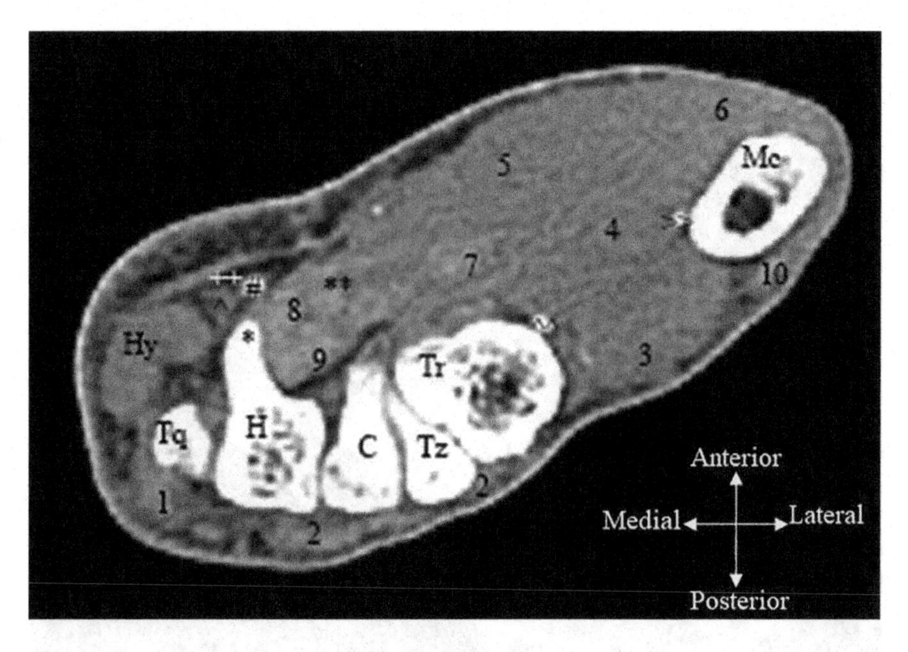

FIGURE 10.9 Axial computed tomography (CT) scan – left distal carpal level.

Mc – first metacarpal	++ – ulnar canal	3 – first dorsal interossei
Tr – trapezium	^ – ulnar nerve	4 – opponens pollicis
Tz – trapezoid	# – ulnar artery	5 – flexor pollicis brevis
C – capitate	** – median nerve	6 – abductor pollicis brevis
H – hamate	^^ – digital branches of the radial artery	7 – flexor pollicis longus tendon
* – hook of hamate	>> – digital branches of the radial artery	8 – flexor digitorum superficialis
Tq – Triquetral	1 – extensor carpi ulnaris	9 – flexor digitorum profundus
Hy – hypothenar eminence	2 – extensor digitorum	10 – extensor pollicis longus

11 Cross-Sectional Anatomy of the Lower Limb

Arjun Burlakoti, Harsha Wechalekar, and Nicola Massy-Westropp
University of South Australia

Lars Kruse
Dr Jones and Partners
Medical imaging

Shayne Chau
University of Canberra

CONTENTS

DOI: 10.1201/9781003132554-15

SUPERIOR PUBIC RAMI LEVEL

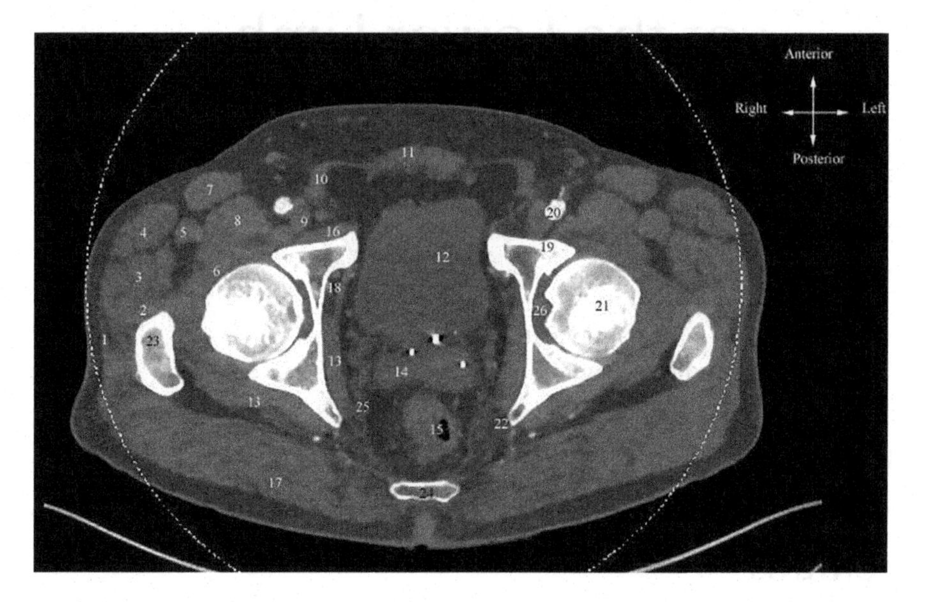

FIGURE 11.1 Axial computed tomography (CT) scan – superior pubic rami level.

1 – iliotibial band
2 – gluteus minimus muscle
3 – gluteus medius muscle
4 – tensor fascia latae muscle
5 – rectus femoris muscle
6 – anterior hip joint capsule
7 – sartorius muscle
8 – iliopsoas muscle
9 – femoral vein
10 – spermatic cord
11 – rectus abdominis muscle
12 – urinary bladder
13 – obturator internus muscle
14 – seminal vesicle
15 – rectum
16 – pectineus muscle
17 – gluteus maximus muscle
18 – obturator canal
19 – superior ramus of pubic bone
20 – femoral artery
21 – head of femur
22 – spine of ischium
23 – greater trochanter (apex)
24 – coccyx
25 – iliococcygeus part of the levator ani muscle
26 – acetabular fossa

ISCHIAL TUBEROSITY LEVEL

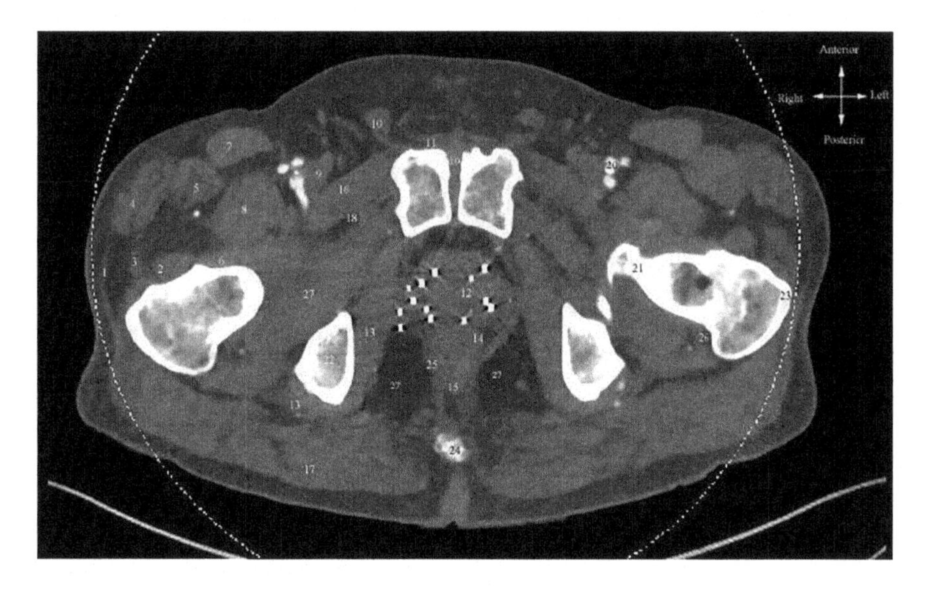

FIGURE 11.2 Axial computed tomography (CT) scan – ischial tuberosity level.

1 – iliotibial band
2 – gluteus minimus muscle
3 – gluteus medius muscle
4 – tensor fascia latae muscle
5 – rectus femoris muscle
6 – anterior hip joint capsule
7 – sartorius muscle
8 – iliacus muscle
9 – femoral vein
10 – spermatic cord
11 – rectus abdominis muscle
12 – prostate gland
13 – obturator internus muscle
14 – seminal vesicle
15 – anorectal junction
16 – pectineus muscle
17 – gluteus maximus muscle
18 – obturator nerve
19 – symphysis pubic (secondary cartilaginous type of joint)
20 – femoral artery
21 – neck of femur
22 – tuberosity of ischium
23 – greater trochanter of femur
24 – coccyx
25 – pubococcygeus part of the levator ani muscle
26 – trochanteric fossa of femur
27 – ischiorectal fossa

BILATERAL MID-FEMORAL LEVEL

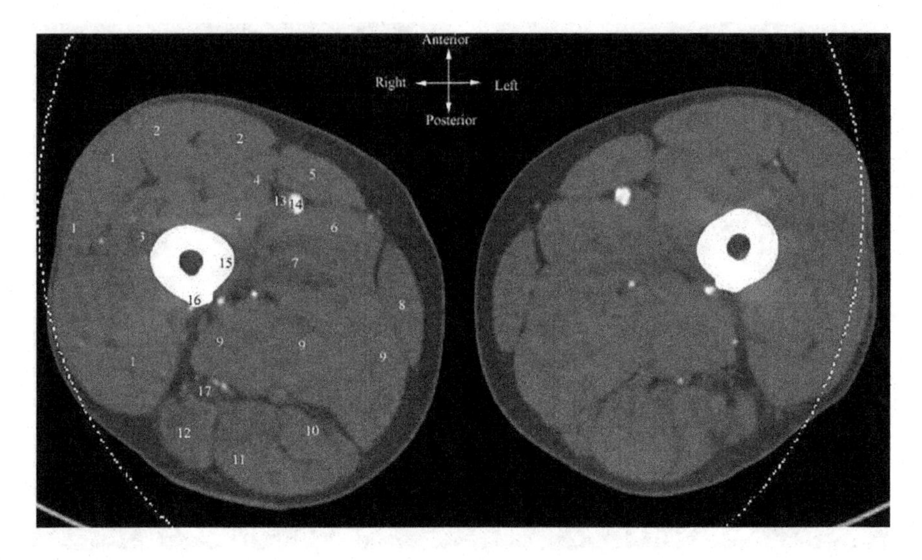

FIGURE 11.3 Axial computed tomography (CT) scan – bilateral mid-femoral level.

---

1 – vastus lateralis muscle (position deep to the iliotibial band)
2 – rectus femoris muscle
3 – vastus intermedius muscle
4 – vastus medialis muscle
5 – sartorius muscle
6 – adductor longus muscle
7 – adductor brevis muscle
8 – gracilis muscle
9 – adductor magnus muscle
10 – semimembranosus muscle
11 – semitendinosus muscle
12 – long head of biceps femoris muscle
13 – femoral vein in the adductor canal
14 – femoral artery in the adductor canal
15 – medial border of femur
16 – lateral lip of linea aspera
17 – sciatic nerve

BILATERAL DISTAL-FEMORAL LEVEL

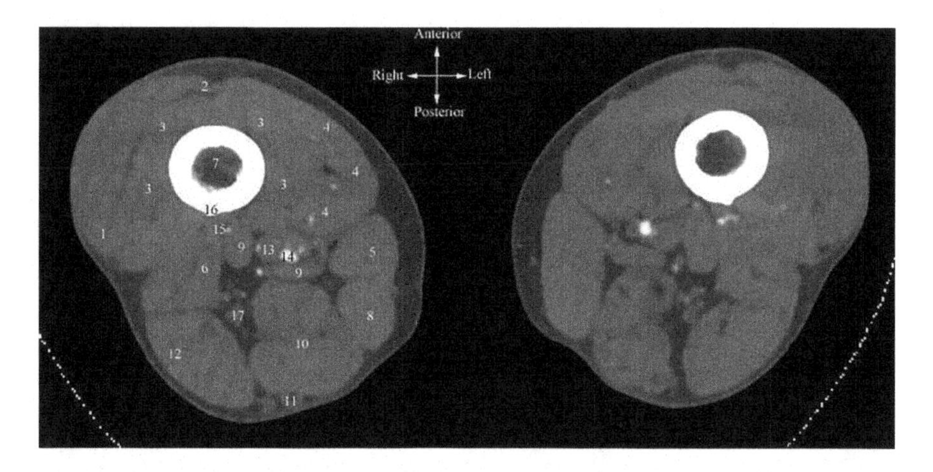

FIGURE 11.4 Axial computed tomography (CT) scan – bilateral distal-femoral level.

1 – vastus lateralis muscle (position deep to the iliotibial band)
2 – rectus femoris muscle
3 – vastus intermedius muscle
4 – vastus medialis muscle
5 – sartorius muscle
6 – short head of biceps femoris muscle
7 – medullary canal of femur
8 – gracilis muscle
9 – adductor magnus muscle
10 – semimembranosus muscle
11 – semitendinosus muscle
12 – long head of biceps femoris muscle
13 – femoral vein in the adductor hiatus
14 – femoral artery in the adductor hiatus
15 – distal perforator artery
16 – lateral lip of linea aspera
17 – sciatic nerve

BILATERAL PATELLOFEMORAL JOINT LEVEL

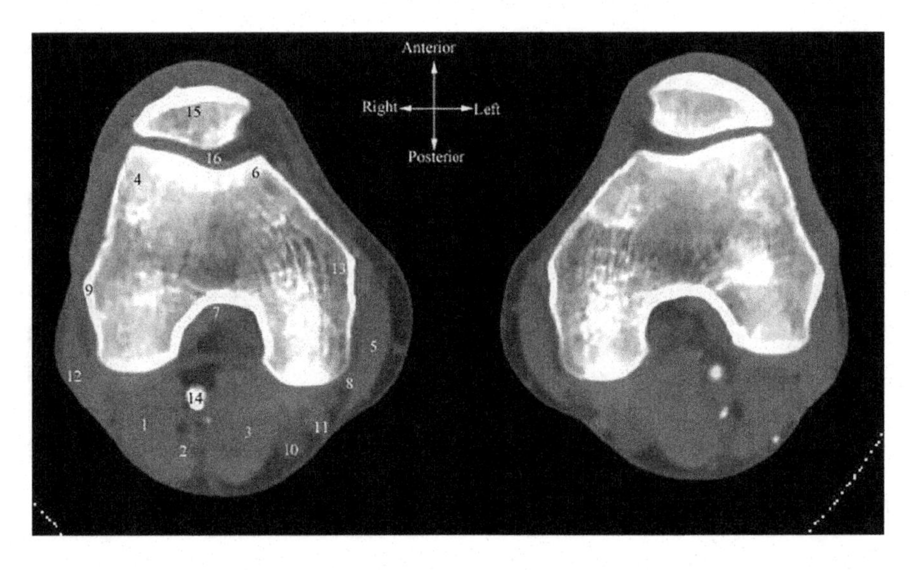

FIGURE 11.5 Axial computed tomography (CT) scan – bilateral patellofemoral joint level.

1 – lateral head of gastrocnemius muscle
2 – plantaris muscle
3 – medial head of gastrocnemius muscle
4 – lateral condyle of femur
5 – sartorius muscle
6 – medial condyle of femur
7 – intercondylar fossa of femur
8 – gracilis muscle
9 – lateral epicondyle of femur
10 – semimembranosus muscle
11 – semitendinosus muscle
12 – biceps femoris muscle
13 – medial epicondyle of femur
14 – popliteal artery in the popliteal fossa
15 – patella
16 – patellofemoral joint cavity

KNEE JOINT LEVEL

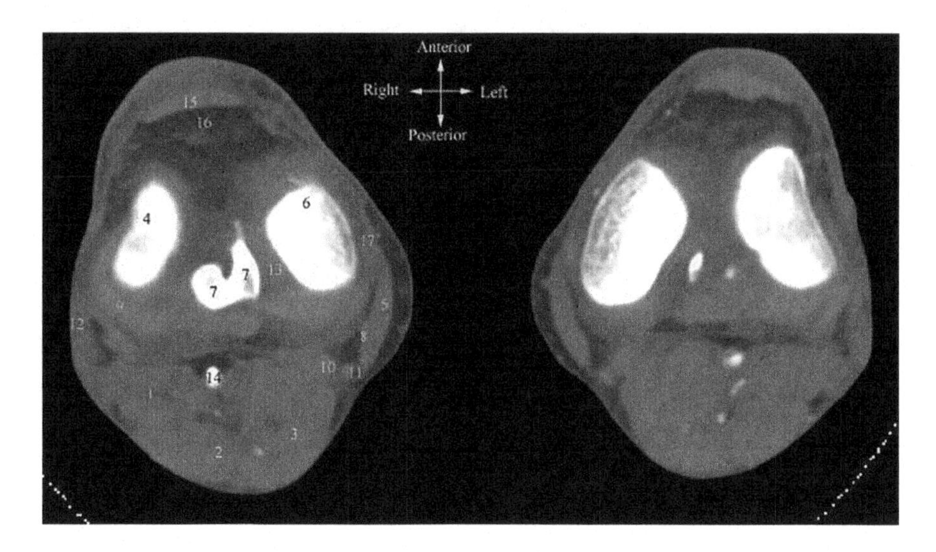

FIGURE 11.6 Axial computed tomography (CT) scan – knee joint level.

---

1 – lateral head of gastrocnemius muscle
2 – plantaris muscle
3 – medial head of gastrocnemius muscle
4 – lateral condyle of femur
5 – sartorius muscle
6 – medial condyle of femur
7 – tubercles in intercondylar eminence of tibia
8 – gracilis muscle
9 – popliteus muscle tendon
10 – semimembranosus muscle
11 – semitendinosus muscle
12 – biceps femoris muscle tendon
13 – lateral meniscus of right knee
14 – popliteal artery in the popliteal fossa
15 – patellar tendon
16 – infrapatellar pad of adipose tissue
17 – medial collateral ligament of right knee

PROXIMAL TIBIOFIBULAR JOINT LEVEL

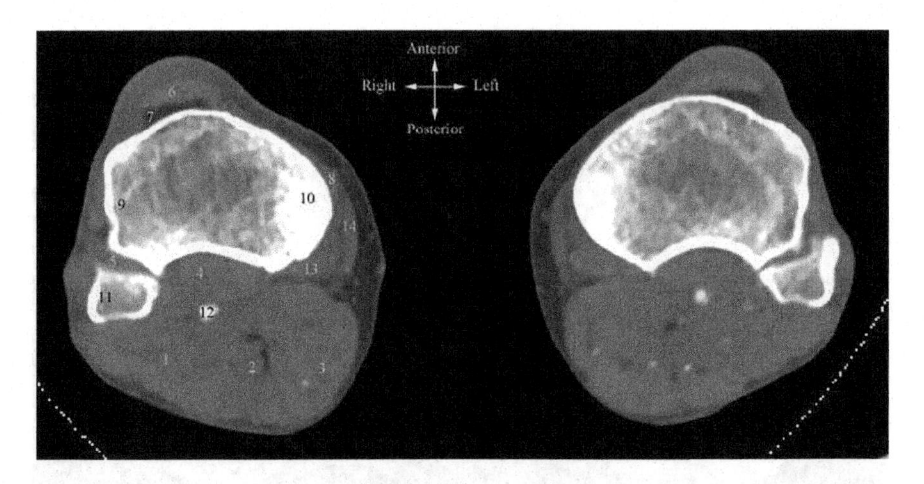

FIGURE 11.7 Axial computed tomography (CT) scan – proximal tibiofibular joint level.

1 – lateral head of gastrocnemius muscle
2 – plantaris muscle
3 – medial head of gastrocnemius muscle
4 – popliteus muscle
5 – proximal tibiofibular joint
6 – patellar tendon
7 – sub-patellar tendinous bursa
8 – medial collateral ligament
9 – lateral condyle of tibia
10 – medial condyle of tibia
11 – head of fibula
12 – popliteal artery
13 – semimembranosus muscle
14 – pes anserine flattened tendon

MID LEG LEVEL

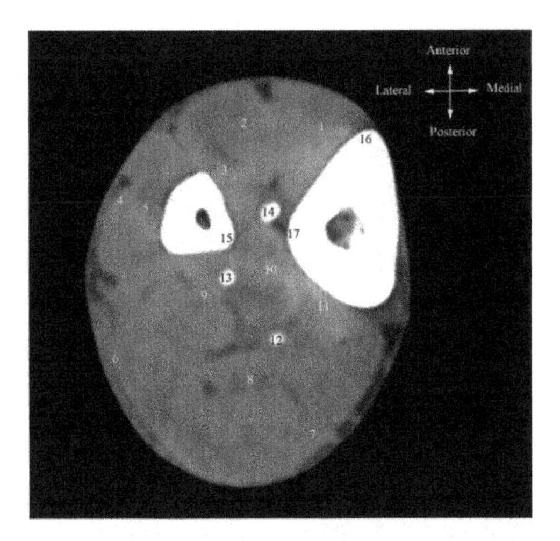

FIGURE 11.8 Axial computed tomography (CT) scan – mid leg level.

1 – tibialis anterior muscle
2 – extensor digitorum longus muscle
3 – extensor hallucis longus muscle
4 – fibularis longus muscle
5 – fibularis brevis muscle
6 – lateral head of gastrocnemius
7 – medial head of gastrocnemius
8 – soleus muscle
9 – flexor hallucis longus muscle
10 – tibialis posterior muscle
11 – flexor digitorum longus muscle
12 – posterior tibial artery
13 – fibular artery
14 – anterior tibial artery
15 – interosseous border of fibula
16 – anterior border of tibia
17 – interosseous border of tibia

DISTAL TIBIOFIBULAR JOINT LEVEL

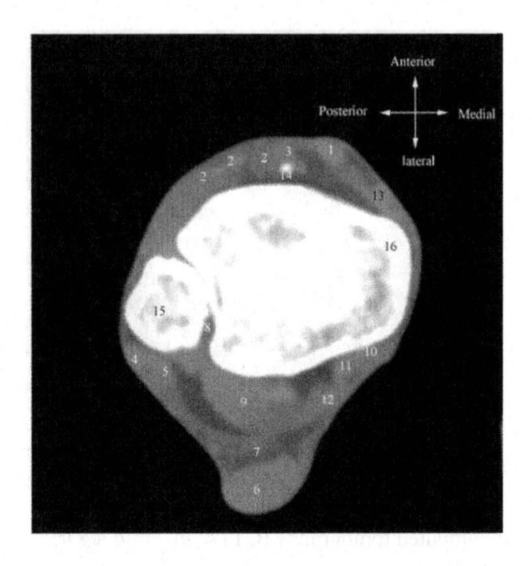

FIGURE 11.9 Axial computed tomography (CT) scan – right distal tibiofibular joint level.

1 – tibialis anterior muscle tendon
2 – extensor digitorum longus muscle tendon
3 – extensor hallucis longus muscle tendon
4 – fibularis longus muscle tendon
5 – fibularis brevis muscle tendon
6 – calcaneal tendon
7 – sub tendinous (calcaneal) bursa
8 – distal tibiofibular joint
9 – flexor hallucis longus muscle
10 – tibialis posterior muscle tendon
11 – flexor digitorum longus muscle tendon
12 – posterior tibial artery
13 – great saphenous vein
14 – anterior tibial artery
15 – distal fibula (proximal to the lateral malleolus)
16 – distal tibia (proximal to the medial malleolus)

ANKLE JOINT LEVEL

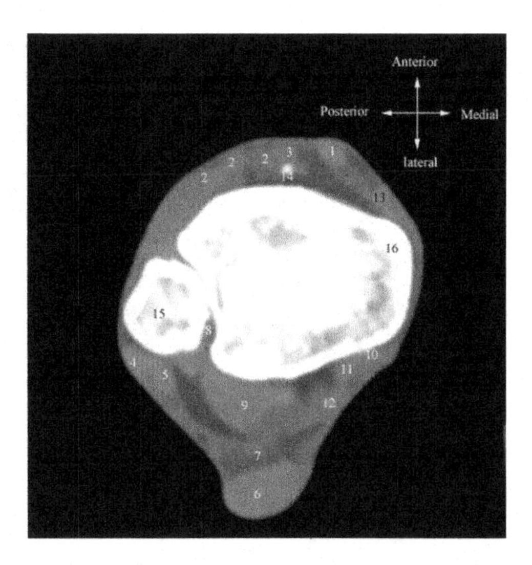

FIGURE 11.10 Axial computed tomography (CT) scan – right ankle joint level.

---

1 – tibialis anterior muscle tendon
2 – extensor digitorum longus muscle tendon
3 – extensor hallucis longus muscle tendon
4 – fibularis longus muscle tendon
5 – fibularis brevis muscle tendon
6 – calcaneal muscle tendon
7 – sub tendinous (calcaneal) bursa
8 – ankle joint cavity
9 – flexor hallucis longus muscle
10 – tibialis posterior muscle tendon
11 – flexor digitorum longus muscle tend-on
12 – posterior tibial artery
13 – great saphenous vein
14 – anterior tibial artery
15 – lateral malleolus
16 – medial malleolus
17 – distal surface of tibia (anterior border)
18 – distal surface of tibia (posterior border)
19 – trochlea of talus

TARSAL BONES (OBLIQUE VIEW)

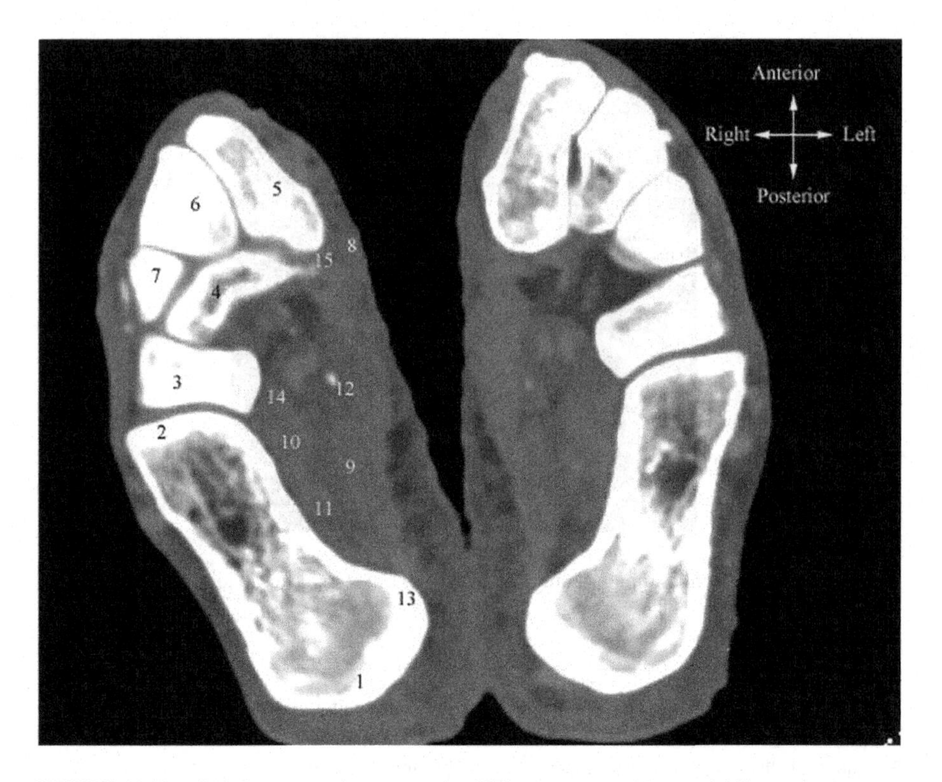

FIGURE 11.11 Axial computed tomography (CT) scan – tarsal bones (oblique view).

1 – calcaneal tuberosity
2 – head of calcaneus
3 – cuboid bone
4 – navicular bone
5 – medial cuneiform bone
6 – intermediate cuneiform bone
7 – lateral cuneiform bone
8 – abductor hallucis muscle
9 – flexor digitorum brevis muscle
10 – quadratus plantae muscle
11 – lateral plantar artery
12 – medial plantar artery
13 – medial process of calcaneal tuberosity
14 – adductor hallucis muscle
15 – flexor hallucis brevis

Section 5

Imaging Procedures

12 Imaging of the Head

Debbie Starkey and Gordon Mander
Queensland University of Technology

Deb Watson
Sunshine Coast University Hospital

CONTENTS

DOI: 10.1201/9781003132554-17

INTRODUCTION

The chapters in this section are not intended to cover the entire range of options for image acquisition. Many departmental imaging procedures are uniquely developed in response to factors which include the type and capability of the CT unit (number of detectors, dual energy capability, etc.); ancillary equipment capability, as well as the case mix and staffing of the setting. Recognising the enormous diversity possible in departmental protocols, the authors have provided examples of standard imaging procedures for the anatomical regions. Examinations are described in a generic manner – the user should consider the detector widths, exposure factors, dose reduction techniques, etc., specific to the CT unit being used, in the application of the techniques described. Discussion is also provided for the modification to standard procedure undertaken in response to patient presentation, and this includes a separate chapter on imaging paediatric patients.

CT equipment is available from a range of vendors – The available range of detector sizes and number vary between vendors and models within the manufactured range. Operating platforms also vary – however, the essential processes are constant. Irrespective of the CT equipment being used, the CT imaging process can be considered under two broad categories: Factors selected prior to image acquisition and post-processing options after acquisition. Contemporary multidetector CT has considerable options in post-processing; however, prudent choice of acquisition factors still holds the greatest impact on the quality outcome of the CT examination. Figure 12.1 demonstrates the relationship between the acquisition factors to post-processing outcomes.

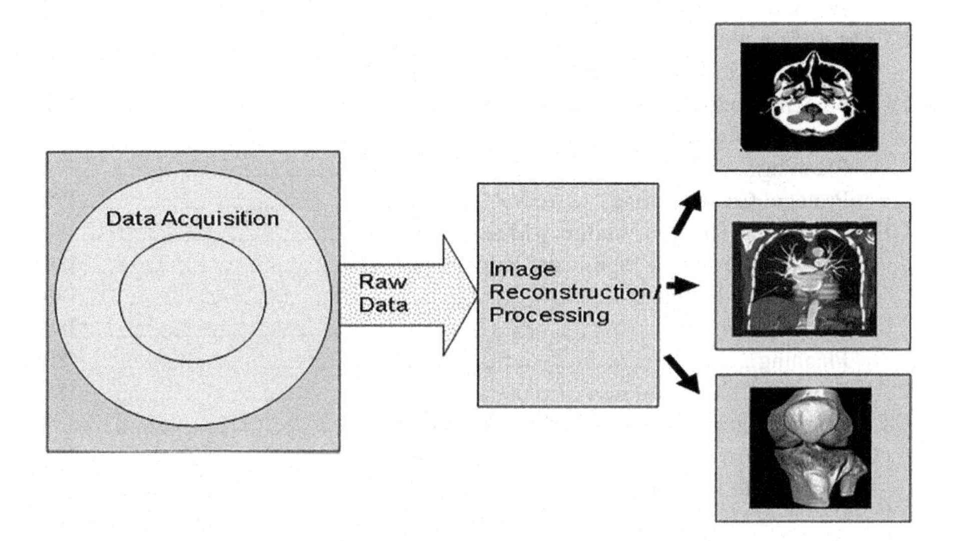

FIGURE 12.1 Relationship between the acquisition factors to post-processing outcomes.

Before any CT scan, as for any radiographic examination, the patient's identity should be checked and consent to undergo the examination should be confirmed. A critical examination into patient considerations can be found in Chapter 5. Here, we should appreciate that CT scanning environments have physical limitations which may prevent some patients from being scanned. Unit weight limits must be adhered to. Additionally, the gantry aperture can be a physical limitation to the ability to scan large patients. It is important to be aware of the physical limits of your specific unit and be able to determine patients who exceed the safe operating limits of the unit.

Where possible, any radio-opaque objects in the body area to be imaged should be removed. All patients should be changed into a gown for any examinations of the neck, chest, abdomen, and pelvis. For examinations where the use of intravenous (IV) contrast may be required, patients should be carefully evaluated for any allergic history, previous radiographic contrast examinations, and presence of any disease/s or medications which may impair renal function. All patients undergoing examination with IV contrast need to be carefully assessed as to their suitability. Guidelines for the use of IV contrast should be strictly adhered to and alternate investigations undertaken on patients deemed unsuitable (see Chapter 5).

The use of multidetector CT has brought a range of options in post-processing as outlined in Chapter 2. Irrespective, prudent choice of pre-acquisition factors still holds the greatest impact on the quality outcome of the scan. Appropriate selection of acquisition factors can also significantly reduce patient radiation dose due to CT Imaging and so the role of the CT radiographer is crucial in ensuring that the examination is performed as an efficient diagnostic aid with minimum radiation dose to the patient.

HEAD

CT of the head is the most commonly performed CT examination (Zarb et al., 2011). Following requests for chest X-ray, it is the most requested imaging in most radiology departments. Whilst the increasing availability of MRI has meant fewer scans are performed for purposes of classification of primary malignancy (for example, studies of the pituitary fossa), CT remains the primary investigation of choice for most clinical neurological concerns in acute care. This is due to its availability, speed, and accuracy in the determination of most acute neurological condition(s).

Imaging of the head in CT is most frequently performed as a non-contrast examination using limited detector post patient collimation coverage and a thin slice image reconstruction to allow for multiplanar reformation (MPRs). Whilst, historically, scans of the head were always performed as axial "step and shoot" type scans, this is almost never the case with recent generation technologies.

Specific other non-contrast examinations are performed within the anatomical region of the head. These include scans of the paranasal sinuses, specific scans of the facial bones or internal auditory meatii and petrous-temporal bones.

Contrast is regularly required to interrogate pathological and traumatic conditions more closely, particularly following the performance of a non-contrast head scan.

Considerations

Neuro imaging in CT often requires adaptive and careful consideration of the patient and their surroundings. Where a patient presents to the scanner acutely confused, uncooperative or aggressive, manipulation to the protocol may be necessary. Often a pragmatic approach is required with these patients, especially where there is reluctance or inability to aid in the form of sedation.

Safety and potential danger to the patient themselves, as well as the staff involved, should always be carefully assessed. Consideration for damage to equipment from patients displaying outwardly violent and aggressive behaviours should also be noted. Where a level of safety cannot be guaranteed following appropriate sedation or with the use of provided restraints (as agreed by patient, their next-of-kin or the treating doctor), then the scan should be discontinued until such time as this is possible.

Where patients are at risk of moving through the scan, care should be taken to ensure the following parameters are optimised:

- Rotation time
- Detector coverage

A "fast" protocol, in addition to a routine head protocol, is useful to allow simple adjustment from routine settings without the need to change multiple parameters at the time of the examination. Where a patient moves significantly through a scan, the scan should be discussed with a radiologist or medical specialist prior to being repeated as the images may hold sufficient information to answer the clinical question.

Additionally, all routine non-contrast scans should be reviewed by the CT radiographer in the first instance and by the radiologist if required, to ensure there is no obvious lesion or pathology visible that would indicate further imaging (with contrast) is necessary. Further to this, radiographers have a duty of care to escalate any unusual findings to a medical professional (MRPBA, 2020). This should be the reporting radiologist in the first instance or to the referrer where this is not possible. The specifics of this process will differ between jurisdictions and institutions and is beyond the scope of this text to define further.

CT HEAD PROTOCOL

Commonly Presenting/Significant Pathologies

Clinical indications for performing a CT head without contrast commonly include both traumatic and atraumatic aetiologies. Appearances of significant cranial pathologies are covered in Chapter 16. CT head acquisitions are likely to investigate clinical suspicion (or follow-up) of the following:

- Skull fracture
- Intracranial haemorrhage (extra-dural, sub-arachnoid, sub-dural or intraparenchymal/petechial)

- Cerebral infarction
- Investigation into organic cause for psychosis
- Tumour (primary or secondary metastases)
- Abscess
- Arteriovenous malformation (AVM)
- Hydrocephalus
- Hypoxic brain injury
- Diffuse axonal injury

Approaches to Imaging

Patient Positioning

For routine CT head scans, patients are positioned supine using the vendor-specified head cradle attachment. Note, scans can be performed with patient flat on the scan couch when there is significant risk of spinal trauma (for example). However, for most scanners, this is less preferred as it increases the attenuation profile of the scanogram image unnecessarily, potentially leading to increased radiation dose or unwanted image noise. The patient should be positioned so that the area of interest is central to the isocentre of the gantry.

The patient should be positioned to minimise the irradiation of the lens of the eye. A radiolucent cushion may be placed behind the patient's head to allow some flexion of the neck, so the chin is tucked down. Where gantry angulation is possible, this should be utilised as required to further reduce the radiation dose to the patient.

For most patients, the preferred movement is to position the patient so that the table movement is out of the scanner; so with the patient positioned in the head cradle, the table movement will be in the caudocranial direction.

Planning

There are two approaches when planning and reformatting axial images. The orbito-meatal baseline is the historically more preferred reformation plane (Yeoman et al., 1992). This baseline emerged historically when scans were performed as axial type scan and translate (or "step and shoot") mode scans. The purpose of this baseline was to reduce radiation dose the lens of the eye and provided a reduction in beam hardening caused by the base of skull. More recently, with the technological improvements associated with larger generator capacity as well as the capability to scan in helical mode, sites more commonly produce images utilising the tuberculum sellae occipital protuberance line. The tuberculum sellae occipital protuberance line is similar to that used in MRI and makes radiological comparison between modalities simpler (Kim et al., 2009). However, both methods are still employed and it is largely a matter of preference at each site.

Scanners will differ significantly on the exposure settings required for head scans as this will depend on a number of factors, such as the generator capacity, the number of detector rows and whether or not tube current modulation exposure control settings are utilised. A 120 kV station will routinely be set by most vendors to mitigate beam hardening in the posterior fossa while allowing for sufficient detail in the images. The tube current and exposure time are heavily dependent on the helical pitch factors.

Window level/centre should be set at approximately 35–45 HU to allow for optimal visualisation of the brain parenchyma. The window width will normally be very narrow 70–100 HU to allow for differentiation between the grey–white matter and to maximise low contrast conspicuity to visualise space occupying lesions, etc.

A second reconstruction is commonly created to review bony anatomy in cases where this is relevant. This should be produced with a sharp reconstruction algorithm and will normally have a window level/centre between about 200 and 400 to centre on bony anatomy, with a broad window width of 2,000–4,000. This is particularly relevant for any patient imaged post -trauma.

Volume rendered images are typically not performed routinely; however, they do provide useful information display for patients with complex fractures or craniosyndesmosis.

Protocol Considerations

Depending on the clinical indications and findings from the initial non-contrast images, an acquisition post IV contrast may be indicated. The specifics of when IV contrast should be used is a matter of departmental protocol and policy; however, it is routine for contrast to be administered where the patient has a known primary malignancy and there is reasonable suspicion that it might have metastasised to the brain, or where a primary malignancy is being investigated further – although more often MRI may be considered at larger clinics. See Chapter 4 for more information on patient preparation for IV contrast usage.

Other occasions where contrast may be administered frequently include the following:

- New space occupying lesion – malignancy vs abscess or other
- High suspicion of AVM
- Venous sinus thrombosis

Where acute ischaemic events are highly suspected, contrast should also be considered, but should be performed as an angiographic and/or perfusion imaging protocol.

Contrast Phase and Timing

IV contrast phase and timing for routine head scans is performed at low rates and may be administered by hand. Fifty millilitre of non-ionic, low- or iso-osmolar iodinated contrast should be used. Although not critical, optimal timing may be as late as 5 minutes following the administration of contrast to allow take up of contrast through the blood brain barrier by lesion of interest (Hou et al., 2014) (Table 12.1).

TABLE 12.1
CT Head Example Protocol

Patient position	Head first, supine
Topogram	Caudocranial, centre on chin Lateral image only
Scan region	PreMonitoring: none Acquisition: include foramen magnum to skull vertex
Contrast	Generally only required for cases with known or highly suspected oncological conditions. Fifty millilitre low or iso-osmolar non-ionic intravenous contrast (hand injection or slow flow rate – recommend approx. 5-minute delay for optimal enhancement)
Breath hold	N/A
Recons	Axial MPRs Coronal MPRs Sagittal MPRs VRT useful for craniosyndesmosis or skull fracture cases

CT SINUSES PROTOCOL

Commonly Presenting/Significant Pathologies

Clinical indications for sinus scans are numerous but are usually related to obstructive infections within the paranasal sinuses which may be either bacterial, viral or fungal aetiology. Polyps are also frequently seen. Difficult dental extraction may lead to infection particularly in the maxillary sinus.

Approaches to Imaging

Patient Positioning

Similar to head scans, patients should be positioned supine in the head cradle. The patient's head should be placed in a neutral position with the hard palate perpendicular with the floor (parallel to the scan plane).

Planning

Planning of a sinuses scan should ensure the range that includes the entirety of the maxillofacial sinuses, from inferior to the maxillary sinus to superior to the frontal sinus. The display field of view (FoV) should include the extent of the maxillary sinuses laterally and ensure the sphenoethmoid sinuses are fully contained posteriorly within the field of view. For some patients, the frontal sinuses can extend significantly superiorly. The topogram should be carefully examined to ensure the acquisition includes the superior aspect of these sinuses.

TABLE 12.2
CT Sinuses Example Protocol

Patient position	Head first, supine
Topogram	Lateral only Caudocranial, centre on chin
Scan region	PreMonitoring: None Acquisition: include dentition immediately below maxillary antra to above frontal sinuses
Contrast	Generally not required, may be indicated for infective processes (e.g. abscess) Fifty millilitre low or iso-osmolar non-ionic contrast (hand injection or slow flow rate – recommend approx. 5-minute delay for optimal enhancement)
Breath hold	Quiet respiration
Recons	Axial MPRs Coronal MPRs Sagittal MPRs Further axial MPR 1.1 mm reconstruction with soft tissue may be created for Stealth protocol.

Protocol Considerations

Reformations are commonly performed in all 3 orthogonal planes with relatively thin slice thickness and intervals, with attention paid to ensure lateral symmetry of anatomy in axial and coronal planes.

Ear, nose and throat (ENT) surgeons may request imaging prior to surgery to be used in conjunction with a stealth surgical guidance protocol. In this case, a second display FoV should be reconstructed using contiguous 1mm slice thickness with a large field of view that includes the ears and tips of the nose and skin margin to the vertex.

IV contrast is rarely required in routine scans of the sinuses. Where contrast is used, to delineate the site of infection, consideration should be given to whether a face and orbits protocol may be more valuable (for example, in the context of periorbital cellulitis) as good soft tissue definition will be more relevant for these clinical situations (Table 12.2).

CT ORBITS/FACE PROTOCOL

Commonly Presenting/Significant Pathologies

Scans of the facial bones and sinuses are usually considered for one of the following general indications:

- Malignancy
- Infection
- Trauma

The former indications will generally require IV contrast to be administered, whereas the latter will not.

Approaches to Imaging

Patient Positioning

The patient should be positioned supine, head first and will have arms resting by side. Care should be taken to remove all dense materials capable of significant artefacts (including earrings, nose rings, necklaces, hearing aids, etc.).

Planning

Topograms/Scanograms should be performed to include from the sternal notch to the vertex of the skull. In some departments, both lateral and anteroposterior topograms will be performed to plan these acquisitions.

A helical scan should be determined based on the type of examination required. That is, for facial bones in the case of trauma, this will usually include the entire mandible through to the frontal sinuses. For scans of the face for infective causes, a scan will normally be performed from below the maxillary antra to above the frontal sinuses. The field of view should be similar including paranasal sinuses and temporomandibular joints as well as superior airways. Less commonly, scans of the orbital region only are required. These scans will only require a limited range to include the bony orbits themselves.

Protocol Considerations

IV contrast will be required for patients with infective causes or neoplasm. A slow flow rate and small bolus is required in this case to define vascularity structures and surrounding tissues.

Where soft tissue contrast is not required, e.g. in the case of trauma for facial bones, a lower tube current can be used to reduce dose. This is due to the attenuation difference between the air filled sinus cavity and the bony structures (Table 12.3).

TABLE 12.3
CT Face Example Protocol

Patient position	Head first, supine
Topogram	Caudocranial, centre on sternal notch
	AP and lateral may be performed
Scan region	PreMonitoring: none
	Acquisition: include below mastoid air cells to include frontal sinuses
Contrast	Indicated for malignant or infective processes
	Fifty millilitre low or iso-osmolar non-ionic intravenous contrast (hand injection or slow flow rate)
Breath hold	Quiet respiration
Recons	Axial MPRs (thin slices)
	Coronal MPRs (thin slices)

CT PETROUS BONE (INTERNAL AUDITORY MEATUS) PROTOCOL

CT of the petrous bones and internal auditory meatii (IAMs) is a commonly performed protocol in most institutions and is particularly important for ENT surgeons. Whilst it does not provide the same level of detail of the soft tissue as MRI, it is valuable in defining the intricate bony details of anatomy in the region.

COMMONLY PRESENTING/SIGNIFICANT PATHOLOGIES

Common clinical indications for CT petrous bones can be broadly classified as infective (such as chronic otitis media, cholesterol granulomas or cholesteatoma), neoplastic (including basal and squamous cell carcinoma, Schwannoma, acoustic neuroma or meningioma) or traumatic (such as dehiscence or base of skull fracture complications).

Additional consideration should be given to the malignancy group to ensure that the correct imaging modality is being used. Many neoplastic pathologies present as isodense with the surrounding tissue in non-contrast CT. Therefore, MR is commonly the preferred modality for this group and CT may be requested in conjunction with an MRI to facilitate detailed visualisation of the bony anatomy. Where MRI is unavailable, post IV contrast imaging is important to visualise neoplasms.

APPROACHES TO IMAGING

Patient Positioning

Patients should be positioned supine and in the specified head cradle for examination of the petrous bones and IAMs. Patients should maintain a neutral head position with hard palate approximately perpendicular to the floor (parallel to the scan plane).

Planning

Scanogram should include from the chin to the vertex of skull.

Helical scans should include from below the mastoid air cells to above the petrous ridges.

Protocol Considerations

For evaluation of infectious and inflammatory conditions of the inner ear or malignant tumours, IV contrast may be warranted. However, contrast is no longer routinely used due to the availability of MRI. This should still be considered at sites without MRI or where the patient has a contraindication to MRI.

Where the request is concerning for dehiscence of the semicircular canals, additional oblique reformats should be considered in the planes of Stenver and Porschl (Barton F. Branstetter et al., 2006) (Table 12.4).

TABLE 12.4
CT Petrous Bones Example Protocol

Patient position	Head first, supine
Topogram	Caudocranial, centre on chin Lateral only
Scan region	PreMonitoring: None Acquisition: include below mastoid air cells to above petrous ridges
Contrast	Generally not required, may be indicated for malignant processes Fifty millilitre low or iso-osmolar non-ionic contrast (hand injection or slow flow rate)
Breath hold	Quiet respiration
Recons	Axial MPRs (thin slices) Coronal MPRs (thin slices) NOTE: further reformats may be included in plane of Porschl/Stenver where superior semi-circular canal dehiscence is suspected

CT HEAD ANGIOGRAM (CIRCLE OF WILLIS) PROTOCOL

Commonly Presenting/Significant Pathologies

Common clinical indications for CT Head angiograms include

- Berry aneurysm
- AVM or connective tissue disorder.

Approaches to Imaging

Patient Positioning

As with other scans of the head, patients should be positioned supine with some head tilt applied.

Planning

Scans should be performed from C1/2 to the vertex of the skull. It is important to ensure the basilar artery is included from the unification of the vertebral arteries.

The range and display field of view in modern CT scanning should include the entirety of the head. This will allow subsegmental branches to be well defined.

Bolus-tracking is frequently utilised for CTA of the cerebral arteries. A pre-monitoring slice may be positioned at the most inferior slice of the helical acquisition to determine flow through the internal carotid arteries. However, it can be challenging to identify these vessels with a ROI without contrast. Therefore, it is common to monitor the area visually, and for the radiographer, to trigger the acquisition when sufficient contrast is visible in the area. An alternative option is to place a pre-monitoring slice at the level of the aortic arch, however, this requires the scanner to move

TABLE 12.5
CTA Head Example Protocol

Patient position	Head first, supine
Topogram	Lateral
	Caudocranial, centre on chin
Scan region	PreMonitoring: place ROI in ICA at level of C1/2 vertebra
	Acquisition: include from C1/2 vertebra to vertex
Contrast	Pressure inject 50 mL low or iso-osmolar non-ionic contrast followed directly by a 40 mL saline.
	Flow rate: 5 mL/s
Breath hold	Quiet respiration
Recons	Axial slab MIPs (10 mm, 3 mm)
	Coronal slab MIPs (10 mm, 3 mm)
	VRT with bone removed or with transparent bone algorithm applied

the scan couch between the initiation of the threshold being reached and the acquisition, which may add a number of seconds to the delay. See Chapter 4 for IV contrast administration.

Protocol Considerations

Cranial angiograms will usually be performed in conjunction with/or following a non-contrast head scan. Head angiograms are often requested following a finding of sub arachnoid haemorrhage to assess the cause (Table 12.5).

REFERENCES

Barton, F. Branstetter, I., Harrigal, C., Escott, E. J. & Hirsch, B. E. 2006. Superior semicircular canal dehiscence: Oblique reformatted CT images for diagnosis. *Radiology*, 238, 938–942.

Hou, D., Qu, H., Zhang, X., Li, N., LIU, C. & Ma, X. 2014. Multi-slice computed tomography 5-minute delayed scan is superior to immediate scan after contrast media application in characterization of intracranial tuberculosis. *Medical Science Monitor: International Medical Journal of Experimental and Clinical Research*, 20, 1556–1562.

Kim, Y. I., Ahn, K. J., Chung, Y. A. & Kim, B. S. 2009. A new reference line for the brain CT: The tuberculum sellae-occipital protuberance line is parallel to the anterior/posterior commissure line. *AJNR American Journal of Neuroradiology*, 30, 1704–1708.

Medical Radiation Practice Board of Australia (MRPBA). 2020. Professional capabilities for medical radiation practice. Available from: https://www.medicalradiationpracticeboard.gov.au/registration/professional-capabilities.aspx.

Yeoman, L. J., Howarth, L., Britten, A., Cotterill, A. & Adam, E. J. 1992. Gantry angulation in brain CT: Dosage implications, effect on posterior fossa artifacts, and current international practice. *Radiology*, 184, 113–116.

Zarb, F., Rainford, L. & Mcentee, M. 2011. Frequency of CT examinations in malta. *Journal of Medical Imaging and Radiation Sciences*, 42, 4–9.

13 Imaging of the Neck

Debbie Starkey and Gordon Mander
Queensland University of Technology

Deb Watson
Sunshine Coast University Hospital

CONTENTS

INTRODUCTION

The neck is a complex region of anatomy, and therefore, there are a number of important considerations required when imaging the neck with CT.

CONSIDERATIONS

Care should be taken to determine whether a request for CT Neck is a request for soft tissue and/or airway or is actually a request for an assessment of the cervical spine. As the area covered in the scans is similar, the acquisition parameters and reconstructions are quite different and should therefore not be confused.

DOI: 10.1201/9781003132554-18

CT CERVICAL SPINE PROTOCOL

Commonly Presenting/Significant Pathologies

- Trauma
- Musculoskeletal problems (e.g. disc protrusion, severe osteoarthritis)

The latter indication is usually only considered where MRI is unavailable or in cases prior to surgery/intervention as requested by neurology and orthopaedics specialists. These protocols will be considered in the relevant chapters.

CT SOFT TISSUE NECK PROTOCOL

Commonly Presenting/Significant Pathologies

Common indications for CT scan of the neck include

- Survey of the neck anatomy
- Infection
- Malignancy

Approaches to Imaging

Patient Positioning

Patients should be positioned supine headfirst with their head in a neutral/comfortable position to allow breathing. Care should be taken to ensure patient is aligned to the midline of the table and the patient's head is not angled to the left or right. The patients' arms should be positioned down by their side to avoid shoulders from tensing and increasing beam attenuation. Patients may benefit from supporting their arms by clasping hands as this will reduce shoulder movement as patients move through the gantry.

Planning

The neck scan will normally consist of a single-time post-intravenous contrast phase from the external auditory meatii to below the arch of aorta.

Protocol Considerations

Reconstructions are created using a soft tissue algorithm and window, with multiplanar reformats (MPRs) created in all three orthogonal planes. Care should be taken to ensure the lateral areas of the neck are reconstructed comparably to allow clear interpretation of structures and more easily determine any space occupying lesion.

Intravenous contrast is commonly used in acquisition scans of the neck. Where a salivary duct calculus is the concern, a non-contrast scan may be warranted. Also, a non-contrast scan should also be considered in the case of foreign body in the airway.

Acquisition following intravenous contrast administration may be timed as a single bolus at or around the 40–50 second mark to attempt to enhance both arteries

TABLE 13.1
CT Neck with Contrast Example Protocol

Patient position	Head first, supine
Topogram	AP and lateral
	Caudocranial, centre on midsternum
Scan region	PreMonitoring: place ROI in descending aorta immediately below aortic arch
	Acquisition: include from arch of aorta to the above petrous ridges
Contrast	Pressure inject 60 mL low or iso-osmolar non-ionic contrast
	Flow rate: 2.5 mL/s
Breath hold	Suspended inspiration, requested not to swallow
Recons	Axial MPRs
	Coronal MPRs
	Sagittal MPRs

and veins with contrast. Some sites utilise a dual-bolus approach, injecting a small amount of intravenous contrast, pausing and then a second bolus at higher flow rate to allow for more clarification of arterial and venous structures.

In the case of parathyroid adenoma and hyperplasia, prior to surgery, ENT may request a multiphase examination of the neck. This should include a pre-contrast scan followed by an arterial, venous and 2-minute washout delay (Malinzak et al., 2017). The range of these scans should be reduced to include the thyroid and surrounding anatomy only (i.e. including from the temporomandibular joint to the sternal notch in each phase).

Modern scanning protocols allow for various additional techniques when scanning. This includes vocalising or breathing during a functional (real-time) assessment of the larynx and laryngopharynx. Although some institutions perform "4DCT" scans of the neck or vocal folds regularly, these are still primarily used in research studies and have not been included in this text as a routine protocol. Note, although commonly requested as "4DCT" neck scans, multiphase scans of the neck should not be confused with this type of functional assessment (Table 13.1).

CT HEAD AND NECK ANGIOGRAM PROTOCOL

Commonly Presenting/Significant Pathologies

CT head and neck angiograms commonly assess

- Stenoses
- Dissection
- Aneurysm
- Definition of anatomy (e.g. prior to surgery)

Approaches to Imaging

Patient Positioning

Patients should be positioned supine, headfirst with their head in a neutral/comfortable position to allow free breathing. Arm should be positioned down by side to avoid shoulders from tensing and increasing beam attenuation. Where patients have a neglect due to stroke, restraint with table straps should be considered to keep patients comfortable and safe during couch movement.

Planning

Scans should be performed from below the aortic arch to the vertex of the skull. Where only the carotid vessels are of interest, the scan can be terminated at the petrous ridges; however, this is rarely the case in contemporary imaging requests.

Protocol Considerations

Images should be reconstructed using maximum intensity projections (MIPs) in the coronal plane to elucidate the carotid and vertebral arteries bilaterally.

Curved MPRs may also be performed to more effectively visualise pathology in each of the four major arteries of the neck. Volume rendered images may also assist in visualising the position and the effect of stenoses in the arteries.

Head neck angiograms may be performed independently or in combination with a brain perfusion scan (Table 13.2).

TABLE 13.2
Head and Neck Angiogram Example Protocol

Patient position	Head first, supine
Topogram	AP and lateral
	Caudocranial, centre on at midsternum
Scan region	PreMonitoring: place ROI in descending aorta immediately below aortic arch
	Acquisition: include from arch of aorta to vertex of skull
Contrast	Pressure inject 60–80 mL low or iso-osmolar non-ionic contrast followed by 40 mL of saline
	Flow rate: 4–6 mL/s
Breath hold	Suspended inspiration, requested not to swallow
Recons	Axial MIPs
	Coronal MIPs
	Sagittal MIPs
	VRT of the head and neck vessels with bone removed or semitransparent
	Curved multiplanar reformats – trace both left and right carotid and vertebral arteries of the neck from the aorta/subclavian artery

REFERENCE

Malinzak, M. D., Sosa, J. A. & Hoang, J. 2017. 4D-CT for detection of parathyroid adenomas and hyperplasia: State of the art imaging. *Current Radiology Reports*, 5, 8.

14 Imaging of Paediatric Patients

Debbie Starkey and Gordon Mander
Queensland University of Technology

Deb Watson
Sunshine Coast University Hospital

CONTENTS

DOI: 10.1201/9781003132554-19

INTRODUCTION

Paediatric patients propose unique challenges when performing computed tomography (CT) examinations, and it is important to remember that they are not just little adults. Most people instantly recognise size as the major difference between adults and children but many fail to recognise the anatomical, physiological and psychological differences. A successful paediatric CT examination requires attention to not only dose optimisation but also patient preparation, environment and justification. All of these elements are pivotal in obtaining a successful paediatric CT examination.

Paediatric patients of varying ages require a different approach in imaging. But first how do we define what is a paediatric patient?

WHAT IS A PAEDIATRIC PATIENT?

The Macquarie dictionary defines Paediatrics as "the study and treatment of the diseases of children" (Macquarie Dictionary 2021, curriculum entry).

However, within the healthcare context, the definition of what is a child is less clear with many variations on access to Paediatric health services and the age of consent. For the purpose of this publication, Paediatrics or children will refer to a person less than 17 years of age.

PAEDIATRIC PATIENTS IN THE MEDICAL IMAGING DEPARTMENT

When undertaking medical imaging procedures, children often do not understand what is happening or why it is happening, especially why it is happening to them. This inherently introduces a feeling of being scared and intimidated. These emotions are often overwhelming for children and can produce a wide range of reactions from quiet compliance to a full meltdown. Children also have a short attention span so examinations, such as a CT scan, that take a little longer and are more complex to explain, can propose more of a challenge.

When dealing with all children, communication is a critical concept and there are some fundamental principles that work across different age groups.

The most important thing to remember when communicating is to always involve the child. When speaking to the family and explaining the procedure, talk to the child and involve them in all of your explanations. If you can engage the child and make them happy, you are already on the way to a successful CT examination. A happy child means happy parents. Explanations need to be thorough but simple. Continue to talk with them through every step of the procedure as the CT scan is being performed.

Be careful of your choice of language, children take things literally. A phrase as simple as "Would you like to lay on the bed now?" can lead to non-compliance. Any hesitant or scared child will say "no, I don't want to lie on the bed". Instead use words like, "It is time to lay on the bed now". By changing your words, you are not giving them a choice in laying on the bed.

However, it is very important to give children choices when having a CT scan. This empowers the child, and the procedure changes from something that is happening to them to something they are a part of. These choices can be very small, such as what reward they get at the end or what toy they hold while having the CT scan.

Always use positive language. When talking about the administration of intravenous (IV) contrast, never mention the word injection. Children and often adolescents associate this word with a needle and pain. Instead of the word injection, depending on the age group, you could use the words:

"I am going to start the magic medicine now"
Or
"I am going to start the dye now".

Always warn the child that they might feel warm and that is ok.

Always keep reassuring the child during the procedure.

Children of different ages require a different approach to achieve a successful CT scan. A good understanding of the developmental stages of children will help you prepare for CT scanning of paediatric patients. However, all children require their own individual assessment to obtain optimum results.

As a general approach, they can be divided into the following different stages of development or age groups:

- Neonate–Infants (0–6 months);
- Toddler–Preschool (6 months–4 years);
- Young Children and Pre-teens (5–12 years);
- Adolescents (13–16 years).

NEONATE–INFANTS (0–6 MONTHS)

The term infant is derived from the Latin word infans which means "speechless" (Encylopedia.com 2021, Mijolla-Mellor). This is the only age group that cannot verbally communicate with you and all your verbal communication must be with the parents or carers. However, your non-verbal communication and preparation are key as infants are generally aware of the world around them.

Feed and Wrap Technique

For this age group, CT scans are best performed using the feed and wrap technique (unless breath holds are required). The aim of the feed and wrap is to settle the baby during a feed and then to place them in a neonate cradle for the CT scan (Figure 14.1).

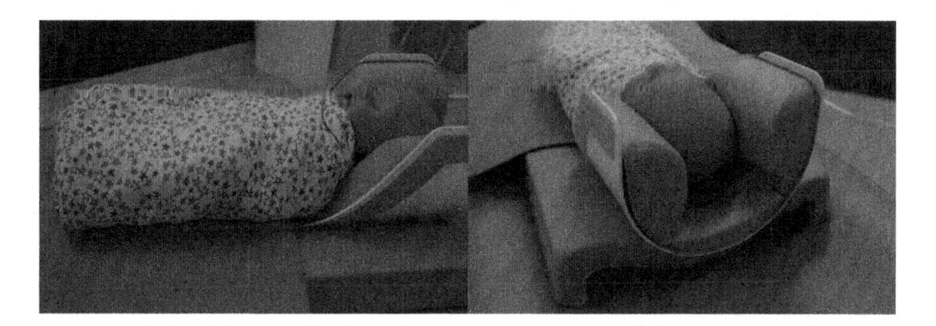

FIGURE 14.1 Preparation of CT scan.

If you have space in the Imaging department, it is best to bring the infant into the medical imaging department 30 minutes prior to the feed. Place the parent/carer in a quiet dark room to feed the infant and then settle the infant to sleep. The infant can then be swaddled and placed in the neonate cradle in a quiet, darkened CT room (Figure 14.2). A warm bunny rug is best to swaddle the baby.

When scanning neonates or infants, you need to be aware that any sudden noises, such as velcro, and movement may alarm them. Before entering the scan room, remove any name tags or keys that you may have on you as these may be a source of noise.

As the patient progresses towards 6 months of age, bright colours, textures and sounds are good distractions; and singing and familiar musical mobiles may comfort them. Neonates and infants respond well to touch so a comforting hand on them during the scan can help maintain cooperation.

If the patient is used to sucking on a dummy, they may be helpful in settling the child. However, dummies need to be used cautiously when scanning for CT of the head as the sucking action can cause motion artefact and disguise possible base of skull pathology.

General Anaesthesia may be used in the age group for studies requiring a breath hold.

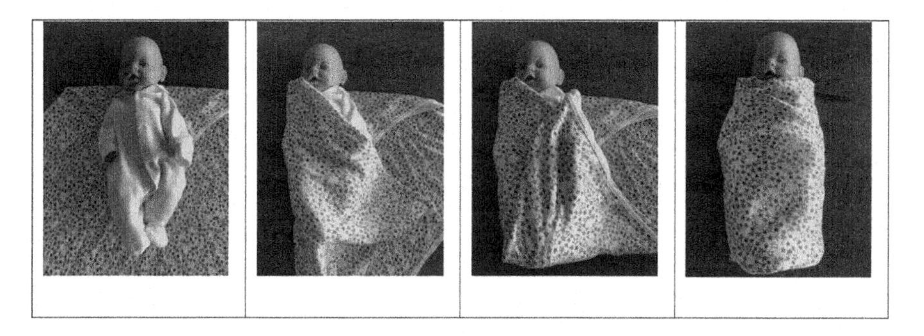

FIGURE 14.2 Feeding and wrapping technique.

TODDLER–PRESCHOOL (6 MONTHS TO 4 YEARS)

Toddlers and Preschool children have limited language and cognitive skills and are unable to understand abstract principles. Explaining a CT scan through audiovisual aids and picture books are very useful with this age group. There are many online videos and an app available to help parents prepare their child for a CT scan. Practice makes perfect, or so they say, so practicing lying still and holding your breath at home makes life so much easier when it comes to having the scan.

Toddlers and preschool children are prone to separation anxiety and will nearly always require a parent to stay in the room with them. They are also rather egocentric. It is often known as the ME, ME, ME and the WHY, WHY, WHY age.

They begin showing signs of independence by not always doing what is asked of them and often throw in a NO, NO, NO for good measure (Miller et al. 2021). Preschoolers and older infants think in terms of cause and effect and often think they are being punished for being naughty. For example, "I must have been bad to have to have this needle".

Preparation is key with this age group. Make sure there are no surprises. Tell the child everything you are about to do. Use positive language and try to avoid instilling fear. Keep the explanation simple. Take time to play with the child. Play is reassuring and familiar and can often relieve anxiety and stress. They learn about their environment through play and allow active participation. They like to know what things look, feel, smell and sound like. Walk around the scanner and show them what it looks like from behind. Kids have a huge imagination and unless they have seen what is behind there, it can be like the monster hiding in the wardrobe. Some kids relate to the idea of the CT scanner being a spaceship that goes up and down and has cool lights and sounds. Some children relate better to it being referred to as a giant donut or cookie.

Tell them it sounds like mum or dads washing machine at home and reassure them that the scanner will not touch them. They may want to watch mum, dad or their favourite toy go for a ride through the "donut" first.

Incentive works well for this age group. Keep choices simple. Make sure they understand they cannot choose whether to have the examination or not, but they can choose which sticker they get, for example:

Beware of delaying tactics with this age group.

Sedation may be used in this age group if scanning is required urgently and the patient is being uncooperative. General Anaesthesia may be required in this age group if breath holds are required. A seat belt/protective belt could be used to immobilize movement as children are unpredicable.

YOUNG CHILDREN AND PRE-TEENS (5–12 YEARS)

The level of maturity can vary significantly across this age group. School age children can also tend to suffer from separation anxiety and the younger children also still experience the ME, ME, ME stage. It is important to explain everything you are going to do. Speak to the child. Involve them in the discussions. Try and earn their trust as this usually results in cooperation.

Young children also benefit from play therapy like the toddler and preschool age group. Involve active participation. This age group tend to respond to TV, movies, books, video games and conversation. Talk about teachers, friends and favourite football teams and TV shows. Talking about things they are familiar with can be both comforting and a distraction from what is going on.

Beware of delaying tactics with this age group.

They usually cope better without sedation as they like to be in control.

ADOLESCENTS (13–16 YEARS)

Teenagers vary significantly in their development. Some you can treat similar to adults while others you will need to adapt your approach. It is important to adapt quickly in your communication with this age group.

With adolescents, self-image is often very important. They may be very self-conscious about their identity and appearance. Try and be sensitive about changing rooms and patient gowns. Speak directly to the teenager and give thorough explanations. Direct any questions to the teenager.

They may not want their parents with them. They are becoming fiercely independent and want to exercise their freedom.

Adolescents respond to conversation, music, video games and social media.

ENVIRONMENT

A child friendly and family-oriented environment is very important. Children and families attending health care facilities and imaging departments are often stressed and scared. This is not only due to the medical illness and treatment but also due to experiencing a foreign environment.

A child centred environment with play areas helps to ease the anxiety for the children and the families. The environment needs to cater for a wide range of age groups and any special needs of patients.

You also need to attend to the needs of the siblings who often spend a lot of time in health facilities whilst their brother or sister is getting treatment. A sticker or two for them for being patient and caring for their sick sibling is well deserved and always well received.

For a non-dedicated paediatric imaging department, it is handy to have a distraction box available. This could include things such as bubbles, vinyl stuffed toys, musical toys, books, puzzles or a tablet device. Everything in the box needs to comply with infection control standards.

Before bringing a paediatric patient into a CT scan room, it is vital that the room and the patient are completely prepared:

- Remove anything from the patient's clothes that may artefact.
- Have any immobilisation devices, such as the neonate cradle, ready for use.
- Have the correct table attachment ready to go.
- Ensure lead gowns are available for use if required.
- Have all distraction devices enabled and ready to use.

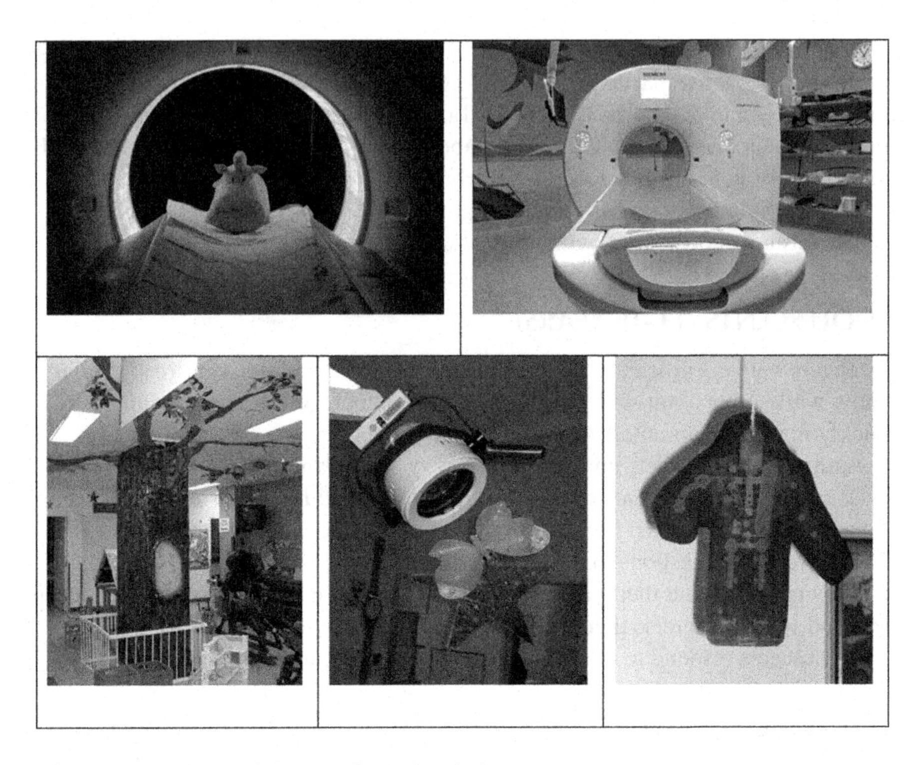

FIGURE 14.3 Distraction examples and techniques.

If the patient requires IV contrast, it is best to cannulate the patient away from the CT scan room. This reduces the association of pain with the actual CT scan and may help with future compliance. The use of a topical anaesthesia or tools, such as "Buzzy bee", which uses ice and vibration, may also be used to minimise the trauma of cannulation (Canbulat et al. 2015).

JUSTIFICATION

Children are more sensitive to radiation due to their rapidly dividing cells and longer life expectancy for any effects of radiation damage to appear (Nievelstein et al. 2010). This combined with the fact that CT is considered a higher radiation dose modality, it is vital that all CT scans undertaken for paediatric patients have been through a thorough justification process. Justification means that the health risk of not having a CT scan outweighs the risk from the radiation exposure (Brenner and Hall 2007, RANZCR 2018, Brady et al. 2012).

When justifying a paediatric CT scan, the following questions must be asked:

- Can the result be achieved by other modalities that have lower ionising radiation dose such as Ultrasound (US), MRI or General Radiography?
- Is the result readily available from previous scans?

- Is a CT scan the appropriate modality/scan to answer the clinical question?
- Do I need to scan as many phases or the same range if it is a follow-up examination?

When undertaking justification, it is important to be as rigorous in justification for all examinations as if it is the patients first.

There are several clinical decision-making guidelines and tools available to help clinicians and radiologists in deciding if a scan is justified. Examples of these are the following:

- ACR appropriateness Criteria (American College of Radiologists 2020);
- CHALICE rules for Paediatric Head CT (Hacking et al. 2021);
- CATCH rules for Paediatric Head CT (RANZCR 2015a).

CONTRAST

IV Contrast

IV contrast is routinely required for paediatric CT just as it is for adults. A non-ionic, low osmolar agent of approximately 300 mg I/mL is most typically used. The standard dose calculation is 2 mL/kg; however, with lower kV capabilities of newer generation scanners, a standard dose of 1.5 mL/kg is possible for some clinical indications (Nievelstein et al. 2010).

When assessing suitability for administration of IV contrast in a paediatric patient, it is important that you are just as rigorous in checking the safety factors, such as renal failure and patients with diabetes who are prescribed metformin. Paediatric patients will most often not have an estimated glomerular filtration rate (eGFR) as part of their routine blood results. An eGFR calculator such as "Schwartz Pediatric Bedside eGFR" is able to be used to calculate an age- and size-related eGFR for patients up to 17 years of age, if required (Wong et al. 2012).

Paediatric patients have the same risk of extravasation as adult patients (Amaral et al. 2006). The difference is that children often struggle to communicate effectively during contrast administration. This may lead to a higher percentage of the volume of contrast being extravasated. The same treatment for extravasation of contrast should be used for paediatric patients as for adult patients (see Section 3).

Oral Contrast

Children have much smaller abdominal organs and lack the intra-abdominal fatty tissue of adults (Nievelstein et al. 2010). This makes the diagnosis of abdominal pathology more difficult for the radiologists. To assist, positive oral contrast is still used routinely in paediatric patients for abdominal imaging. The oral contrast agents may be either diluted iodinated or barium-based contrast agents. It may be administered orally or through a nasogastric tube and may be mixed with apple juice or flavoured cordial to improve the taste. As with adult patients, if you are imaging for a suspected bowel perforation, do not administer barium-based contrast agents.

TABLE 14.1
Example of an Oral Contrast Protocol

Age	90 Minutes Prior (mL)	60 Minutes Prior (mL)	30 Minutes Prior (mL)	Total Dose (mL)
0–6 months	40	40	40	120
6–12 months	60	60	60	180
1–3.5 years	80	80	80	240
3.5–6 years	120	120	120	360
6–10 years	150	150	150	450
>10 years	200	200	200	600

A sample paediatric oral contrast protocol for diluted iodinated contrast can be seen in Table 14.1.

If a young patient is required to have a General Anesthetic for their abdominal CT scan, the normal oral contrast regime is not compatible with fasting requirements for the anaesthetic. For these cases, a compromise is often used and is negotiated with the local anaesthetic team. An example is where barium-based contrast is administered as a total bolus up to 2 hours prior to the CT scan. Barium-based contrast is used as iodinated oral contrast agents are a known bowel irritant often causing the contrast to transit swiftly through the gastrointestinal system. Barium, on the other hand, is not a bowel irritant. It coats the bowel and stays in the gastrointestinal system for longer. This permits the administration of the oral contrast agent much earlier for those patients requiring an anaesthetic.

There is some evidence of low-density oral contrast agents such as milk being used as an alternative oral contrast agent for paediatrics. The applications of this are limited to very specific pathologies, and positive oral contrast is still used as the oral contrast of choice by most paediatric radiologist (Nievelstein et al. 2010).

PROTOCOLS

Paediatric imaging requires adaptability in both protocols and technique. There are many variables with patient size, age and anatomy, as well as cannula size and placement. Every CT should be tailored to meet the individual requirements of each patient to answer the clinical question. Each of the following areas needs to be addressed in the planning of your paediatric CT.

Vascular Access and Contrast Timing

Vascular access can often be difficult to obtain in a paediatric patient, and cannulating a child is often incredibly traumatic. As a result, the size and location of the cannula may vary significantly. CT scans for paediatric patients are often performed with what would commonly be considered a sub-optimal cannula and re-cannulating is avoided where possible.

The size and location of the vascular access, patient size, heart rates and the smaller volume of circulation will all impact your scan timing. A one size fits all approach does not work.

There are several different techniques used to time contrast on children's CT scans. When using bolus tracking, it is important not to start the monitoring scans too early, or in fact, too late. For arterial bolus tracking, a good starting point is the patient's age. For example, if the patient is 5, start your bolus tracking scans at 5 seconds. If your patient is 10, start your bolus tracking at 10 seconds. The minimum delay for this technique is 3 seconds, as there is always a small amount of time taken for the contrast to be administered and travel to the mediastinum. The maximum delay used for this technique is 15 seconds. If the cannula is in the foot, a slightly longer delay may need to be considered, and if there is a central access device, such as a Peripherally Inserted Central Catheter, then a shorter delay should be considered.

Test bolus can also be used to time contrast for paediatric CT scans; however, for the very young children, you may be limited by the total volume of contrast you are able to administer (Nievelstein 2010).

The flow rates for contrast administration in paediatrics are limited by the cannula size, the same as for adult scanning. Table 14.2, Injection flow rates based on cannula size is an example of recommended flow rates.

Scan Speed

Children have short attention spans and can be unpredictable. The faster you can obtain the scan, the more likely you are to have a successful scan free from motion artefact. To achieve this, there are three options to consider:

1. Utilise the fastest rotation time possible.
2. Use the widest detector coverage possible (taking into consideration the patient size and area of interest).
3. Use higher pitch values, preferably greater than 1.

Whilst all of these will make your scan acquisition faster, changing any or all of these will have implications for image quality. It is important to understand how your scanner works and to understand what effect any protocol changes will have on both image quality and radiation dose (see Section 1).

TABLE 14.2
Injection Flow Rates Based on Cannula Size

Cannula Size	Maximum Injection Rate (mL/s)
20 gauge (Yellow)	1
22 gauge (Blue)	2.5
18 gauge (Pink)	4
16 gauge (Green)	6
14 gauge (Grey)	6

Scan Direction

For many patients, the act of the CT table driving into the gantry is terrifying. This is particularly the case for children. To help overcome this fear, take the opportunity to plan your scan so that the patient is positioned feet first into the gantry wherever possible. This way you can keep eye contact as you drive them into the scanner and provide positive reinforcement that they are ok. Programming the topogram so that the patient travels out of the gantry is another valuable tool. It is far less intimidating coming out of the gantry then going in.

Dose Optimisation

The key to dose optimisation is a clear understanding of all the technical parameters and how they interact. When optimising protocols, it is important to consider the ALARA principle in keeping radiation dose, "As Low As Reasonably Achievable", whilst maintaining appropriate image quality for each specific clinical investigation (Nievelstein et al. 2010, RANZCR 2018). The radiation dose selected should be relevant to the patient size and the body area being examined.

When reviewing paediatric CT examinations, radiologists typically accept more noise in the images than for adult CT scans. In paediatric specialist centres, with specialist trained Paediatric radiologists, the level of noise accepted in the CT images is often higher than that found in other medical imaging practices. It is important to work closely with the radiologists and physicists in your department to optimise the appropriate level of noise for an acceptable radiation dose.

This chapter will not address in detail the specifics of dose optimisation. We will however discuss broadly the considerations for paediatric CT using the principles discussed in Chapter 4.

When optimising radiation dose for a paediatric CT, the following elements of the examination need to be considered: the topogram, bolus tracking or test bolus scans, the scan acquisition and post-processing.

Topogram

It is important that the radiation dose is optimised for the topogram as it may represent a greater percentage of the total overall dose for paediatric patients than for adults. It is recommended that the kV should be at the lowest possible setting. However, you need to be aware of how your particular scanner uses the topogram for CT dose modulation as there may be some restrictions depending on the technology/vendor you are using. The topogram length should be minimised to the area of clinical concern.

Bolus Tracking or Test Bolus

Bolus tracking/test bolus, when not optimised, has the potential to significantly contribute to the overall patient dose, and in some cases, the radiation dose may be higher than the acquisition dose. This is because the current technology generally does not have dose modulation capability for bolus tracking or test bolus scans. They require individual manipulation of the kV and mA based on patient size.

Contrast timing also plays a role in the optimisation of the bolus tracking/test bolus. Starting your bolus tracking/test bolus scans too early results in additional scans acquired to time the bolus correctly, thus increasing the radiation dose. Both of these factors are enhanced in paediatric imaging with significant change in patient sizes and contrast timing. Thus, bolus tracking and test bolus require heightened attention when scanning paediatric patients.

Scan Acquisition

It is important to tailor your scan acquisition to the patient size. This includes not only the kV and mA but also the scan length and the detector collimation.

With the introduction of CT Automatic Exposure Control (CT AEC), the voltage and tube current adjust to the patient size and thickness, with respect to a programmed acceptable level of noise. CT AEC is an excellent resource to optimise radiation dose, however, oversight checking the proposed parameters and DLP is required before acquisition. For those scans where CT AEC is not available, reducing the kV and mA based on patient size is crucial to dose optimisation. kV ranges significantly in modern generations of CT scanners, from 70 to 150 kV. Adjusting your kV appropriate to patient size is critical in dose optimisation. Reduction in mA is also a crucial factor in reducing patient dose. This dose reduction is particularly achievable in areas of low attenuation, such as the chest, where a large reduction of mA can be achieved without a significant loss of image quality. In areas of low contrast attenuation, such as the abdomen, noise is a limiting factor when reducing mA.

The scan range should be customised individually for each examination to answer the specific clinical question for that patient.

The detector collimation should also be tailored to the area of interest and to answer the clinical question. Whilst a wide detector collimation is recommended for a faster scan, a balance is required between a faster scan, z-axis resolution, the noise level and radiation dose. If your detector collimation is wider than area required, this is known as overscanning, this will increase radiation dose without any contribution to patient care. This is more critical in paediatrics as the scan lengths are often shorter (Nievelstein 2010).

When performing scans that traditionally require multiple phases, liaising with the radiologist can help minimise the number of acquisitions. Ask the question, can you adapt the technique and use a dual bolus technique instead?

If the patient moves significantly throughout a scan, the scan should be shown and discussed with a radiologist prior to being repeated as the images may hold sufficient information to answer the clinical question.

Understanding the principles behind the choices in the dose optimisation procedure will help improve the decision-making process.

Patient Positioning

Positioning the patient correctly in the centre of the gantry is important for two reasons:

1. CT AEC
2. Bowtie filters

As discussed in Section 2, it is important to ensure the patient is centred at the correct height in the gantry to avoid over or under exposure (Barreto et al. 2019, Habibzadeh 2011).

It is also important to ensure the patient is centred with the mid-sagittal plane directly in the centre of the gantry. This is to ensure not only the correct exposure with the CT AEC but also the correct use of the bowtie filter. As paediatric patients are smaller, it is easier for them to lie off centre on the bed. Bow tie filters are designed to even the exposure at the periphery of the patient. If the patient is not in the centre of the gantry, then this may lead to increased and uneven exposure to the patient.

Shielding

The use of Bismuth Shielding is no longer recommended as there are alternate techniques that produce the same dose reduction at a similar or improved image quality. This is supported by the 2017 statement from the American Association of Physicist's in Medicine (AAPM 2017).

Reconstruction

Paediatric CT scans are generally produced with a greater level of noise. The noise in a CT image can always be reduced by using a smoother algorithm/reconstruction kernel and thicker reconstruction slices. This may seem a logical way to help reduce noise in a lower dose CT acquisition. However, you are limited by the size of the anatomy and potential pathology in paediatric imaging. Ensure your reconstruction slice thicknesses are tailored to the size of the patient and the particular anatomic area.

Choosing the appropriate algorithm for the clinical question is critical. Some vendors offer paediatric specific algorithms due to the anatomical differences between paediatrics and adults. This is particularly the case for brain examinations where the myelination process continues after the patient is born. This means there is less grey/white differentiation and a focused algorithm/kernel is required. There may also be specific torso algorithms to improve the contrast as paediatrics have less visceral fat.

Before you start scanning paediatric patients, it is important to know your particular CT scanner and how it works. Be aware of any changes to protocols and the resulting dose/image quality implications.

The following are a guideline for the most commonly performed paediatric examinations.

HEAD AND NECK IMAGING

CT Head

CT head is the most commonly performed paediatric CT examination. It is usually performed as a non-contrast examination, with any requirement for post contrast CT head imaging preferred to be examined using MRI. However, in regions with decreased or no access to MRI, post contrast head examinations may also be performed.

The paediatric skull changes significantly as the child grows with rapid development from birth to 6 or 7 years of age. The most significant growth occurs in the first 2 years until the fontanelles close and most of the adult features are present. At 7 years of age, all of the adult features of the skull are fully formed. After 7 years of age, the growth slows down with a small growth spurt again in the teens. The skull continues to grow and change throughout life, but most of the growth has occurred by the early 20s (Standring 2016).

As a result, the radiation dose required for a head CT will change significantly from birth then plateau from seven until the teenager years.

As the skull is rapidly developing, so too is the white matter. The myelination process undergoes a significant growth in the first 2 years then slows and continues into adulthood (Timmler and Simons 2019). Thus, when scanning a neonate, the head scan appears very different to an adult CT, with greatly reduced grey–white differentiation, as can be seen in the axial acquisitions (Figure 14.4). As a result, there is decreased level of contrast in the brain, and lower image noise levels are required. This is a limiting factor in reducing radiation dose for this cohort.

Non-contrast head scans for paediatric patients are often classified into two different protocols: a standard non-contrast head and a low dose non-contrast head protocol.

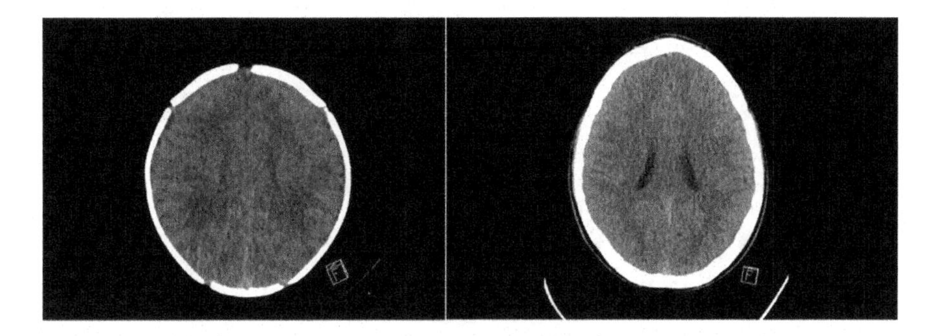

FIGURE 14.4 Neonate axial (a) and adult axial images (b).

Non-Contrast CT Head Protocol

Commonly Presenting/Significant Pathologies

The two most common indications for undertaking a non-contrast CT head in a paediatric patient are trauma and investigating a clinical suspicion of an atraumatic intracranial haemorrhage. These include

- ruptured arterio-venous malformation,
- subarachnoid haemorrhage,
- subdural haemorrhage,
- extradural haemorrhage,
- intracerebral haemorrhage,
- diffuse axonal injury and
- skull fracture.

CT is the preferred modality over MR for these clinical suspicions due to the ability to its availability, speed and accuracy, enabling the expedition of treatment options.

Pre-Acquisition

Patient Positioning

Patient is positioned head first, supine wherever possible.

Neonates and infants should be swaddled and placed supine in the neonate cradle (Figure 14.5).

Toddlers and preschool patients should be placed supine using the head cradle attachment with cushions to pad either side of the head. An alternative if they will not settle in the head cradle is to use a hollowed-out head cushion on tabletop. They often find this more comfortable and settle easier, however, it may increase the radiation dose slightly.

School age and above should be laying supine head first with head in the head cradle table attachment.

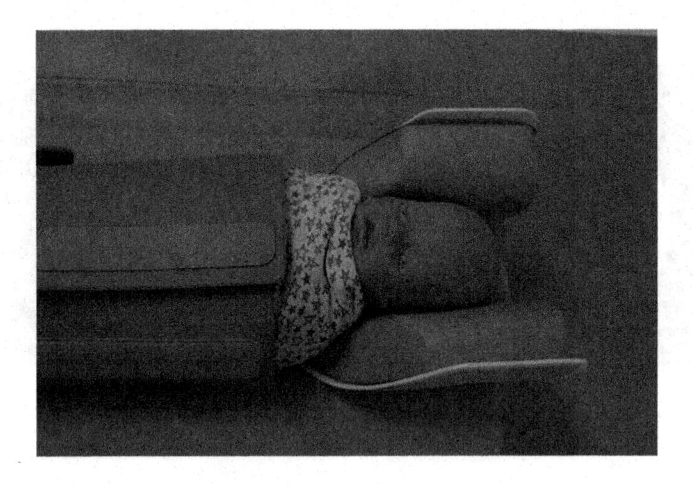

FIGURE 14.5 Example of swaddling in CT.

Any patient with suspected spinal injury should be imaged flat directly on the table top maintaining spinal precautions.

The patient should be in the centre of the gantry with the mid-sagittal plane perpendicular to the scan plane. The orbito-meatal line should be parallel to the scan plane to reduce radiation to the orbits and to reduce the overall scan length. Using gantry angulation, tilting head cradle attachments or positioning cushions will help you achieve this.

If the patient is uncooperative, you may try lying the patient on their side or use a head cushion instead of the head cradle attachment. It is best to adapt your technique to obtain the scan rather than persist with perfect positioning. Remember to change your patient position and angle of the topogram in the protocol if you are scanning the patient on their side.

Planning

A lateral topogram is acquired.

The scan range is from the base of skull to include the vertex.

Protocol Considerations

The kV selection will depend on the vendor and the type of CT scanner. A lower kV ranging from 80 to 100kV for neonates and toddlers should be sufficient. Once the patient is over 7 years old and the skull is fully formed and roughly 90% of adult size, an adult kV will be required.

A fast rotation time of 0.5 seconds is recommended particularly for the younger cohorts that are liable to move.

Image Reconstruction

Some vendors offer specific paediatric algorithm/kernels for neonate, infant and toddler brains due to different grey white differentiation. It is highly recommended to utilise these.

Axial, coronal and sagittal reformats are required in both a brain and bone algorithm. The brain reformats are usually 3 mm, while the bone reformats are 1.5–2 mm thick.

Window width is usually very narrow to give better contrast between the grey and white matter. This is usually somewhere around 60–90 HU.

The window level/centre is usually slightly lower than that of adults and is set at around 25–35 HU.

Soft tissue thin slice volumes are required for volume rendered reconstructions. These are performed for any patient that has a depressed skull fracture or a significant cranial injury.

Low Dose Non-Contrast CT Head

Commonly Presenting/Significant Pathologies

Some studies of the paediatric head can be performed at a reduced radiation dose and with a higher level of noise as the detail is not required to answer specific clinical questions.

These are

- craniosynostosis,
- ventricular peritoneal shunt patency and
- hydrocephalus.

The protocol may include both a reduced kV and mAs, or if using CT AEC, an indicator that you are willing to accept a higher level of noise.

Contrast CT Head Protocol

When to perform a contrast-enhanced CT head instead of an MR brain is a complex decision-making process that should involve a radiologist or senior clinician. There are many reasons why this may occur, including difficulty in accessing an MR service or the patient is not suitable for MR.

Always confirm with the radiologist prior to scanning if both a non-contrast and post contrast phase is required to minimise the radiation dose. The post contrast head CT scan should be performed in the same manner as a non-contrast head CT with IV iodinated contrast administered. The contrast should be delivered at 1.5–2 mL/kg up to a maximum of 50 mL. It can be administered by hand or pressure injected at 0.5–1 mL/s. Scan time should be approximately 3–5 minutes post injection depending on the age of the child.

Soft Tissue Neck

Commonly Presenting/Significant Pathologies

The most common presentation requiring a soft tissue neck in children is for infection. They are prone to three main types of infection. These are

- retrophayrngeal abscess,
- parapharyngeal abscess and
- peritonsillar abscess.

Soft tissue necks may also be imaged for malignancy. These, however, are almost exclusively examined in conjunction with scans of the torso. This will be addressed in the multi-region studies section.

Pre-Acquisition

Patient Positioning

The patient is positioned head first, supine. The head cradle attachment may be used or a hollowed cushion for head support may be used. As there may be swelling and/or a neck mass, it is important to ensure the patient is comfortable and the airway is patent. A general anaesthetic is commonly used for patients under 3 years of age for this examination as they find it difficult to lie flat.

The patient should be in the centre of the gantry with the mid-sagittal plane perpendicular to the table.

Planning

The topogram is performed in a AP view. The acquisition should include from the aortic arch to the above the petrous temporal bones.

Protocol Considerations

Before the acquisition, the patient should be asked to suspend respiration and requested to not swallow.

Contrast Phase and Timing

Contrast would be visualised in both the arterial and venous vessels, with contrast enhancement of any potential infection. To achieve this, there are generally two different methods of administration of IV contrast for a soft tissue neck examination.

The first method is a single injection of contrast, 1.5–2 mL/kg, with a maximum volume of 75 mL. This can be administered either by hand injection or at 1–1.5 mL/s using a pressure injector.

The second method is a dual bolus injection using a pressure injector with maximum bolus of 75 mL. The volume of contrast is split into two, and the first injection is completed and the injection paused, then the second injection is commenced so that it finishes immediately prior to the 40-second scan time. This ensures adequate contrast enhancement of the carotid and vertebral arteries, as well as the venous anatomy.

Image Reconstruction

The soft tissue neck CT should be reconstructed using a soft tissue algorithm/kernel in the axial, coronal and sagittal planes. The reconstruction slice thickness should be contiguous at 3 mm. A mediastinal window width and centre of approximately 300–350 W and 40–50 C is recommended.

Cervical Spine

CT of the cervical spine is primarily performed after trauma; however, injury in the paediatric cohort is uncommon (RANZCR 2015). The anatomy of the cervical spine in children differs significantly from adults and puts children at risk with different types of injuries. Children heads, particularly infants and those under 8 years of age, are larger relative to the body. This results in a higher centre of gravity and fulcrum. This cohort also has more horizontal facet joints and lax ligaments. These patients under 8 years of age are more likely to have injuries involving the cervical vertebrae 1–3. However, also due to these anatomic differences, the younger patients are more likely to result in a neurological injury rather than musculoskeletal (Baumann et al. 2015, Delaney et al. 2013).

After 8 years of age, the centre of gravity and fulcrum have moved to cervical vertebrae 5 and 6, the facet joints are more vertical in orientation and the ligaments are no longer lax. As the patients age increases, it progressively becomes more likely

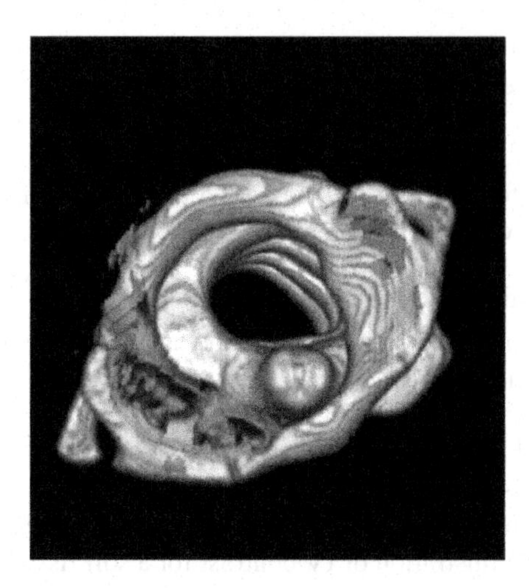

FIGURE 14.6 Subluxation.

that the patient will have a musculoskeletal injury, and the site of that injury is more likely to be in the lower c-spine (Baumann et al 2015, Delaney et al. 2013).

Another presentation seen in paediatrics is atlantoaxial rotatory subluxation or traumatic torticollis (Figure 14.6). This is where one vertebra displaces in relation to another vertebrae. The patient presents with ipsilateral rotation and contralateral tilt of the head. Subluxation occurs due to ligamental damage and may result from neglected torticollis or trauma (Powell et al. 2017, Crook and Eynon 2005).

Patient Positioning

The patient should be positioned head first supine on the table top. The cervical spine should be immobilised during transfer on and off the CT table and during the scan. Do not use sandbags to immobilise the cervical spine during acquisition. They will increase the radiation dose significantly.

Planning

A lateral topogram should be performed from the EAM to T2–3. The patient should be in the centre of the gantry, with the patient table height at the posterior margin of the EAM.

Scan ranges from base of skull to the inferior margin of T1.

If scanning for atlantoaxial rotatory subluxation, check with the radiologist if you can minimise your scan range to include only base of skull to C4.

Image Reconstruction

Images should be reconstructed in axial, coronal and sagittal planes in both bone and soft tissue algorithm/kernel. All reconstructions should be contiguous, with a slice thickness of 2 mm for bone and 3 mm for soft tissue images.

A volume rendered image should be reconstructed for patients with atlantoaxial rotatory subluxation.

TORSO IMAGING

Chest

CT is the cornerstone of imaging for airway disease and is one of the most commonly performed CT examinations for paediatric patients (Nievelstein 2010). The most common indications for CT chest are trauma, malignancy, infection and congenital abnormalities.

Breath holds are necessary particularly when assessing for interstitial lung disease. Coaching young children on holding their breath prior to an appointment can contribute to a successful examination. This may include practicing holding your breath "like going underwater" or "blowing out birthday candles" for expiratory acquisitions. Children 2 years and under will generally require a general anaesthetic for this examination.

Non-Contrast Chest

Commonly Presenting/Significant Pathologies

There are a number of indications for a non-contrast CT chest in paediatrics. They include

- langerhans cell histiocytosis;
- follow-up examinations for bone tumours, e.g. osteosarcoma and Ewing sarcoma;
- follow-up examinations for solid organ tumours, e.g. Wilms tumour and hepatoblastoma (This is for chest imaging only, when abdominal imaging is followed up using US or MR. If the chest is being imaged at the same time as a CT abdomen for solid organ tumours, contrast should be administered).

Chest with Contrast

Commonly Presenting/Significant Pathologies

This is the most common CT chest examination. There are a number of indications which include

- trauma,
- malignancy,
- infection,
- lung sequestration,
- tracheomalacia,
- congenital cystic adenomatoid malformation and
- recurrent pneumonia and collapse.

Pre-Acquisition

Patient Positioning

Patient should be supine feet first with arms resting above their head. They can hold on to a favourite teddy or toy above their head if desired.

Planning

An AP topogram is acquired from just above the shoulders to include the entire lung field.

Scan acquisition to include apices and just past the costophrenic angle inferiorly.

Low osmolar, IV contrast (if required) is administered via a pressure injector using 1 mL/kg up to a maximum of 50 mL. Bolus tracking is utilised with the pre-monitoring slice at the level of the descending aorta just below the aortic arch. The Region Of Interest, ROI, is placed in the descending aorta. The contrast timing will vary with age of the patient and the vascular access. Change the monitoring scan delay according to their age, e.g. 1 second per year up to 10 years of age. So, if the patient is 7, then the monitoring scan delay is 7 seconds.

Scan is performed on full inspiration.

Image Reconstruction

Thin slice, axial, coronal and sagittal should be reconstructed in both a soft tissue, mediastinal algorithm/kernel and a sharp lung algorithm/kernel. A bone algorithm/kernel may be used for the lung reconstructions with some vendors, as it is also a sharp algorithm/kernel. The soft tissue reconstructions should be contiguous at 3–5 mm thick, and the lung reconstructions should also be contiguous at 2 mm. A paediatric specific lung algorithm/kernel may be used for the younger cohort less than 2 years of age. This is due to the underdeveloped nature of the lungs in very young children.

Thick axial maximum intensity projection, or MIP, reconstructions should be produced for all oncology patients. These need to be adapted for the patient size. For patients under 5 years of age, MIPs should be reconstructed approximately 16 mm thick and 2 mm apart. For patients older than 5 years of age, the MIPs should be reconstructed approximately 20 mm thick and 2 mm apart. These MIP reconstructions are for the detection and monitoring of lung nodules.

HRCT (High-Resolution Computed Tomography) Chest

Commonly Presenting/Significant Pathologies

High-Resolution Computed Tomography (HRCT) is used primarily for interstitial lung disease. This includes

- cystic fibrosis,
- bronchiectasis,
- bronchiolitis and
- congenital lobar emphysema.

Patient Positioning

Patient should be supine feet first with arms resting above their head. They can hold on to a favourite teddy or toy above their head if desired.

Planning

An AP topogram is acquired from just above the shoulders to include the entire lung field.

A helical acquisition from the apices to include the costophrenic angle is performed as outlined in the chest CT section previously. HRCT inspiratory helical acquisition may be performed with or without contrast. Seek advice from the radiologist regarding their desired protocol. In addition to the helical acquisition, expiratory scans are required to detect air trapping which may indicate early peripheral airway obstruction. These are performed as axial sequential acquisition. An example is shown in Table 14.3.

The scan range for the expiratory imaging may be reduced to start at the carina and extend through the costophrenic angles. Confirm the expiratory scan range with your radiologist. For the younger children, you may need to turn the automatic voice off for the expiratory acquisition and manually trigger the scan following your breathing instructions.

Image Reconstruction

The expiratory images are reconstructed in both soft tissue and lung algorithms.

Portal Venous Phase Abdomen

Paediatric abdominal CT is becoming less common as US and MR have become the first avenues for imaging of the abdomen for most indications except trauma. It is still performed for reasons other than trauma, but they are becoming less frequent. Most often, the CT abdomen will be performed as part of a multi-region study for malignancy and major trauma. The abdomen may be imaged on its own for trauma when mechanism of injury is a direct trauma to the abdomen only, e.g. direct blunt trauma such as a bicycle handlebar.

Commonly Presenting/Significant Pathologies

The most common indications for a CT abdomen include

- malignancy,
- trauma and
- infection.

TABLE 14.3
Example of Expiratory HRCT Protocol

Patient age	Patient ≤ 4 years of age	Patient > 4 years of age
Scan interval	1 mm slices at 10 mm intervals	1 mm slices at 20 mm intervals

Patient Positioning

Patient should be supine feet first with arms resting above their head. They can hold on to a favourite teddy or toy above their head if desired.

Planning

Positive oral contrast is used routinely for malignancy in abdominal CT. In the interest of expediting the scan, it is generally not administered in trauma patients. However, some radiologists may request positive oral contrast for right upper quadrant trauma to better visualise the duodenum and pancreas.

An AP topogram is acquired from above the diaphragm (nipple level) to the inferior margin of the symphysis pubis.

The scan acquisition is from the top of the dome of the diaphragm to the inferior margin of the symphysis pubis.

Contrast Phase and Timing

Trauma:

For all abdominal trauma, a small volume of low osmolar, IV contrast is given to the patient approximately 5 minutes prior to the CT acquisition. This IV contrast should be 5 mL for a patient under 45 kg or 10 mL for a patient over 45 kg. This can be delivered as a hand injection, generally prior to the topogram. This is to highlight the renal pelvis identifying any potential renal injury that might result in a urinoma. Giving the small volume of contrast prior to the acquisition minimises the potential radiation exposure of a delayed acquisition.

For the main acquisition, low osmolar, IV contrast is administered as a bolus via a pressure injector. Contrast is administered at 1.5–2 mL/kg up to a total of 100 mL. For trauma CT, an arterial and portal venous phase acquisition is often desired to visualise the arterial vasculature and the solid organ perfusion. This increases the radiation dose to patient twofold. To reduce the radiation dose, a dual bolus technique may be used to allow a single acquisition. Two-thirds of the total volume is injected for the portal venous phase, then the injection is paused. The final third of the injection is administered to provide contrast enhancement in the arterial vasculature. The total injection duration should be 45 seconds for patients under 10 years of age and 70 seconds for patients 10 years of age and over.

For example: A patient weighs 30 kg and is less than 10 years. The total volume is at 2 mL/kg = 60 mL contrast. The patient has a 22 g cannula permitting an injection rate of 2.5 mL/s. The following calculation will provide the volumes and the timing for the scan:

Portal Venous 2/3 of 60 mL = 40 mL
Arterial 1/3 of 60 mL = 20 mL
Portal Venous injection time = 40 mL @ 2.5 mL/s = 16 seconds
Arterial injection time = 20 mL @ 2.5 mL/s = 8 seconds
Portal Venous injection time + Arterial injection Time + pause = scan delay
16 seconds + 8 seconds + pause = 45 seconds
45 seconds – (16 + 8) seconds = a pause of 21 seconds.
Scan at the completion of the injection.

TABLE 14.4
Recommended Time Delay for Portal Venous Abdomen

Age	Time Delay for Portal Venous Abdomen Scan
< 10 years	45 seconds
> 10 years of age	70 seconds

This injection protocol is only suitable for trauma. It is designed to minimise radiation dose.

Malignancy or Infection:

When undertaking a CT abdomen for malignancy or infection, a portal venous phase is usually sufficient. Low osmolar, IV contrast is administered as a bolus via a pressure injector. Contrast is administered at 1.5–2 mL/kg up to a total of 100 mL. Bolus tracking is utilised with the pre-monitoring slice at the level of the descending aorta, just above the diaphragm. The ROI is placed in the descending aorta. The contrast timing will vary with the age of the patient and the vascular access. Change the bolus tracking and monitoring scan delay according to their age. For example, 1 second per year up to 10 years of age. So if the patient is 5, then the monitoring scan is 5 seconds. A scan delay of 45 seconds after trigger is prescribed in the protocol to ensure a portal venous phase acquisition.

Some prefer to use a manual approach to contrast timing for paediatric abdominal CT to reduce radiation dose by eliminating the bolus tracking acquisitions. Using this method, the same volume of contrast is administered by pressure injector and a timed delay for the acquisition is used. Suggested time delays are shown in Table 14.4.

Abdominal CT scans are usually performed on full inspiration to improve compliance. Most children have difficulty with expiratory instructions.

Image Reconstruction

Children have a very different deposition of body fat to most adults. They are born with a large amount of subcutaneous fat, however, they have very little visceral fat. This lack of visceral fat reduces the contrast between the organs and makes diagnosis more difficult. Positive oral contrast is used to assist in diagnosis. Specific paediatric algorithms are also available from some vendors and they should be applied to the infants and young children's scans for reconstruction.

MULTI-REGION STUDIES

Head, Neck, Chest, Abdomen and Pelvis – Malignancy

CT of the head, neck, chest, abdomen and pelvis is primarily performed to diagnose or stage malignancy. With MR and US, this type of examination is becoming increasingly rare, especially scanning the head. This scan may also be adapted to a neck, chest, abdomen and pelvis, by removing the head from the protocol, or just a chest, abdomen and pelvis scan. To minimise radiation dose, if scanning the head, this is usually just a post contrast head.

Patient should be supine with their head in a head cushion, arms are above their head.

An AP topogram of the chest, abdomen and pelvis is performed. To minimise radiation dose, the main acquisition is often performed as a single acquisition of the entire torso at the portal venous timing. With a longer injection of 2 mL per kilo, the thorax is still sufficiently enhanced in a late arterial phase.

For young children under 10, with small shoulders, the neck can be included in the single acquisition to reduce radiation dose due to overlap. If the child is over 10 and/or has broad shoulders, a separate neck acquisition is required. For a separate neck acquisition, the arms should be lowered and a soft tissue neck examination followed. Sufficient contrast volume would need to be allocated from the total contrast volume permitted for the neck acquisition. The neck should always be reconstructed separately.

If a post contrast head is required, the arms are by the patients side and this should be scanned at 3–5 minutes post contrast administration.

Head, C-Spine, Chest, Abdomen and Pelvis – Multi-Trauma

CT of the head, c-spine, chest, abdomen and pelvis is primarily performed after trauma. The head and c-spine should be imaged first without contrast. This is to detect any intracranial injuries and c-spine fractures. If there are c-spine fractures involving the vertebral foramina, a carotid angiogram may be required after the chest, abdomen and pelvis acquisition. Check with the radiologist before removing the patient from the table.

Pre-Acquisition

Patient Positioning

The patient should be positioned head first supine on the table top. The cervical spine should be immobilised during transfer on and off the CT table and during the scan. Do not use sandbags to immobilise the cervical spine during acquisition. They will increase the radiation dose significantly.

After the head and c-spine imaging, if possible the arms should be repositioned above the head.

Planning

A lateral topogram of the head and c-spine is performed as one acquisition.

The head and c-spine are then acquired as individual acquisitions.

An AP topogram of the chest, abdomen and pelvis from above the shoulders to the inferior margin of the symphysis pubis is acquired.

A single acquisition from above the first rib to the inferior margin of the symphysis pubis is acquired. Scanning should be on inspiration or free breathing if unable to follow breathing instructions.

Contrast Phase and Timing

For all trauma CT examinations, a small volume of low osmolar, IV contrast is given to the patient approximately 5 minutes prior to the CT acquisition. This IV contrast should be 5 mL for a patient under 45 kg or 10 mL for a patient over 45 kg. This can be delivered as a hand injection generally prior to the topogram. This is to highlight the renal pelvis identifying any potential renal injury that might result in a urinoma. Giving the small amount of contrast prior to the acquisition minimises the potential radiation exposure of a delayed acquisition.

For the main acquisition, low osmolar, IV contrast is administered as a bolus via a pressure injector. Contrast is administered at 1.5–2 mL/kg up to a total of 100 mL. For trauma CT, an arterial and portal venous phase acquisition is often desired to visualise the arterial vasculature and the solid organ perfusion. This increases the radiation dose to the patient twofold. To reduce the radiation dose, a dual bolus technique may be used to allow a single acquisition. Two-thirds of the total volume is injected for the portal venous phase, then the injection is paused. The final third of the injection is administered to provide contrast enhancement in the arterial vasculature. The total injection duration should be 45 seconds for patients under 10 years of age and 70 seconds for patients 10 years of age and over.

For example, 50 kg patient that is 13 years old will require 2 mL/kg = 80 mL contrast with a 20 g cannula access permitting an injection rate of 3 mL/s.

Portal Venous 2/3 of 80 mL = 53 mL
Arterial 1/3 of 80 mL = 27 mL
Portal Venous injection time = 53 mL @ 3 mL/s = 18 seconds
Arterial injection time = 27 mL @ 3 mL/s = 9 seconds
Portal Venous injection time + Arterial injection Time + pause = scan delay
18 seconds + 9 seconds + pause = 70 seconds
45 seconds – (16 + 8) seconds = a pause of 43 seconds.
Scan at the completion of the injection.

This injection protocol is only suitable for trauma. It is designed to minimise radiation dose.

AXIAL SKELETON

Thoracic and Lumbar Spine

These scans are most commonly performed for scoliosis and hemivertebrae. They are usually performed in a paediatric specialists centres where the surgeons perform the corrective surgery.

APPENDICULAR SKELETON

Extremities (Non-contrast)

CT examinations of extremities in paediatric patients are commonly examined, particularly for injuries involving the physes. It is important to only scan the region of interest. If possible, position the patient so that the area of interest is not overlapping with other anatomical areas, for example, raise the arm above the head for imaging of the elbow or wrist.

REFERENCES

Amaral J, Traubici J, BenDavid G, Reintamm G, Daneman A, 2006, Safety of power injector use in children as measured by incidence of extravasation, *American Journal of Roentgenology*. Vol. 187, pp. 580–583

American Association of Physicists in Medicine, 2017, AAPM position statement on the use of bismuth shielding for the purpose of dose reduction in CT scanning, https://www.aapm.org/org/policies/details.asp?type=PP&id=431, accessed online 20 January 2021.

American College of Radiologists, 2020, ACR appropriateness Criteria, https://www.acr.org/Clinical-Resources/ACR-Appropriateness-Criteria, accessed January 20, 2021

Barreto I, Lamoureux R, Olguin C, Quails N, Correa N, Rill L, Arreola M, 2019, Impact of patient centering in CT on organ dose and the effect of using a positioning compensation system: Evidence from OSLD measurements in postmortem subjects, *Journal of Applied Clinical Medical Physics*, Vol. 20(6), pp. 141–151.

Baumann F, Ernstberger T, Neumann C, Nerlich M, Schroeder GD, Vaccaro AR, Loibl M, 2015, Pediatric cervical spine injuries: A rare but challenging entity, *Journal of Spinal Disorders & Techniques*, Vol. 28(7), pp. E377–E384.

Brady Z, Cain TM, Johnston PN, 2012, Justifying referrals for paediatric CT. *Medical Journal of Australia*, Vol. 197(2), pp. 95–99.

Brenner DJ, Hall EJ, 2007, Computed tomography—An increasing source of radiation exposure, *New Journal of Medicine*, Vol. 357(22), pp. 2277–2284.

Canbulat N, Ayhan F, Inal S, 2015, Effectiveness of external cold and vibration for procedural pain relief during peripheral intravenous cannulation in pediatric patients, *Pain Management Nursing: Official Journal of the American Society of Pain Management Nurses*, Vol. 16(1), pp. 33–39.

Crook TB, Eynon CA, 2005, Traumatic Atlantoaxial rotatory subluxation, *Emergency Medicine Journal*, Vol 22, pp. 671–672.

De Mijolla-Mellor S, Infans, February 2021, Encyclopedia.com, https://www.encyclopedia.com/psychology/dictionaries-thesauruses-pictures-and-press-releases/infans, accessed 17 February 2021.

DeLaney M, Booton J, 2013, Pediatric spinal trauma. *Pediatric Emergency Medicine Reports*, Vol. 18(6).

Habibzadeh MA, Ay MR, Kamali Asl AR, Ghadiri H, Zaidi H, 2011, Impact of miscentering on patient dose and image noise in x-ray CT imaging: Phantom and clinical studies, *Physica Medica*, Vol. 28(3), pp. 191–199.

Hacking C, Dempsey P, 2021, *Chalice Rule*, https://radiopaedia.org/articles/chalice-rule, accessed January 20 2021.

Macquarie Dictionary online, 2021, Macquarie Dictionary publishers, an imprint of Pan Macmillan Australia Pty Ltd, https://www.macquariedictionary.com.au/features/word/search/?search_word_type=Dictionary&word=paediatric, accessed 17 February 2021.

Miller S, Church E, Pool C, *Ages & Stages: All About Me*, Scholastic inc., https://www.scholastic.com/teachers/articles/teaching-content/ages-stages-all-about-me/, accessed 17 February 2021.

Nievelstein R, Dam I, van der Molen A, 2010, Multidetector CT in children: Current concepts and dose reduction strategies, *Pediatric Radiology*, Vol. 40(8), pp. 1324–1344.

Powell EC, Leonard JR, Olsen CS, Jaffe DM, Anders MD, Leonard JC, 2017, Atlantoaxial rotatory subluxation in children, *Pediatric Emergency Care*, Vol. 33(2), pp. 86–91.

Royal Australian and New Zealand College of Radiologists, 2015a, RANZCR Education Modules for appropriate imaging referrals – Clinical Decision Rule Summary Paediatric Head Trauma, RANZCR.

Royal Australian and New Zealand College of Radiologists, 2015b, RANZCR Education Modules for appropriate imaging referrals – Paediatric Cervical Spine Trauma, RANZCR.

Royal Australian and New Zealand College of Radiologists, 2018, Computed Tomography and Radiation Risks, Version: 2.0 Faculty of Clinical Radiology Council, accessed online January 20 2021.

Standring S, 2016, *Gray's Anatomy the Anatomical Basis of Clinical Practice*, 41st Ed. Elsevier, Chapter 27, pp. 416–428.

Timmler S, Simons M, 2019, Grey matter myelination, Glia, Special Issue Edition, accessed online 17 February 2021.

Wong CJ, Moxey-Mims M, Jerry-Fluker J, Warady BA, Furth SL, 2012, CKiD (CKD in children) prospective cohort study: A review of current findings. *American Journal of Kidney Diseases*, Vol. 60(6), pp. 1002–1011.

15 Imaging of the Thorax

Debbie Starkey and Gordon Mander
Queensland University of Technology

Deb Watson
Sunshine Coast University Hospital

CONTENTS

DOI: 10.1201/9781003132554-20

INTRODUCTION

High-resolution computed tomography (HRCT) scanning of the chest has been possible since body CT was available. Resolution has increased considerably since that time. High resolution of the chest was historically performed using an axial (step-and-shoot) scan mode. Helical scanning is now routinely performed with reconstructions applied to produce the requisite imaging.

CT angiography of the thoracic region is performed either in the emergency clinical setting or routinely to follow up or investigate vascular anomalies. CT Aortogram examinations are a relatively non-invasive study to rule out dissection as a cause of a patient's chest pain in the emergency department. CT pulmonary angiography (CTPA) has become the gold standard for the assessment of pulmonary embolism, overtaking ventilation/perfusion (V/Q) imaging and traditional angiographic assessments due to its ease and availability (Moore et al., 2018).

Electrocardiogram (ECG) gating has been increasingly incorporated to improve image quality both for CT aortography as well as for use in dedicated CT coronary angiography (CTCA). The latter use has expanded significantly since improvement in the temporal resolution of scanners, initially with the advent of 64-slice scanners and then more recently following the iteration of current generation >128 slice scanners. These incorporate dual source scanners.

CT CHEST PROTOCOL

Commonly Presenting/Significant Pathologies

Specific clinical indications for performing a CT scan of the chest are numerous. Commonly, routine CT imaging of the chest is for the following indications:

- Trauma,
- malignancy and
- infection

Approaches to Imaging

Patient Positioning

For routine scans of the chest, patients are positioned supine and generally enter the scanner feet first. This allows the patient to be positioned without moving fully through the scanner gantry, reduces the amount of time the patient's head is close to the gantry and allows close proximity for access to intravenous contrast delivery.

Planning

For routine imaging of the chest, a scanogram (topogram) should be performed to include from above the mid neck to the iliac crests. Departmental protocol may include a scanogram in two planes. Planning for helical acquisition should include from above the lung apices (suprasternal notch) to the mid pole of the kidneys to include the adrenal glands. Adrenal glands should routinely be included for chest examinations as they are a common site for metastases from lung cancers (Popper, 2016).

Protocol Considerations

Clinical indications for CT imaging of the chest may include patients presenting with shortness of breath. Some patients are likely to find extended breath hold challenging. It is important to consider acquisition factors which minimise the time required for breath hold. Taking the time to provide clear instruction and opportunity for the patient to practice are important ways to support quality acquisition. It may also be prudent to consider the direction of acquisition. For patients with severe dyspnea, acquisition from below the diaphragm to the apices of the lung will limit the impact of breath hold challenges.

It is important that the patient undertakes a moderate breath for the inspiration. Excessive inspiratory effort impacts the intravascular thoracic pressure gradients and can alter the blood flow in the inferior and superior vena cava. This in turn impacts the contrast opacification particularly in investigations for the pulmonary arteries (Bauer, 2012).

Use of Intravenous Contrast

For routine chest scans, intravenous contrast is administered where suitable. A 20-gauge cannula positioned in the antecubital fossa is preferred for contrast administration. A high flow rate of 2.5–4 mL/s assists in opacification of vascular structures. This should be performed via bolus-triggered acquisition to allow contrast visibility through the arterial phase of enhancement.

Two methods have been described to determine timing. Most commonly, a triggered tracking technique is incorporated. Each vendor will have a proprietary name for the product, but they perform the same process. A preliminary monitoring slice is placed at the relevant level. A region of interest is positioned to measure the baseline value at that position. Once contrast is administered, the location will be continuously monitored (usually every second approximately) to sample the Hounsfield Unit (HU) within the Region of Interest (ROI); once a preset threshold is reached, the acquisition is triggered. The acquisition may also be triggered manually.

CT scans of the chest are frequently performed in conjunction with scans of the abdomen and pelvis. In these circumstances, a scan of the chest is acquired as described above and then a further delay is included to acquire images of the abdomen and pelvis during portal-venous phase timing.

Acquisition and Reconstruction

Acquisition should be at the thinnest detector width. Images will be reconstructed to both thin slices (detector width to 1 mm) and thicker summary slices (6–10 mm). The use of thicker summary slices provides a succinct series for review. Acquisition data should be reconstructed to demonstrate soft tissue/mediastinal structures, lung and bone structures as required. Each series will require separate window settings and kernel/algorithms. Edge enhancement should be used for both the lung and the bony series.

Patient position	Feet first, supine, arms raised above head
Topogram	Craniocaudal table movement, align above the superior skin margin of the shoulder. Include above the level of the iliac crest
Scan region	Acquisition: Include from lung apices to the posterior costophrenic angles (When imaging for suspected lung cancer – include the adrenal glands in the acquisition)
Contrast	As indicated
Breath hold	Yes – Suspended respiration with a comfortable inspiration (not a large breath in)
Image display	Soft tissue/mediastinum Window: Level 40–60; width 400–500 Lung Window: Level −500 to −800; width 1,200–1,800 Bone Window: Level 300–500; width 2,000–3,000
Image reconstruction	Reconstruction in the following planes should be undertaken in soft tissue, lung and bone formats – with both thin and summary slice widths Axial plane Coronal plane Sagittal – as required – may not be routinely performed

High-Resolution CT (HRCT) of the Chest

The term "high resolution" imaging is somewhat obsolete in today's world of sub-millimetre isotropic resolution and high-definition monitors. High resolution scanning was historically performed as incremental fine slice axial scans sampled over the thorax to maximise the resolution of the lung parenchyma. With contemporary scanners, helical scanning of the entire region is performed with reformatted edge enhancement images to demonstrate the lung parenchyma. This approach avoids the slice misregistration issues historically associated with variable inspiratory effort of axial scanning.

Commonly Presenting/Significant Pathologies

- Interstitial lung disease,
- asbestos lung disease/mesothelioma
- Langerhans cell histiocytosis,
- idiopathic pulmonary fibrosis,
- nonspecific interstitial fibrosis,
- hypersensitivity pneumonia,
- chronic eosinophilic pneumonia,
- drug-induced lung disease,
- rheumatoid lung disease,
- scleroderma,
- sarcoidosis and
- silicosis.

Approaches to Imaging

Patient Positioning

The patient should be positioned supine as for standard CT chest acquisition.

Planning

High resolution scanning is generally performed without intravenous contrast, as the purpose of the scan is to visualise the lung parenchyma rather than vascular anatomy.

Scans should be performed from above the lung apices to include entirety of lung bases distally.

Protocol Considerations

High resolution scans are traditionally performed without intravenous contrast. There may be a need to perform additional acquisitions. Performing a second scan with the patient in the prone position allows differentiation between atelectasis and solid opacities (Gotway et al., 2007). Additional acquisitions performed on holding expiratory effort can also be employed. This may assist differentiation between diffuse interstitial lung diseases (Gotway et al., 2007).

In all scans, reconstructions are performed using a lung window. A lung algorithm with edge enhancement aids visualisation of the lung parenchyma. Axial images are traditionally performed at 1 mm slice thickness with a 10 mm slice interval, although with helical scanning, the reconstructed slice interval is less important. In practice, HRCT scans of the chest differ from routine chest imaging protocols more in how they are performed than the quality of the lung resolution they offer.

Patient position	Feet first, supine, arms raised above head Subsequent imaging with the patient prone may be performed
Topogram	Craniocaudal table movement, align above the superior skin margin of the shoulder. Include to below costophrenic margin
Scan region	Acquisition: Include from lung apices to the posterior costophrenic angles
Contrast	As indicated – Not usually required
Breath hold	Yes – Suspended respiration with a comfortable inspiration (not a large breath in)
Image reconstruction	Reconstruction should be undertaken with edge enhancement and displayed in lung windows Axial plane Coronal plane Sagittal – Not routinely performed

CT PULMONARY ANGIOGRAPHY (CTPA)

CTPA has grown considerably in its use of the past few decades. Whilst the test has excellent proven sensitivity and specificity in the detection of pulmonary emboli, there are several factors that have been suggested considerably alter the test effectiveness. These include (Chaturvedi et al., 2017)

- patient size,
- cardiac output and blood pressure,
- flow rate and timing of contrast,
- cannula size and position and
- acquisition kV used.

Commonly Presenting/Significant Pathologies

The most common presenting pathology investigated by CTPA is pulmonary embolus. Where the clinical indications on a request suggest multiple differential diagnoses, a routine contrast scan should be considered as an alternative to a dedicated CTPA.

Approaches to Imaging

Patient Positioning

Patients should be positioned supine as for a standard CT chest acquisition. Consideration should be given to the position of the patient's arms, particularly with regard to cannula location. Care should be taken not to overextend a patient's arms at the shoulder, as there is a risk of partially obstructing the flow of the contrast into the brachiocephalic region. An additional pillow or vendor provided arm rest may facilitate a preferred arm position. Likewise, attention should be given to clothing that might act as a tourniquet. This includes blood pressure cuffs, tight sleeves or jewellery.

Planning

A scanogram should be performed to include the entire chest from chin to above the iliac crests. Planning should include from above apices to lung bases. Inclusion of the whole of the lung fields allows identification of other pathologies with a similar differential (pneumonia, tumour, interstitial lung disease) as well as assisting in determining any associated pleural effusion present secondary to a pulmonary embolism.

Protocol Considerations

CT pulmonary angiography is always performed with intravenous contrast. A high bolus rate is required usually between 4.5 and 6 mL/s, but may be higher when required, e.g. where cardiac output is poor.

Timing in CTPA acquisition is critical. Most commonly, a triggered tracking technique is incorporated. A preliminary monitoring slice is placed at the level of the pulmonary trunk. A region of interest is placed in the pulmonary trunk and will measure the baseline value at that position. Once contrast is administered, the location will be continuously monitored (usually every second approximately) to sample the HU within the ROI; once a preset threshold is reached, the CTPA acquisition is triggered. The acquisition may also be triggered manually. Some sites may perform an *a priori* timing bolus of contrast to determine the time of peak enhancement within the pulmonary trunk. This is then entered in as the start of the acquisition time. There is currently limited published evidence to determine which of the two methods is more effective in providing optimal pulmonary enhancement and therefore should be based on an individual site's preferences.

Several technical issues are important to understand to optimise the chance of producing an accurate result. In their 2017 paper, Chaturvedi et al. (2017) describe several challenges to achieving diagnostic scan result, and these can be considered as extrinsic or intrinsic. Extrinsic factors include technical factors relating to the way in which the scan was performed, such as choice of scan parameters, the type of cannula and flow and timing of the contrast.

Intrinsic factors include patient related factors. The position of the patients arms as paramount to achieve an effective result. Patients should always be supported and coached on the importance of correct breath hold. Respiratory motion during the scan causes significant problems in the images themselves.

Furthermore, recent guidance from the society of cardiovascular CT recommends the use of ECG gating for certain patient cohorts as this will mitigate cardiac motion. It is unlikely this is routine practice at this stage due to the large volume of requested scans and the relative specialist nature of ECG gating techniques.

Further consideration should be given to obese or pregnant patients, where increased intrabdominal pressure is likely to create further difficulties.

Patients should be coached to suspend respiration rather than take a large inspiratory effort. This limits the changes to the intravascular pressure gradients.

Patient position	Feet first, supine, arms raised above head
Topogram	Craniocaudal table movement, align above the superior skin margin of the shoulder. Include above the level of the iliac crest
Scan region	Acquisition: Include from lung apices to the posterior costophrenic angles
Contrast	Yes – High bolus rate (4–6 mL/s) Appropriate bolus tracking for start of acquisition Tracking slice at the level of carina with ROI in pulmonary trunk
Breath hold	Yes – Suspended respiration with a comfortable inspiration (not a large breath in)
Image display	Soft tissue/mediastinum Window: Level 40–60; width 400–500 Lung Window: Level −500 to −800; width 1,200–1,800 Bone Window: Level 300–500; width 2,000–3,000
Image reconstruction	Reconstruction in the following planes should be undertaken in soft tissue window settings Axial plane – Both thin and summary slice width Coronal plane – Maximum Intensity Projection (MIP) reconstructions Lung formats in coronal and axial planes Bone formats – As required

Identification pulmonary emboli represents a medical emergency and should be escalated immediately.

CT Calcium Score

CT calcium scoring has been possible since the development of electron-beam CT; however, the limitations in temporal resolution of traditional third generation scanners has meant that this scan was not widely provided until more recent generations of scan technology were introduced. Standardisation of the acquisition technique is important for comparison with previous and future calculations. It is important that the radiation dose is minimised for all CT examinations. CT calcium score is used as a screening assessment, so all radiation dose minimisation strategies should be implemented. Where possible acquisitions should be acquired with prospective ECG gating.

Commonly Presenting/Significant Pathologies

CT calcium score is utilised to determine an estimate of the calcium burden of the coronary arteries and provide an age and sex risk assessment based upon the previously calculated epidemiological data. The study should not be used in isolation. It is not possible to exclude coronary artery disease alone from a calcium scoring scan, as an Agatston score of zero (0) does not necessarily equate to zero disease (Holvoet et al., 2007). Calcium score calculation scans are often performed in conjunction with CTCA.

Approaches to Imaging

Pre-scan

As the study will be ECG gated, patients should have ECG leads placed on their chest as recommended by vendor. This will usually involve a lead placed on at least the right upper (placed on the midshaft of the right clavicle), left upper (placed on the midshaft of the left clavicle) and left lower (placed on the lower costal margin anteriorly).

Patient Positioning

Patents should be positioned supine with arms extended above head.

Planning

A scanogram should be performed to include the entirety of the mediastinum.

Scan range should include from the carina to below the base of the heart. The field of view should include the entirety of the heart laterally, the sternum anteriorly and the descending aorta posteriorly.

For most scanners, 120 kV must be used regardless of patient size or other factors. Scans should be reviewed using a 3.0 mm reconstructed image thickness. These parameters will ensure that the scans are consistent with historical data and therefore comparable.

Protocol Considerations

As the aim of a calcium score is to determine the amount of calcium within the coronary artery vessels, calcium score scans are performed without intravenous contrast.

The reconstructed images should be reviewed using a vendor-specific analysis package for calcium scoring. The radiographer will review these predefined areas and select the specifically determined areas that match the calcium deposited within each of the right coronary artery, left anterior descending artery and the circumflex artery.

Patient position	Feet first, supine, arms raised above head ECG leads
Topogram	Craniocaudal table movement, align above the superior skin margin of the shoulder. Include to the lower costal margin (to include costophrenic angles)
Scan region	Acquisition: Include from just below carina to below the apex of the heart
Contrast	Nil
Breath hold	Yes – Suspended respiration with a comfortable inspiration (not a large breath in)
Image display	Soft tissue/mediastinum Window: Level 40–60; width 400–500
Image reconstruction	Images reconstructed to ECG gating for minimised cardiac motion Axial plane 3 mm Reviewed using analysis software for Coronary Calcification

Each area that has been determined as including coronary calcium is then summarised to produce a volume and Agatston score (Agatston et al., 1990). This score can be compared to epidemiological data in order to determine the patient's total plaque burden in comparison with a historic population (Holvoet et al., 2007). Whilst it should be stressed that this is by no means a definitive test in determining the patient's risk of a future ischaemic event, it gives important information to the referrer in determining (in conjunction with other indicators, such as cholesterol and lifestyle factors) the value of drug therapy to reduce risk.

CT CORONARY ANGIOGRAPHY (CTCA)

Perhaps the most notable implementation in CT applications in recent decades is the capability in CTCA or cardiac CT. Whilst the concept of CT imaging of the coronary arteries is not new, the last decade or so has brought several important technological advancements to make the visualisation of these vessels as well as other heart structures much more effective.

Commonly Presenting/Significant Pathologies

CTCA is most employed to rule out coronary artery disease and its excellent negative predictive value in outpatient populations gives this significance. It is also employed in investigating chest pain.

Approaches to Imaging

Pre-scan

The pre-preparation for cardiac CT is of utmost importance. Care must be taken to ensure patients have appropriate heart rates for the test wherever possible. Optimum heart rate is between 65 and 70 bpm. Patient preparation should include avoiding caffeine for a minimum of 12 hours before the study. It is recommended that patients are cannulated outside the scanner and ECG leads are connected beforehand. This may assist to reduce any anxiety patients may have and the associated impact on heart rate.

Once an initial assessment of the patient's heart rate and blood pressure has been performed, a decision by the Radiologist based on these results and other factors will guide whether the patient requires heart rate lowering medication prior to the scan. The most utilised medication in this scenario is beta-blockers, which may be administered intravenously or orally as preferred. Oral medication requires the patient to wait for an hour or so prior to scan to allow the medication to have full effect. Intravenous administration may be preferred as the effects are far quicker via this route; however, there is some evidence to suggest it is less reliable than oral via route. Patients contraindicated to beta-blockers may receive a sinus node inhibitor. Alternatively, some sites may administer a calcium channel blocker. An awareness of the patient's heart rate prior to the scan is important to identify the best way to approach the scan.

Patient Positioning

Patients should be positioned supine on the scan couch with arms extended above head. Care should be taken to ensure ECG leads are adequately positioned so as not to interfere with scan table movement, injector line or irritate the patient. Time should be spent with the patient, ensuring they understand the test and what is required of them. In addition to the standard explanation of CT scans (contrast, verbal consent), the patients should be coached on the expectations around

- an explanation of the test,
- the duration of the test,
- importance of holding still,
- the purpose of ECG gating and why the ECG leads are necessary,
- the purpose and side effects of GTN administration (and beta-blocker if administered on table),
- the purpose and side effects of iodinated contrast,
- the length and timing of breath hold instructions and
- any further questions the patient may have.

Planning

The specifics of the protocol selected will depend on specifics of the model of the CT scanner. However, there are several steps in common when planning a CTCA. A scanogram should be performed to include the entirety of the lung fields.

The range of the scan for a dedicated scan of the coronary artery tree will include from a couple of centimetres distal to the carina to the base of the heart. Where a calcium score is performed in conjunction with the CTCA, the z-position of the most proximal and distal slices should be noted and reproduced for the CTCA.

Where the patient has had previous coronary artery bypass grafts or there is a requirement to include the aortic arch in the scan, the range should be extended to include the sternal notch proximally. This will allow visualisation of the subclavian artery and will provide evidence of the patency of internal mammary artery grafts.

The field of view will need to include the heart laterally and should visualise the sternum anteriorly and the descending aorta posteriorly. Additional reconstructed field of view of the lung fields to review extracardiac findings is recommended in scanning guidelines (Abbara et al., 2016).

The amount of temporal padding included in the scan will need to be addressed. Contemporary scanner technology is able to assist in this decision-making process and individual practices will have their own determining arguments. However, care should be taken to ensure the ALARA principle is being adhered to and the padding is only increased where there is substantial risk of motion due to high heart rate or significant heart rate variability. Generally speaking, padding should routinely include the end diastolic temporal window, normally between 70% and 80%. An extension in padding to include the mid-systolic window (30%–80%) may be necessary where heart rates are highly variable, such is atrial fibrillation cases. For current generation scanners, retrospective ECG gating should not be required.

Protocol Considerations

As with CTPA, the determination of contrast timing may be made either via a conventional bolus tracking technique or use of a timing bolus. Both methods have advantages and disadvantages.

Patient position	Feet first, supine, arms raised above head ECG leads
Topogram	Craniocaudal table movement, align above the superior skin margin of the shoulder. Include to the lower costal margin (to include costophrenic angles) Perform a CT calcium score acquisition initially
Scan region	CTCA acquisition: Include from just above the sternoclavicular joints to 2 cm below the apex of the heart
Contrast	Yes – Times to aortic root (Bolus timing)
Breath hold	Yes – Suspended respiration with a comfortable inspiration (not a large breath in)
Image display	Soft tissue/mediastinum Window: Level 40–60; width 400–500
Image reconstruction	Images reconstructed to ECG gating for minimised cardiac motion Axial plane Then multiplanar and three-dimensional reconstruction to demonstrate each of the coronary vessels

CT GATED AORTOGRAM

CT aortogram is a valuable test and may be performed with or without ECG gating. The former is preferable with a more useful assessment of the aortic root, especially when dissection is a significant concern.

Commonly Presenting/Significant Pathologies

CT aortogram is commonly performed for excluding or determining degree of aortic dissection, stenosis, coarctation or aneurysm. Scans of the aorta are usually indicated for patients with a complicated vascular pathology history, connective tissue disorders (such as Marfan's syndrome), aortitis (aortic vasculitis) or other lifestyle risk factors (history of diabetes, smoking, etc.).

Aortic dissection may be classified as traumatic or non-traumatic. Patients presenting with non-traumatic dissections may have a wide variety of presenting signs and symptoms and there are no well-advised non-imaging tests to assess pre-test probability. Patients at risk of dissection may present with "tearing" chest pain through to the back or into the jaw, significant differences in left and right limb blood pressure, cold or discoloured limbs, nausea, headache or vomiting, or syncope (Strayer et al., 2012). However, none of these are definitive signs of dissection.

Due to the central location of the aorta, patients may also present with symptoms of stroke or myocardial infarction. Identification of an aortic dissection represents a medical emergency and should be escalated immediately.

Approaches to Imaging

Pre-scan

ECG leads should be connected to the patient.

Patient Positioning

Patients should be positioned supine and feet first where possible. Care should be taken not to overextend the patients' arms due to the risk of reducing the effectiveness of the contrast flow into the brachiocephalic region.

Planning

The nature of the scan will determine the extent of the scan range. Occasionally, cardiology referred examinations of the aorta will only require inclusion of the thoracic aorta, for example. In this case, the range should extend to the diaphragm to include the heart. More commonly however, a scan of the entire aorta is required. This should be performed to include from above the apices of the lungs to below the pubic ramus. This will allow visualisation of the major arterial supply that the aorta provides including the base of the common carotid arteries of the neck, the subclavian arteries, the common femoral arteries of the legs. Classification of certain aortic pathologies such as dissection requires this anatomy to be included to establish severity.

The field of view should include chest and abdomen to the skin line, or if not possible, muscle line.

Protocol Considerations

Consideration should be given to performing a non-contrast scan immediately prior to the CT angiogram. This will allow assistance in identifying subtle mural or pericardial haematoma associated with aneurysmal dissection of the thoracic aorta (Holloway et al., 2011). Where dual-energy scanners are used, consideration should be given to including a virtual non-contrast dataset.

CT aortograms are always performed with intravenous contrast. A flow rate between 3 and 5 mL/s is necessary to adequately opacify the aorta. To accommodate this, a 18 or 20 gauge cannula should be inserted (ideally in the right antecubital fossa).

Reconstructions should be performed and may include MIPs to better delineate smaller vessels. A vascular window should be used to sufficiently differentiate calcium from contrast. Volume rendered images are also useful to determine stenotic or obstructed regions. Curved MPRs may add value also.

REFERENCES

Abbara, S., et al. (2016). SCCT guidelines for the performance and acquisition of coronary computed tomographic angiography: A report of the Society of Cardiovascular Computed Tomography Guidelines Committee: Endorsed by the North American Society for Cardiovascular Imaging (NASCI). *J Cardiovasc Comput Tomogr* 10(6) 435–449.

Agatston, A. S., et al. (1990). Quantification of coronary artery calcium using ultrafast computed tomography. *J Am Coll Cardiol* 15(4) 827–832.

Bauer, S., B., Beeres, M., Wichmann, J. L., Bodelle, B., Vogl, T. J. and Kerl, J. M. (2012). High-pitch dual-source computed tomography pulmonary angiography in freely breathing patients. *J Thoracic Imag* 27(6) 376–381. doi:10.1097/RTI.0b013e318250067e.

Chaturvedi, A., et al. (2017). Contrast opacification on thoracic CT angiography: challenges and solutions. *Insights Imag* 8(1) 127–140.

Gotway, M. B., M. M. Freemer and T. E. King, Jr. (2007). Challenges in pulmonary fibrosis. 1: Use of high resolution CT scanning of the lung for the evaluation of patients with idiopathic interstitial pneumonias. *Thorax* 62(6) 546–553.

Holloway, B. J., D. Rosewarne and R. G. Jones (2011). Imaging of thoracic aortic disease. *Br J Radiol* 84(3) S338–S354.

Holvoet, P., et al. (2007). The relationship between oxidized LDL and other cardiovascular risk factors and subclinical CVD in different ethnic groups: The Multi-Ethnic Study of Atherosclerosis (MESA). *Atherosclerosis* 194(1) 245–252.

Moore, A. J. E., et al. (2018). Imaging of acute pulmonary embolism: An update. *Cardiovasc Diag Ther* 8(3) 225–243.

Popper, H. H. (2016). Progression and metastasis of lung cancer. *Cancer Metast Rev* 35(1) 75–91.

Strayer, R. J., P. L. Shearer and L. K. Hermann (2012). Screening, evaluation, and early management of acute aortic dissection in the ED. *Current Cardiol Rev* 8(2) 152–157.

Section 6

Image Evaluation

16 Introduction to CT Image Interpretation

Lynne Hazell
University of Johannesburg

CONTENTS

INTRODUCTION

This chapter provides the background to assist CT radiographers in interpreting the CT images they produce. Radiographers are in an ideal position to provide an initial interpretation of CT images as they are viewing the images during the procedure. Radiographers can look at the images and assist in recognising the need for further imaging or a change in protocol. In the Society of Radiographers document outlining the role of the radiographer in CT, they emphasised the need for the CT radiographer to be proactive and ensure they provide effective service delivery to the patient and referring clinician (Johnson, 2017). For this to be achieved, all CT radiographers need the skills to offer a patient-centred, safe and efficient service. Thus, it is important that all CT radiographers have an understanding of pattern recognition of CT

DOI: 10.1201/9781003132554-22

imaging, cross-sectional anatomy and physiology and the application of clinical history to the CT examination.

CT imaging includes trauma, the diagnosis and planning of cancer treatment, cardiac disease diagnosis, orthopaedic imaging and brain pathology. These will be discussed further in the subsequent chapters. This chapter outlines the methods that should be incorporated into image interpretation for any CT image.

- The learning outcomes from this chapter will be
- understanding the need for a systematic approach to image interpretation;
- understanding cross-sectional anatomy;
- understanding the level of the pathology in the body and its significance;
- understanding the normal and abnormal patterns on CT imaging;
- understanding the normal variants in each anatomical area and
- understanding the clinical history as it applies to the CT examination.

When interpreting an image, the term pattern recognition can be used. Corr (2001) defined pattern recognition as:

> being able to recognise normal anatomical and physiological appearances on an image and those variations of appearances, which may indicate pathology.

From this, we can understand that familiarity with normal appearances of all anatomical structures is essential. Without this knowledge, undertaking image interpretation is challenging. To become proficient in image interpretation, it is important to spend as much time as possible looking at CT images, both normal and abnormal. Image interpretation cannot be taught in the conventional sense. Books can provide the tools for interpreting images, but only experience can provide the mental pictures to compare normal and abnormal images. Thus, visual experience enables the knowledge to become concrete, as Higgs and Jones (1995) stated, "pattern recognition involves comparing mental images of patterns, (anatomical and pathological), to arrive at a diagnostic opinion". The information provided in the book will provide the guidance to improve your efficiency in interpreting and evaluating images in clinical practice.

CLINICAL HISTORY

Radiographers may need to consider the clinical history before undertaking any examination, however, with a CT scan, the need to consider the clinical history should be at the forefront (Davies et al., 2018). A CT scan has an associated high dose of radiation, and therefore, an examination must always be justified (Lampignano and Kendrick, 2021). In addition, the possible administration of contrast media either oral or intravenous is often dictated by the clinical history. Clinical history for specific pathologies will be discussed in future chapters.

No radiology examination should be undertaken without a full clinical history, and as a radiographer, the importance of your verbal and non-verbal interaction with the patient will enhance your understanding of the patient's clinical history. Verbal communication with your patient will ensure your knowledge of the onset of the symptoms, possibly what triggers the symptoms and the length of time the patient has had the symptoms (Maizlin and Somers, 2019). Non-verbal communication could involve the appearance of the patient: Do they look pale, flushed, are they able to keep still, is one side of their body affected, etc. There are many visible signs of diseases that should not be overlooked.

Again, radiographers are often be in the best position to communicate with the patient and patient's often communicate more with the radiographer. All the information provided should be noted and will assist with possible diagnosis at a later stage. There should be a correlation between the clinical history and the pathological findings (Brady, 2017); therefore, an evaluation should not be performed without the clinical history. Previously, the lack of medical training by radiographers has been noted as a knowledge gap (Donovan and Manning, 2006) for understanding the correlation between clinical history and pathology. However, radiographers' visual experience with imaging modalities should be considered and training has been seen to enable radiographers to report on images to a high standard.

SYSTEMATIC METHODS

When interpreting CT images, it is important to consider a systematic method by using the same methods every time. There should be consistency in the evaluation of the image. When referring to a system, the Collins dictionary defines it as: A system is a way of working, organising, or doing something which follows a fixed plan or set of rules, (https://www.collinsdictionary.com). If you have an organised way of evaluating images, you will not fall into some of the pitfalls which can occur when a more random non-specific method is used to view images. Some of these are "failure to search" and having "tunnel vision." These will be discussed in more detail later in the chapter.

Humans have a tendency to see what they want to see and not always observe the nuances of an appearance. Therefore, a systematic approach can overcome this trait enabling the viewer to look at the entire structure methodologically. A disciplined approach will improve accuracy. The use of an acronym can assist in ensuring the same routine is followed every time. Chan (2013) used the ABCDES method of interpreting an image and this is a good place to start with image interpretation. The method Chan (2013) describes may need adaptation, but a simple acronym is very useful. The acronym is not used in exactly the same way for every area of the body or every system. However, ABCDES provides an easy way to remember the method to interpret images. The A has a generic aspect common to all areas and all modalities within the radiology field. Adequacy and Anatomy are always an essential point of analysis before the interpretation of the examination in the context of the clinical history can take place. These two areas will be discussed below as your first point of analysis of your image.

A

ADEQUACY

As with any imaging technique, it is essential to confirm the identity of the patient ensuring the patient's data correlate with the referral letter. A CT image should be checked for the patient's name and often an identifying number such as a hospital number. The date of birth and the age of the patient appear on the image. This information should again be confirmed and can be very useful when considering and identifying pathology as certain pathologies are more prevalent in certain age groups. Age can also assist in the identification of anatomy and the orientation of anatomical structures. Gender is also provided on a CT image which could also assist in the types of pathology relevant to the gender, and naturally, the anatomy of male and female reproductive organs.

When considering the adequacy of a CT image, the position of the patient should be assessed to establish if the area of interest is included in the examination. In the case of a CT scan, it is important to ascertain how the patient was scanned and whether the patient was scanned in the supine or prone position. The orientation of the patient will impact on the anatomical markers which although selected on a CT protocol can still be impacted by human error. For example, the CT radiographer uses a supine protocol for a patient lying prone. The orientation of the patient must correlate with the anatomical markers and should be confirmed before evaluation continues. When considering the orientation of the patient, this will impact on any fluid levels identified within the patient and how they present.

If contrast media has been administered, it should be identified on the image itself and were the correct phases captured on the imaging. Motion needs to be considered. Is there any patient movement during the scan: this would be of particular relevance in the chest and abdomen. Artefacts on the image: are they impacting on the quality of the image and could they be removed. If not, could the scanning protocol be adjusted to enable better visualisation of the anatomy.

Anatomy

When undertaking image interpretation, an essential aspect is a good knowledge of the anatomy of the area under examination. In CT, this would mean cross-sectional anatomy is important when interpreting images. When considering cross-sectional anatomy, it is also important to understand the normal orientation of organs and the level in the body that particular anatomical structures should be visualised. In the previous chapters, the cross-sectional anatomy has been discussed. Use this for a reference when looking at CT images. A pattern of the normal position, outline, density and orientation of organs as seen on a CT scan will assist with detecting abnormalities.

Understanding the normal position and anatomical level of a structure, if you are interpreting the chest or abdomen, can be useful in providing a clinician with an indication of the changes you have seen and their position in the context of normal patterns. If we look at the structures in the image below and consider the anatomy seen at a specific level, you will understand the requirement.

In Figure 16.1, both kidneys are seen. The left kidney is demonstrated at the renal pelvis; however, as the right kidney lies anatomically slightly lower than the left, the right renal pelvis is not demonstrated. The conclusion would be the kidneys are orientated normally and then the size of the kidneys could also be assessed if they are within normal limits. The right lobe of the liver and gall bladder are also seen in the image in Figure 16.1. In addition, a section of the large intestine and the abdominal

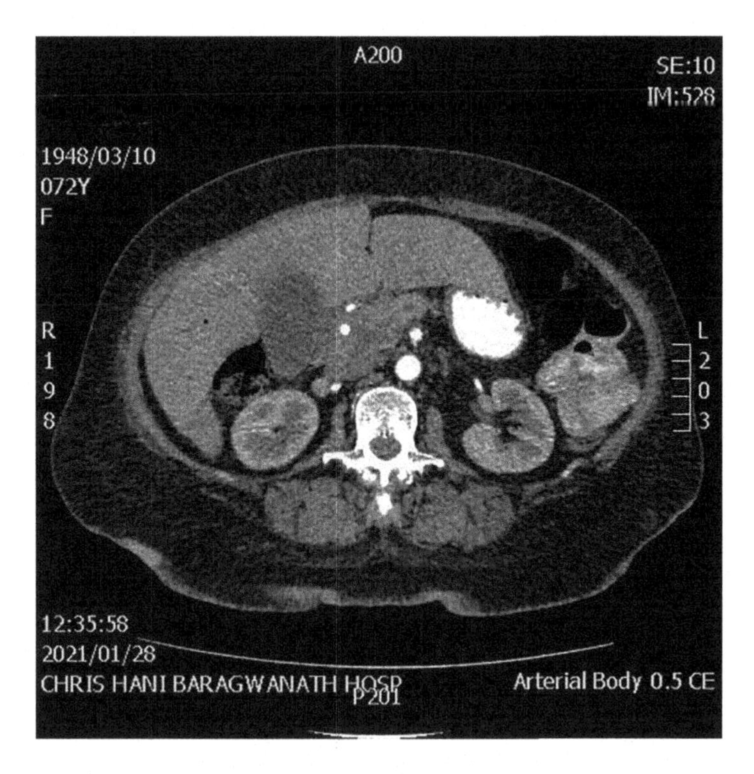

FIGURE 16.1 Cross section through the abdomen.

aorta are visualised. With this information in a normal abdomen as seen here, the vertebral body seen is lumbar vertebra 2. This can assist us should we for example see an abdominal aortic aneurysm and we can orientate the position of the abnormality from the surrounding anatomy visualised. When interpreting images, location is key to providing a written or verbal comment. The scout view can also assist with the level that the anatomy is being seen as we can orientate the image to the scout particularly if pathology or an abnormality is identified.

Window Level/Width

When interpreting an image, the window level and width must be adjusted to enable the reviewer to identify different anatomical structures. Window levels and widths are standardised for many procedures and protocols. The window level will affect the brightness of the image and the window width changes the contrast of the image. See Table 16.1 below for average window levels and widths per examination.

Although these are suggested levels, it may be necessary to change these window widths/ levels depending on the patient's habitus and the pathology.

Reconstruction

An advantage of CT imaging compared with conventional imaging is that the images can be reconstructed in different formats. Different reformatting techniques can also assist in identifying anatomy if there is some doubt in the axial plane. The use of

TABLE 16.1
Window Widths and Levels for CT Examinations

Examination	Anatomy	Window Width	Window Level
Chest	Lung	1,500	600
	Mediastinum	350	50
Abdomen	Soft tissue	400	50
	Liver	150	30
Spine	Soft tissue	250	50
	Bone	1,800	400

multiplanar reformats provides a different perspective for interpretation. Similar to an additional view in conventional radiography, a 3D image or a maximum intensity projection or a volume-rendered image can provide additional information necessary to make a diagnostic comment.

In conventional radiography we refer to requiring two views in CT, a reformatted image could provide similar information to a second view. CT enables the radiographer to reconstruct in different planes and axial scan could be enhanced by the reconstruction in the sagittal or coronal plane. Thus, if you are unsure of a diagnosis, consider a reformat to assist with the report.

Hounsfield Units

Another useful tool for the CT radiographer is the use of Hounsfield units (HU) to identify a mass or structure. Table 16.2 below provides the average HU for various tissue types.

The HUs can assist in the interpretation of the image and could differentiate between a benign and a malignant structure. HUs can also assist with the bone mineral density measurements.

TABLE 16.2
Hounsfield Units for Various Tissue Types

Tissue Type	Hounsfield Units
Air	−1,000
Lung	−700 to −500
Soft tissue	−300 to −100
Fat	−100 to −50
Water	0
CSF	+15
Blood	+30 to +45
Muscle	+10 to +40
Liver	+40 to +60
Bone	+700 to +3,000

The two aspects of image evaluation that are common to all examinations and modalities that are adequacy and anatomy have now been discussed, and below, the other corresponding letters will be briefly outlined, further details will be noted in the subsequent chapters.

A

Dependent on the examination, A will represent different aspects of image evaluation. If the examination is in the chest, then A will be *Airway* as the position and patency of the airways is vital in the chest. In the abdomen, A would just be *Air* as free air within the abdominal cavity is indicative of abnormalities. Finally, in the evaluation of musculoskeletal images, A would represent *Alignment* as in the alignment of a fracture. In addition, the alignment of a joint can be assessed in terms of possible dislocation or narrowing or widening of the joint space.

B

In a CT chest, B is *Breathing* evaluating the lung fields for any abnormalities. With the lung fields and the brain where there are two lung fields or two hemispheres, it is important to always consider the symmetry of the structures and this will be discussed further under the specific anatomical areas.

Bowel gas is the CT abdomen B. This is important for identifying air/ fluid levels in the abdomen and also distension of the bowel due to bowel obstruction or ascites.

For musculoskeletal image evaluation, B is for *Bone* and any changes in the bone such as periosteal reactions, fractures and the type of fracture seen.

C

In a CT chest or abdomen, C for *Circulation* is an important aspect of the image evaluation and is also dependent on whether contrast media has been administered. When evaluating the vessels and the flow again, it is important to revise the vascular structures and understand the blood flow.

Calcifications are important to understand the normal and the abnormal appearances. In the abdomen, calcifications are often stones, for example, gallstones, renal stones and urinary tract stones. All of these would have a pathological significance. However, calcifications, such as phleboliths in the pelvic area, are common normal vessel calcification. Here is an example of understanding the normal pattern of a calcified vessel compared to the ureteric or bladder calcification appearances.

In addition, calcifications should be considered in conjunction with the age of the patient as during our natural life span certain structures are more likely to calcify. For example, calcification of the abdominal aorta, the intercostal cartilage and the osteophytes that form on the bones.

In the context of the musculoskeletal system, the *Cortical* outline of the bone should always be evaluated. Cortical margins can be lost or expanded depending on the pathology.

D

When evaluating the chest, the *Diaphragms* should be assessed on CT specifically due to its cross-sectional nature, herniation of any organs can be properly assessed. Pleural effusions can be evaluated on a CT scan and smaller quantities of fluid can be seen than on CT compared to a conventional chest X-ray, again due to the cross-sectional appearances. If the entire span of the diaphragm requires evaluation, then the opportunity for reconstructing the images in various planes will assist here. Always remember the normal structure of the hemi-diaphragms and that the right hemi-diaphragm is higher than the left.

When considering the musculoskeletal system, the changes in *Density* of the bone should be considered. Again, it is important to recognise the normal appearances of the bone first before considering abnormal appearances. The increase in bone density could be sclerotic changes and the appearance of osteophytes. A decrease in bone density would appear as lucent areas.

E

The *Extras* seen on images such as lines should be assessed. This will require knowledge of the placement of lines. Particularly, this is important in the chest, but can be relevant in the abdomen as well.

S

Soft tissue should be assessed on all CT images looking for swelling, air in the tissue and calcification. Symmetry of the tissue should also be evaluated.

NORMAL VS ABNORMAL AND NORMAL VARIANTS

From the initial definition of pattern recognition, it can be seen that the understanding of normal is vitally important. Often the normal can be far harder to confidently comment on than the abnormal. Therefore, the evaluation of normal CT images is going to provide that visual memory to compare each image too. Normal variants such as an azygous lobe in the lung could mimic pathology. In the abdomen, understanding that the organs in the body vary in position and size due to the habitus of the body of the patient. When considering the spinal level of a pathology, take into consideration of a sixth lumbar vertebra or a cervical rib all of which can impact the accurate evaluation of the image.

FAILURE TO SEARCH

In the context of image evaluation, it is important to always look at the entire image and not to have "tunnel vision." It has been recognised that failure to search is a factor in radiographers image evaluation. This means once an abnormality has been identified, then the image evaluation ceases. In addition, the way the novice scans, the images have been shown to be central looking at the centre of the image and not scanning (Donovan and Manning, 2006). The radiologist has been shown to use a circumferential method of scanning; this enables the viewer to include the whole image (Donovan and Manning, 2006). Thus, the eye needs to be trained to move around the entire circumference of the image to ensure nothing is missed.

LANGUAGE USED FOR REPORTING

Finally, it is important to consider that if you are conducting an image evaluation there is a requirement to communicate these findings. Often a challenge has been found for radiologists that the language used has not been understood by the clinician due to poor vocabulary and the organisation or structure of the report being difficult to interpret (Brady, 2017). Therefore, a template could be useful to assist the novice in reporting their image evaluation with organ system headings for the chest and abdomen (Brady, 2017). The research by Brady (2017) identified that the requirements for a report to assist with the patient's diagnosis and treatment are to provide an opinion regarding the underlying cause of abnormalities and guidance as to other investigations that would be beneficial to the patient's diagnosis.

When undertaking image evaluation, the need for experience has been mentioned. Spending time observing the methods used by experienced reporting radiographers and radiologists can be useful. However, there is a limit to the time that should be spent in evaluating images to prevent burnout. Literature has indicated that for radiologists to function optimally, 20 CT examinations are a maximum to report on in a day (Brady, 2017). Thus, there is time to gain experience versus quality time to have that experience.

CONCLUSION

In summary, it is important to use the same method of evaluating an image every time by having a systematic review tool that you use. Train yourself to scan images to optimise your ability to see everything included on the image. Before starting an evaluation, ensure you have correlated the patient's demographic details with the images and you have the clinical history. To improve your skills, spend as much time as possible observing images, watch others and learn from their experience and find a mentor to assist you with the unusual cases. Practice may not make perfect, but it will allow you to build confidence in your own abilities.

REFERENCES

Brady, A.P. (2017). Error and discrepancies in radiology: Inevitable or avoidable? *Insights in Imaging*. Vol 8. doi:10.1007/s13244-016-0534-1.

Chan, O. (2013). *ABC of Emergency Radiology*. 3rd ed. BMJ Books, London.

Corr, P. (2001). *Pattern Recognition in Diagnostic Imaging*. World Health Organization, Switzerland.

Davies, S., George, A., Macallister, A., Barton, H., Youssef, A., Boyle, L. & Sequeiros, I. (2018). "It's all in the history". A service evaluation of the quality of radiological requests in acute imaging. *Radiography*. Vol 24, 252–256.

Donovan, T. & Manning, D.J. (2006). Successful reporting by non-medical practitioners such as radiographer, will always be task-specific & limited in scope. *Radiography.* Vol 12, 7–12.

Higgs, J. & Jones, M. (1995). *Clinical Reasoning in the Health Professions.* Butterworth. Heinemann, Oxford.

https://www.collinsdictionary.com

Johnson, L. (2017). *The Role of the Radiographer in Computed Tomography Imaging.* Society of Radiographers. https://www.sor.org/learning/document-library/role-radiographer-computed-tomography-imaging.

Lampignano, J.P. & Kendrick, L.E. (2021) *Bontrager's Textbook of Radiographic Positioning and Related Anatomy.* 10th ed. Elsevier Inc. St Louis.

Maizlin, N.N. & Somers, S. (2019). The role of clinical history collected by diagnostic imaging staff in interpreting of imaging examinations. *JMIRS.* Vol 50. Issue 1. doi:10.1016/j.jmir.2018.07.009.

17 CT Head Image Evaluation

Flamur Sahiti
Queen Elizabeth Queen Mother Hospital

Christopher M Hayre
University of Exeter

CONTENTS

INTRODUCTION

Despite advances in magnetic resonance imaging (MRI) and availability of scanners, computed tomography (CT) remains the key imaging modality in the majority of hospitals for intracranial scanning, especially in the acute setting. CT provides a quick and highly accurate diagnosis for the vast majority of intracranial pathologies,

DOI: 10.1201/9781003132554-23

hence its use clinically. When looking at a CT head scan, there are many internal structures that need to be scrutinised in order to avoid missing pathology, big or small. As with any image evaluation criteria, it is important to know our anatomy and be able to identify the norm. The three main structures of the brain include the cerebrum, cerebellum and brainstem. These structures can then be further subdivided. The cerebrum is divided into two hemispheres, containing a frontal lobe, temporal lobe, occipital lobe and parietal lobe. The surface of the cerebrum is called the cortex which has a folded appearance. Each folding of the cortex is called a gyrus with subsequent 'grooves' between folds called the sulcus. White matter tracts are seen connecting the lobes with one another and to the rest of the brain. Further, deep structures are observed in the cerebrum and include the hypothalamus, pituitary gland, pineal gland and basal ganglia. The brain contains fluid-filled cavities, known as ventricles, of which two are lateral (one on each side of the cerebrum), the third ventricle is positioned along the midline of the brain and, finally, the fourth ventricle is observed in the cerebellum. Within the lateral ventricles, we find the choroid plexus, which is responsible for producing cerebrospinal fluid (CSF). CSF flows throughout the ventricles and around the brain, within the subarachnoid spaces, cisterns and spinal cord.

The cerebellum is a structure seen inferior to the cerebrum and considerably smaller in size. The brain stem comprises midbrain, pons and medulla oblongata, and attaches to become the spinal cord. The brain and spinal cord are covered with three layers of tissue called the meninges. These layers are commonly referred as the dura mater, arachnoid mater and pia matter. The dura mater is the outermost layer, lining the inside of the skull. This consists of two layers – the periosteal and meningeal dura – which are fused and separated when forming the venous sinuses. Two of the most important folds upon examining CT head scans is considering the tentorium and falx. The falx divides the cerebrum into two hemispheres and the tentorium separates the cerebrum from the cerebellum. The arachnoid mater is a web-like membrane covering the entire brain. The space between the dura and arachnoid mater is called the subdural space, and upon examination of pathology, it is important to determine if it is subdural or intracranial. The pia mater, which is the innermost layer of connective tissue, hugs the surface of the brain containing blood vessels. The space between the arachnoid and pia is called the subarachnoid space and this space contains CSF, acting as a cushion for the brain. Blood supply to the brain is carried via the internal carotid and vertebral arteries. The vertebral artery supplies the cerebellum and brainstem with the internal carotid supplying most of the cerebrum. The vertebral arteries bifurcate to form the basilar artery. The basilar artery and internal carotid arteries form with one another at the base of the skull, forming what is known as the circle of Willis. For pathologies, such as strokes, it is important to understand what vessel is affected to help determine the part of the brain affected. The venous circulation is different from arterial circulation in the brain whereby the venous sinuses become the major collector of venous blood, which is transferred to the internal jugular veins. The superior and inferior sagittal sinuses drain the cerebrum, with the cavernous sinuses draining the anterior skull base. All sinuses eventually drain to the sigmoid sinuses, which exit via the jugular veins.

The skull encapsulates the brain and acts as a protective structure. It consists of eight bones that fuse along suture lines (not to be confused with fractures). These bones are the frontal, parietal, temporal, sphenoid, occipital and ethmoid. Other structures, which can sometimes be visualised on head scans and worthy of note include, but not limited to, maxilla, zygoma, nasal, mandible, mastoid air cells, foramen magnum and sinuses (maxillary, frontal, ethmoid and sphenoid). Inside the skull, there are three areas often used when describing the location of brain pathology: anterior fossa, middle fossa and posterior fossa. The orbits, neck and other soft tissue structures should not be scanned during a CT head scan; however, due to patient condition, it may sometimes be visualised with structures requiring evaluation if included on the scan. There is no correct way of interpreting a head scan, however, it requires looking at all internal structures mentioned above and within axial, sagittal and coronal planes. Before evaluating a head scan, it is good to know what structures should look like in relation to their density. For example, CSF will appear black and white matter should appear grey. The Hounsfield units, which describe the radio density of structures, should also be known (Grumme et al., 1998, p. 6). As a beginner, it is important to establish a firm baseline of 'what a normal CT head looks like' bearing in mind factors such as age affect how a brain may appear and as to whether it can be deemed normal or not. Once you have a good understanding of the major structures of the brain, you can begin to scrutinise the scan and look for pathology. A good place to start is by first scrolling through the scan looking at both sides of the brain and looking for symmetry. If we draw an imaginary line down the middle of the falx cerebri, it should cut the lateral ventricles in half. There should be symmetry with neither side of the cerebral hemispheres pushing to the opposite side. When this happens, it is called midline shift and often due to pathology. It is very rare to have symmetrical pathology and this will be our first starting point.

We may then start to look at different lobes: frontal, temporal, parietal and occipital. When looking at each lobe, it is important to note other structures such as the sulci, gyrus and white matter (which appears grey). It is important to critique the ventricular system and pay attention to the size and shape of the ventricles. Are they symmetrical, enlarged, small or a different density to what they should normally be? The white matter should also be visible with special attention paid to the basal ganglia (caudate nucleus, putamen and globus pallidus) and thalamus. These structures can sometimes be difficult to visualise but should be clear and symmetrical. Then, examination into the CSF structures, including the cisterns and subarachnoid spaces, making sure they can be visualised, are symmetrical and not being compressed or depict pathology within them. It is important to look at the blood supply to the brain. While smaller vessels may not always be visible, you should be able to identify the basilar artery, circle of Willis and sagittal sinus. Note the density shape and size of these vessels by examining previous imaging and understanding anatomy in order to identify any pathological change. Following this, we begin by looking at the cerebellum and brain stem, in which we should be able to clearly identify symmetry with CSF spaces, with these being identical on both sides. It is important to take note of the foramen magnum and the cerebellum. You should be able to visualise CSF spaces in the foramen magnum and not see the cerebellum completely filling it. The fourth ventricle is also located within the cerebellum; however, it is also good practice to examine the ventricular system, as a whole, and follow it through the brain to identify pathology. At this stage, most structures have been evaluated, thus our critique turns to the skull, orbits, sinuses and mastoid air cells. The sinuses and mastoid air cells should be well aerated with air demonstrated as black and represented with its according HU value; however, CT head scans are not the correct imaging for these structures if pathology is specifically queried in these regions instead specialist protocols should be used. The skull should be viewed on bony windowing, which may demonstrate fractures or lesions, appearing lytic or dense. Caution should be made to demarcate skull sutures with fractures. The orbits are not routinely scanned; however, if included, they should be examined for symmetry. The orbital globe should remain circular with the optic nerve visualised, superior ophthalmic vein, coupled with the rectus muscles. If one side is with observable difference, then this may indicate pathology.

When viewing a CT head scan, it is very important to note that pathologies are best visualised under their according windowing techniques. For instance, skull pathology – bony windowing (W2500, C480); stroke windowing (W40, C40), haemorrhage (W170, C70), pneumocephalus (air in the cranial cavity) lung window (W1500, C-500). Pathologies that may occur within the brain are vast and remain outside the scope of this chapter, however, some of the more common pathologies will be explained. These include haemorrhages, strokes, space-occupying lesions, obstructive hydrocephalus, aneurysms, skull fractures and atrophic changes. Upon deciphering brain pathology, it can be difficult to assess the pathology based on the clinical symptoms alone. The reasoning behind this is that regardless of the pathology observed within the brain, the patient's symptoms depend on the location within the brain and how it interacts with it. Some of the effects of underlying brain pathology reflect midline shift and effacement/mass effect of surrounding structures; hydrocephalus and cerebellar tonsil herniation into the foramen magnum coupled with oedema may also be present. When reporting head scans if pathology is observed, the abovementioned should be explored with appropriate commentary in order to help dictate treatment for the patient/outcome (Xiao et al., 2010). For instance, if cerebral oedema is caused by a space-occupying lesion, then steroids will be prescribed in the short term to reduce oedema and help relieve symptoms prior to further treatment being planned. It is also important to describe pathology by explaining the structure, for example, irregular shaped or density – hyperdense (brighter than surrounding brain tissue); isodense (same density as surrounding brain tissue) and hypodense (darker than surrounding brain tissue). If pathology has been detected, it is important not to presume another pathology is not present in order for the 'satisfaction of search' to be complete (Ashman et al., 2000). A pertinent question should always be asked: Am I happy that no more pathology is identified on the scan and have I looked at all structures adequately?

WRITING A REPORT

Each practitioner will have a different approach to writing their report. From experience, some will write short reports mentioning only key findings, e.g. 'No intracranial/extra-axial haemorrhage, no space-occupying lesion, no acute infarction. No acute findings.' Other reports may demonstrate greater detail describing individual structures, e.g. 'The ventricular system is of normal morphology. The cisterns, sulci and ventricles are clear. Grey white matter differentiation is preserved.' When writing a report, it is important to consider whether the clinical question has been answered. Can this question be answered on CT alone? If, for example, CT is not adequate in detecting a certain pathology should another imaging modality be considered? Next, the report should identify whether the scan is normal or whether there are abnormal findings. These findings may be unsuspected. The reporter must also be clear with their wording in order to prevent confusion with practitioners reading the report. It is important to remember that this remains a legal document, thus central to communicate findings in a way that helps limit misinterpretation. If pathology is demonstrated, describing its appearance is pivotal in order to help provide a firm diagnosis for the patient. In some cases, a differential diagnosis may be offered, if you feel it is relevant. It is important, however, to ensure the report does not become ambiguous, leading to further confusion. If urgent findings are identified, highlighting the need for a specialist referral is important to document and is often stated at the end of the report (or conclusion). The reporter should consider immediately communicating with the clinician or department and inform them of findings if deemed urgent. If the report is unusually too extensive, in light of observed pathology, it is often helpful to offer a condensed conclusion with key points highlighted. This may prevent clinicians or other healthcare professionals from overlooking key information in what may be deemed 'a lengthy report'.

RADIOLOGICAL ERRORS

Errors are not uncommon within radiology, yet, the reduction of errors remains of great importance in relation with associated morbidity and potential preventability (Croskerry, 2003). Within medicine, there are three major types of error: no-fault errors, system errors and cognitive errors (Graber et al., 2002). Cognitive errors are one of the most common errors seen in reporting which result in faulty data collection or interpretation (Graber et al., 2002). These errors often arise from such issues as failures in perception, poor technique, misjudgement and/or lack of knowledge (Robinson, 1997). Failures in poor technique and lack of knowledge can be improved with search strategies and further education in pathologies and appearance. One area in relation to perception and misjudgement is the use of (or lack of) clinical information, previous imagining and previous reports. A study by Leslie et al. (2000) found that correct clinical information improved the radiology report with inaccurate information detrimental to the accuracy of the overall report. The Royal College of Radiologists (RCR) accept that doctors, including radiologists, make errors, but effective processes should be in place to ensure errors are not only identified, but recurrent errors addressed.

HAEMORRHAGES

Haemorrhages can be described as blood, be it fresh (acute), or remnants of old blood (chronic) within the skull. This may present as intra-axial, subdural or within subarachnoid. When reporting, it is imperative that the location of the haemorrhage is described alongside other features including its size and density. Causes of haemorrhage can be vast, perhaps due to trauma, hypertensive haemorrhagic strokes and burst aneurysms. Acute haemorrhages on CT will appear hyperdense (bright) with a respective HU of 50–80 (Grumme et al., 1998, p. 94). The older the haemorrhage, the darker and less dense (hypodense) it appears. The appearance should always be described as it can help inform treatment and management of the patient. Different types of traumatic haemorrhages include extradural, subdural, intracranial, contusions and subarachnoid haemorrhage (SAH). A patient may present with either one of the abovementioned, or in some cases, all at the same time.

Intra-axial Haemorrhage

This type of haemorrhage is, by definition, a bleed within the brain itself. These can be caused by many factors, such as trauma, hypertension and vascular malformations. They will appear hyperdense to surrounding brain tissue in the acute phase and can vary in size. The larger the area of the bleed, the more impact it will have on the brain with regard to mass effect, midline shift and effacement of surrounding structures, thus causing an increased morbidity risk (Emre Kumral et al., 1995). Often, surrounding oedema can also be visualised around the bleed, highlighting a slightly hypodense region.

Extradural Haemorrhage

An extradural haemorrhage is a collection of blood between the inner surface of the skull and outer layer of the dura called the endosteal layer. These types of injuries are associated most commonly with direct trauma to a specific point of the skull. Often, these types of haemorrhages will contain an underlying skull fracture, so bony review remains paramount. In most cases, these types of haemorrhages are bi-convex in shape and will appear hyperdense in the acute phase moving towards isodense subacute and hypodense in the chronic phase.

Subdural

A subdural haemorrhage/collection is an accumulation of blood (acute/subacute/chronic) or other fluid that accumulates within the subdural space between the dura and arachnoid mater of the meninges. They often present unilateral, however, have been observed bilaterally, affecting the falx and tentorium. They may also be shallow in appearance, thus subdural windowing remains beneficial. In the acute phase, subdural haemorrhages appear as a homogenously hyperdense crescent shape with extra-axial collection. They may differ in size and may also cause mass effect, midline shift and effacement of surrounding structures. In some cases, they are observed to contain mixed densities, both hyperdense and hypodense, which is often termed 'acute on chronic'. As the subdural haemorrhage ages, it becomes increasingly isodense, which is termed subacute (Runge et al., 2015, pp. 40–41). Following this, a subdural haemorrhage will become chronic in nature and appear hypodense. These phases of subdural bleeds can differ in size, presenting, unilaterally or bilaterally and have similar effects on the brain, including mass effect, effacement of surrounding structures and midline shift. It is also important to note that subdural collections can be of mixed density indicating the presence of acute blood.

Subarachnoid Haemorrhage (SAH)

A SAH is the presence of blood within the subarachnoid space. Common symptoms include a 'thunderclap headache', sudden onset of headache that is often described as 'the worst headache of the patient's life'. Causes can be due to many factors. The common cause is a ruptured berry aneurysm. Other causes include, but are not limited to, trauma, arteriovenous malformations, cerebral amyloid angiopathy and venous infarction. The sensitivity for SAH using CT depends on the amount of blood present within the subarachnoid spaces at the time of scanning. A lumbar puncture may be performed to look for the presence of blood within the CSF if a head scan is reported normal. Provided no other contraindications are demonstrated, such as cerebellar tonsil herniation, the appearance of a SAH will appear hyperdense, filling subarachnoid structures within the brain. With burst aneurysms being one of the most common causes, they are often identified around the circle of Willis or within the sylvian fissure region. Treatment and prognosis are dependent on the cause of the SAH and severity. With all of the abovementioned haemorrhages, it is important to note that multiple types of haemorrhages can be detected on the same scan.

STROKES

Strokes are a clinical diagnosis resulting in neurological deficit with presumed vascular origin (Kanekar et al., 2012, p. 63). They can be subdivided into 'haemorrhagic' and 'ischaemic' strokes. The former is often caused by reasons such as uncontrolled hypertension, cerebral amyloid angiopathy, or perhaps an underlying lesion such as vascular malformation. A study by Miller et al. (2004) found that in America more than 60% of patients with acute stroke had an elevated blood pressure on initial examination in A&E. The latter are most common types identified clinically and have various appearances. In the acute setting, patients with suspect strokes are predominantly imaged using CT in response to the often accessibility and safety issues arising from MRI, in particular with patients whose clinical history is, perhaps, not fully understood. That said, MRI is highly sensitive, and with the variability of imaging sequences, it identifies hyperacute ischaemic infarcts extremely well. In CT, a non-contrast examination will be performed followed by a CT angiogram of both carotids and circle of Willis (CTA). The benefit of a CTA is that the clinicians will be able to fully visualise the occluded arteries (Lev et al., 2012, p. 1). Some centres may choose to undertake a CT perfusion examination, seeking to identify brain tissue that has not been permanently damaged. This type of study is useful when determining if thrombolysis treatment remains useful following an unknown time of onset. Haemorrhagic strokes are similar in appearance to intra-axial haemorrhages. They can be of any size with acute findings demonstrating hyperdensities, coincided with mild surrounding oedema. The more chronic (or older) the haemorrhage becomes, it will naturally alter its appearance to isodense and, lastly, hypodense. Ischaemic infarcts can be classified into three phases – hyperacute/acute, subacute and chronic.

Hyperacute/Acute Phase

At this stage, it is important to note that a CT head scan may look normal in appearance. This does not mean an ischaemic infarct is not present but likely too early to detect on initial CT imaging. In these instances, clinical correlation alongside other imaging such as CT angiography, CT perfusion or even MRI will be used. It is important to note that MRI Diffusion Weighted Imaging (DWI) alongside Apparent Diffusion Coefficient is highly sensitive to hyperacute ischaemic changes and is visualised as high signal intensity on DWI (Runge et al., 2015). This phase usually occurs within the first few hours from initial onset of symptoms. Typical appearances in the hyperacute/acute phase are hyperdense vessels, e.g. hyperdense middle cerebral artery (MCA) and hyperdense basilar artery (Grumme et al., 1998). It can, however, be difficult to notice hyperdense vessels in the abovementioned scenario as they appear slightly hyperdense in normal findings so accurate/adequate clinical information is imperative. However, sound clinical information and history, such as location of limb weakness, can help enhance the diagnostic accuracy. For example, if a patient came in with left-sided weakness and radiologically presented with a right hyperdense MCA in relation to the other vessels, this would be a good indicator of a hyperacute/acute infarction. If the reporter was still unsure, the HU of the vessel in question could be measured against other vessels within the brain at a similar level. What should be demonstrated is the HU of the affected vessel to be minimally increased compared to unaffected vessels. Other appearances reside in the subtle loss of grey/white matter differentiation, effacement of brain structures such as sulci, insular ribbon, lentiform nucleus and sylvian fissure. Hypodense wedge-shaped areas can also correspond with vascular territory involved. In summary, within this acute phase, the vascular vessels should be thoroughly scrutinised, paying attention to densities and appearance of these vessels. Further to this, stroke window techniques should be used to look for loss of differentiation to normal brain tissue, however, subtle, support correlations with clinical information provided.

Subacute Phase

This phase corresponds to 24–48 hours of affected brain tissue and accordingly corresponds to the vascular territory, which starts to become visible and hypodense in appearance. It will generally be easier to visualise on plain CT.

Chronic Stage

This final stage will occur over a period of months post insult. Appearances of chronic infarcts will be consistent with well-defined regions of hypodensity, similar to CSF in appearance. A term commonly used for such regions is encephalomalacia irrespective of it being originally haemorrhagic or ischaemic.

BRAIN TUMOURS

A large number of space-occupying lesions can occur within the brain and it is outside the scope of this chapter to describe them all. For this reason, some of the most common brain tumours in adults are discussed, notably meningioma, glioma and cerebral metastases. It is important to note that whilst some brain tumours have improved prognosis than others, all brain tumours are potentially life-threatening. By the time a patient presents with symptoms, the mass has already occupied a sufficient amount of space within the skull vault and occupied a large volume of brain tissue.

Meningioma

A meningioma is a primary brain tumour and is often classified as the second most common space occupying lesion. They arise from within the arachnoid cells of the meninges and nerve roots. Because of this, they are, by definition extra-axial lesions, not intra-axial. They can be found near dural surfaces such as frontal, parietal, cerebellopontine angle and falx cerebri (Lockwood, 2011). This type of lesion is not malignant and has a slow growth, with improved prognosis for patients. Due to the slow growth rate, patients often present with these lesions later in life. Typical appearances include a well-defined extra-axial dome-shaped lesion with a hypo-iso dense appearance. They often have calcification within it. Following intravenous contrast, it should be enhanced and appear hyperdense. Depending on the size of the lesion, they may cause mass effect, effacement of surrounding structures and midline shift.

Glioma

These lesions are a type of brain tumour made up from the glial cells. Gliomas often account for 50% of adult brain tumours. There are different groups of gliomas such as astrocytoma, ependyomas, oligodendrogliomas and mixed gliomas. These types of lesions are often aggressive with poor prognosis for patients. Lesions are highly vascular, hence need for intravenous contrast in order to show hyperdense enhancement with uneven shaped ring with a hypodense centre (Lockwood, 2011). Often surrounding oedema will be present with mass effect depending on the size of the lesion.

Metastatic Tumours

Metastatic brain tumours are a common finding and most common when compared with brain tumours. Tumours commonly known to metastasise to the brain involve the lung, breast, colon, melanoma and kidney (Hayat, 2014). The most common route for metastatic spreads via the vascular system. Often, these types of lesions present within the brain as multiple lesions, however, they can also be large solitary lesions that vary from iso–hypodense in appearance. Most commonly, they show ring enhancement following intravenous contrast. They can have a hypodense centre with surrounding oedema and can become haemorrhagic with bony invasion/erosion present. When haemorrhagic, these lesions will show higher density on the unenhanced scan (Naidich et al., 2013). Prior to intravenous contrast, larger lesions may only be identifiable but following contrast multiple smaller lesions become visualised. It is important to have good clinical history when determining radiological features. If a patient with a known tumour elsewhere presents with these findings, it is likely these lesions are cerebral metastases. However, we must consider the differential diagnoses as often multiple pathologies will have similar appearances.

OBSTRUCTIVE HYDROCEPHALUS

Obstructive hydrocephalus is a term used to describe the build-up of CSF within the ventricular system at any particular point due to an obstructive cause (Corns and Martin, 2012, pp. 142–148), such as a congenital malformation or pathology within the brain which may be causing mass effect and compress or occluding aspects of the ventricles. The number of pathologies that cause this is profound, but remains an important consideration because, regardless of the pathology causing obstructive hydrocephalus, it should be identified for clinicians. The brain has limited space within the skull, thus concerns causing compression and according intracranial pressure are potentially life-threatening, requiring urgent attention. It is also important to note that some patients may have 'normal pressure' hydrocephalus and not be caused by obstructive pathology. The overproduction of CSF within the choroid plexus will lead to excessive enlargement of the ventricular system and thus should question whether this is obstructive hydrocephalus. This is perhaps easier to visualise if a patient, with a large brain tumour causing significant mass effect and midline shift, occludes the third ventricle and thus enlarging the lateral ventricles significantly.

ANEURYSMS

Aneurysms are often referred to as focal dilation of blood vessel walls. They vary in size and with the most commonly located in the circle of Willis, anterior cerebral artery, internal carotid artery, posterior cerebral artery, MCA and basilar artery. Often, if found incidentally and not of significant size, close monitoring will be applied. Aneurysms are at risk of rupturing and thus become problematic causing a SAH within the CSF spaces, intraventricular haemorrhage and intra-axial haemorrhage. Unruptured appearances will be iso–hypodense, often with calcification surrounding the wall of the aneurysm. Following intravenous contrast, it will demonstrate hyperdense enhancement, which can be followed via the normal vascular path. If ruptured, appearances appear hyperdense in the acute setting, as described earlier in relation to haemorrhages.

SKULL FRACTURES

Skull fractures are common findings in traumatic head injuries. Detecting a skull fracture using CT is an important marker denoting the severity of the head injury and often an indicator of other intracranial pathology. They can be visualised as fractures within the bone and can be displaced or undisplaced. It is important to recognise normal suture lines within the skull. They are best visualised under bony windowing with CT departments automatically reconstructing these at the time of scanning. When a skull fracture is demonstrated, it is important to review the data set under lung windowing to identify if air has entered the skull vault, commonly known as pneumocephalus. If air has entered the brain, bacteria may also enter, giving rise to the risk of infection.

CEREBRAL ATROPHY/AGEING OF THE BRAIN

As we age, our brain may best visualise this with a generalised prominence of the CSF structures, including the cisterns, ventricles and sulci. If prominence of these structures exists across the brain but does not appear to be correlated with specific regions of the brain or deemed unusual given the patients age, it is often termed as 'generalised involutional changes'. However, such changes can be more specific to key areas such as enlarged ventricles, frontal–temporal predominance and hypodensities within white matter (small vessel disease) to name a few. This can be symmetrical on both sides or specific to certain parts of the brain. It is important to describe these regions of interest by using the term 'atrophic change'. Some conditions closely linked with atrophy of the brain include dementia, Parkinson's, Binswanger disease and Huntington's chorea. Upon examination of a head scan, it is important to decide if there appears to be a generalised prominence of CSF spaces or atrophy. Atrophy within the brain alone is not sufficient enough information to diagnose the above-mentioned conditions and further tests alongside cognitive assessments are required. You should also consider any previous clinical history or current information provided as both alcohol and drug misuse can lead to atrophy of the brain.

Age-related changes are important as vascular cognitive impairment can be caused by cortical and subcortical infarcts and diffuse white matter injury related to small vessel disease (Banerjee et al., 2016). This can potentially explain to the clinician the cause of cognitive impairment as patients will not always present as acute strokes but rather sometime after the event. While they will explain the origin or any cognitive decline, patient management would not have changed significantly if at all.

CONCLUSION

This chapter has both described and evaluated the practice of a reporting radiographer specialising in CT imaging of the head. This chapter sought to provide insight into the clinical thinking and decision-making practiced by a reporting radiographer in the United Kingdom, a role generally not practiced elsewhere transnationally. Here, the premise has been to not only simply appreciate the value, knowledge and understanding of this clinical service but also hint at the celebratory components of reporting radiographers performing these tasks on a daily basis. We have also identified that making a firm diagnosis may not always be possible nor achievable, requiring support from other imaging modalities. This chapter has captured the uniqueness by which radiographers have 'moved on' from simply image acquisition in CT and clearly providing a reporting service that strives to enhance patient outcomes. Whilst this chapter has sought to capture this and provide insight for prospective reporting radiographers in CT, there is, perhaps, wider questions that stem from such works.

For instance, it would be insightful to gauge the practice of reporting itself in the clinical environment and how reporting radiographers in CT (or in general) are supported, appreciated or even celebrated for their work.

REFERENCES

Ashman, C. J., Yu, J. S. & Wolfman, D., 2000. Satisfaction of search in osteoradiology. *American Journal of Roentgenology*, 175(2), pp. 541–544.

Banerjee, G., Wilson, D., Jäger, H. R. & Werring, D. J., 2016. Novel imaging techniques in cerebral small vessel diseases and vascular cognitive impairment. *Biochimica et Biophysica Acta*. doi:10.1016/j.bbadis.2015.12.010.

Corns, R. & Martin, A., 2012. *Hydrocephalus*, Surgery (Oxford), 30(3), pp. 142–148 [Online]. Available at: http://www.sciencedirect.com.chain.kent.ac.uk/science/article/pii/S0263931911002717(Accessed: 9th September 2015).

Croskerry, P., 2003. The importance of cognitive errors in diagnosis. *Academic Medicine*, 78(8), pp. 775–780.

Graber, M., Gordon, R. & Franklin, N., 2002. Reducing diagnostic errors in medicine: What's the goal? *Academic Medicine*, 77(10), pp. 981–922.

Grumme, T., Kluge, W., Kretzchmar, K. & Roesler, A., 1998. *Cerebral and Spinal Comupted Tomography*. 3 ed. Berlin: Blackwell Science.

Grumme, T., Kluge, W., Kretzschmar, K. & Roesler, A., 1998. Vascular diseases, in T. Grumme, W. Kluge, K. Kretzschmar & A. Roesler (eds.) *Cerebra and Spinal Computed Tomography*. Berlin: Blackwell Science, pp. 6–94.

Hayat, M. A., 2014. *Brain Metastases from Primary Tumors* Volume 1. 1 ed. London: Elsevier.

Kumral, E., Kocaer, T., Ertübey, N. Ö. & Kumral, K., 1995. Thalamic hemorrhage a prospective study of 100 patients. *Stroke*, 26(6), pp. 964–970 [Online]. Available at: http://stroke.ahajournals.org/content/26/6/964.full(Accessed: 9th September 2015).

Leslie, A., Jones, A. J. & Goddard, P. R., 2000. The influence of clinical information on the reporting of CT by radiologists. *The British Journal of Radiology*, 73(874), pp. 1052–1055.

Lev, M. H., Smith, W. S., Payabvash, S., Harris, G. J., Halpern, E. F., Koroshetz, W. J., Dillon, W. P., Furie, K. L., Goldmacher, G. V., Camargo, E. C. S. & González, R. G., 2012. Improved outcome prediction using CT angiography in addition to standard ischemic stroke assessment: Results from the stop stroke study. *PLoS One*, 7(1), pp. e30352 [Online]. Available at: http://dash.harvard.edu/bitstream/handle/1/9709719/3262833.pdf?sequence=1(Accessed: 06/09/2015). P1

Lockwood, P., 2011. *CT Head: Diagnosis A Radiographers Guide to Reporting - Part Two Chronic Pathologies*. UK: Createspace, pp. 86–114.

Miller, J., Kinni, H., Lewandowski, C., Nowak, R., Levy, P., 2014. Annals of emergency medicine. *Management of Hypertension in Stroke*, 64(3), pp. 248–255 [Online]. Available at: http://www.sciencedirect.com.chain.kent.ac.uk/science/article/pii/S0196064414001966(Accessed: 11th September 2015).

Naidich, T. P., Castillo, M., Cha, S. & Smirniotopoulos, J. G., 2013. Imaging of the brain: Elsevier inc., p. 54 (Christopher Paul Hess Derk D. Purcell).

Robinson, P. J., 1997. Radiology's Achilles' heel: Error and variation in the interpretation of the Röntgen image. *The British Institute of Radiology*, 70(839), pp. 1085–1098.

Sangam, G., Kanekar, T. Z. & Roller, R., 2012. Imaging of stroke: Part 2, pathophysiology at the molecular and cellular levels and corresponding imaging changes. *American Journal of Roentgenology*, 198(1), pp. 63–74 [Online]. Available at: http://www.ajronline.org/doi/abs/10.2214/AJR.10.7312 (Accessed: 06/09/2015). P1

The Royal College of Radiologists, 2008. Errors in radiology. [Online] Available at: https://www.rcr.ac.uk/audit/errors-radiology [Accessed 23 March 2016].

Val, M. R., Smoker, W. R. K. & Valavanis, A., 2015. Neuroradiology: The Essentials with MR and CT, Thieme Medical Publishers, p. 38, pp. 40–41.

Xiao, F., Liao, C.-C., Huang, K.-C., Chiang, I.-J., Wong, J.-M., 2010. Automated assessment of midline shift in head injury patients. *Clinical Neurology and Neurosurgery*, 112(9), pp. 785–790 [Online]. Available at: http://www.sciencedirect.com.chain.kent.ac.uk/science/article/pii/S0303846710001976(Accessed: 9th September 2015).

18 CT Thoracic Image Evaluation

Lynne Hazell
University of Johannesburg

CONTENTS

INTRODUCTION

The evaluation of the CT chest image is complex and all chest pathologies cannot be covered in this chapter. This chapter aims to provide the tools to enable the reader to apply the methods taught here to CT chest images. Pathology covered will be the more common of the chest pathologies.

The learning outcomes for the chapter would be

- understanding the application of a systematic approach to CT image evaluation for the CT chest and
- applying the systematic approach to common pathologies of the chest.

As has been outlined in the introduction to CT image interpretation, it is important to have a good anatomical knowledge of the structures. When carrying out image interpretation, a systematic method should be undertaken to ensure nothing is missed. The system chosen should be easy to implement and remember, and this is why the ABCDS acronym is often used (Chan, 2013).

DOI: 10.1201/9781003132554-24

When using an acronym, this is not the only systematic requirement. It is important to undertake your image evaluation by scanning the image in the same way for each aspect of the acronym. The method used to scan the image tends to be the reviewer's preference. For example, you could start at the top of the image and scan down or start at one lateral border and then cross to the opposite border or you could scan from one lateral border to the midline and then from the other lateral border to the midline. The method requires consistency rather than one size fits all.

CLINICAL HISTORY

In this chapter, individual cases will be presented and discussed. Each study will have a clinical history provided. All these cases are from clinical practices and the reports have been sourced, and therefore, the findings have been substantiated by a radiologist's report.

The clinical history is essential and no radiology examination should be undertaken without a clinical history. In addition, should contrast media be administered for the examination, it is important to have the appropriate laboratory results available to assess the risks and benefits of administering contrast media for the patient.

SYSTEMATIC REVIEW

Using the ABCDES System

Evaluating Adequacy of the image was discussed in the introduction chapter and will not be discussed in depth again in this chapter. The images are required to fulfil all the technical requirements of a radiology examination. The important aspects to consider are that the medico-legal requirements of an image are correct and they have been checked against the referral letter for patient identification before continuing with the assessment. The entire area of interest must be included in the scan. This would include the patients' position within the field of view and imaging from the thyroid to the upper abdomen using the correct scanning protocol

However, as a radiographer, you are aware not all images that require evaluation will be adequate. Patient movement is possibly the most obvious factor that cannot always be eliminated. In CT chest examinations, often a breath hold would be the optimum imaging technique; however, all patients will not be able to do this adequately particularly with underlying chest pathology. Thus, adequacy needs to be evaluated in the context of the patient condition and the risks and benefits of repeating images.

CT also provides the opportunity to reconstruct the images in different planes; therefore, if a patient has been scanned in the axial mode, reconstruction in the coronal and sagittal planes could assist in image interpretation. The other capabilities of CT are 3D reconstruction and the use of region of interest to analyse the type of tissue seen within the structure scanned. When performing image evaluation, it is important to consider different reconstructions available to assist with diagnosis.

The Airways should be assessed for patency and position observe the position of the trachea, which should be centrally located and consider whether there is any deviation from the norm. In Figure 18.1, the apices of the chest can be evaluated and the patency of the trachea is seen within normal limits. When assessing for patency, consider the aerated appearance: the trachea will be air filled and therefore black and the appearance of the walls of the trachea will be smooth and well defined. The position of the trachea is also seen centrally with no deviation.

Figure 18.2 is of the same patient as in Figure 18.1; the bronchi can now be assessed and the patency can be seen; and the left and right bronchi can be evaluated.

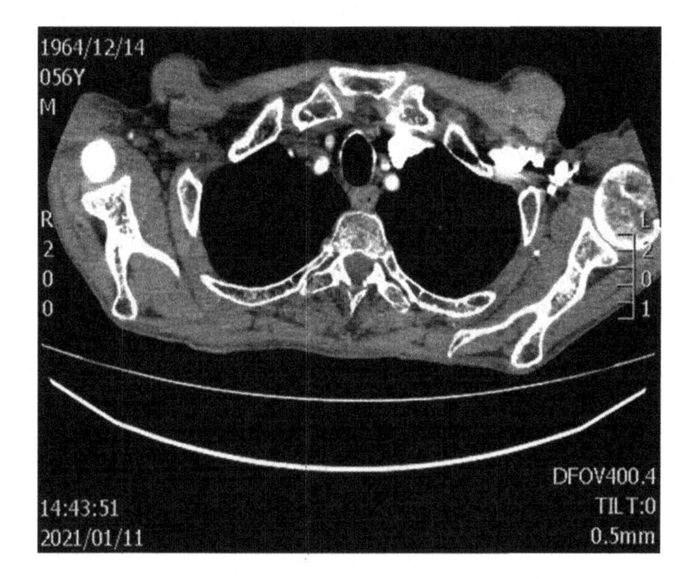

FIGURE 18.1 CT chest assesses airways.

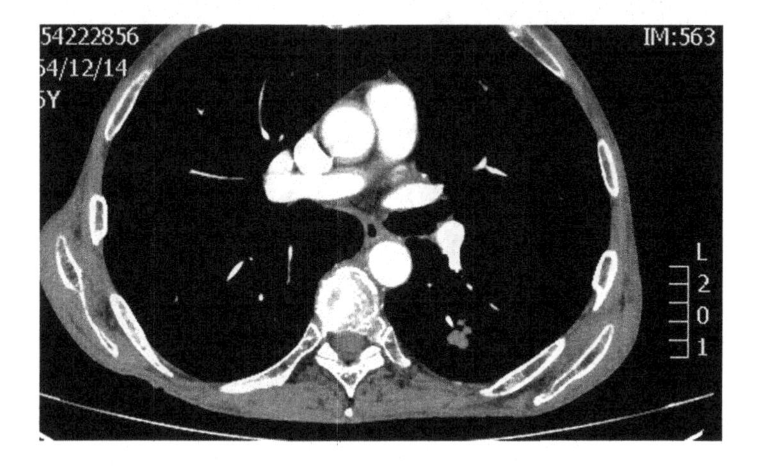

FIGURE 18.2 CT chest assesses airways.

The appearances should be well defined with no narrowing or deviation. The airways can be seen to be normal.

Assessing the airways looking at the images from the apices through the chest would be optimal to ensure the entire structure was evaluated. Consider scrolling through the images from the top to the bottom evaluating the airway in its entirety.

Returning to Figure 18.1 to consider breathing, the two lung fields should be assessed for any abnormalities. Symmetry of the lung fields should be considered in Figure 18.1 though the window levels are not that of the lung fields but of the mediastinum; however, lung fields may still be evaluated for symmetry, fluid and reticular patterns. To evaluate the septal changes, nodular patterns and consolidation, the window in Figures 18.1 and 18.2 is required. In Figure 18.1, the lung fields appear symmetrical and well inflated. In Figure 18.2, there is septal thickening seen in both lung fields and there is an asymmetrical appearance in the left posterior region of the left lower lobe. Systematically scanning the images from the apices enables the viewer to locate the pathology accurately within a specific lobe. Location is particularly important when describing abnormal patterns seen.

The Circulation is evaluated in Figures 18.2 and 18.3. In Figure 18.2, the aorta and major vessels are seen to be patent and normal in size. There are no filling defects or stenoses visualised and no aneurysms seen. In Figure 18.3, the heart is seen in the normal position and orientation. The cardiothoracic ratio is within the normal range and there is no pericardial effusion. The circulatory system for the patient has been evaluated and is seen to be normal.

Figure 18.4 demonstrates the lung bases, and there are no pleural effusions visualised and the lung bases appear normal. In Figure 18.4, the skeletal structures appear to have normal bone density with no fractures seen. In all images of Figures 18.1–18.4, there are no abnormal soft tissue appearances seen.

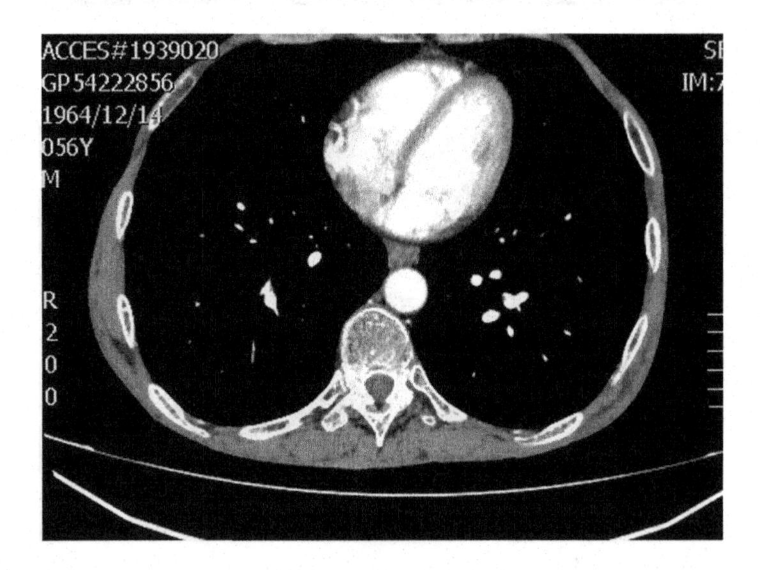

FIGURE 18.3 CT chest assesses the circulation.

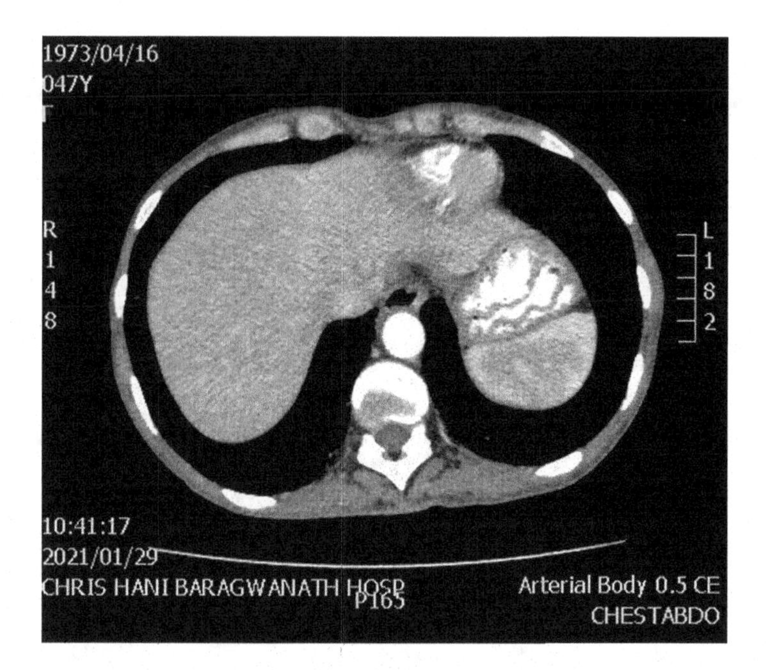

FIGURE 18.4 CT chest assess lung bases.

These images are important to provide the patterns for which further evaluations can be made against. As previously stated, it is necessary to have the normal patterns as pictures to compare and assess whether there are abnormalities present.

EMPHYSEMA

Emphysema is the distension of the airspaces and the destruction of the alveolar walls with associated obstruction of small airways (Eisenberg & Johnson, 2020). On CT, this is characterised by bullae formation with destruction of the lung parenchyma.

A patient was referred for a CT pulmonary angiogram (CTPA) and a high-resolution CT (HRCT) chest. The clinical history was a 73-year-old male with a 40 pack a year smoking history. The patient has shortness of breath and a new onset of rapid atrial flutter. He was COVID negative and was seen in January 2021. The patient has been a smoker over an extended time period, and therefore, the correlation between emphysema and smoking is well documented. The CT examinations are justified for a patient with this history. The patient should provide informed consent and the laboratory results should be assessed before the contrast media is administered as a CTPA was requested.

The images in Figure 18.5 and of the HRCT have been taken on inspiration unenhanced CT which is recommended for Chronic Obstructive Airways Disease (COPD) (Lynch et al., 2015). The CT imaging is adequate; the patient has held their breath for full inspiration during the scan and the anatomy is visualised.

The airways are evaluated, the trachea is seen in a central position and the main bronchi are patent if slightly narrowed. For the breathing, the lung fields appear

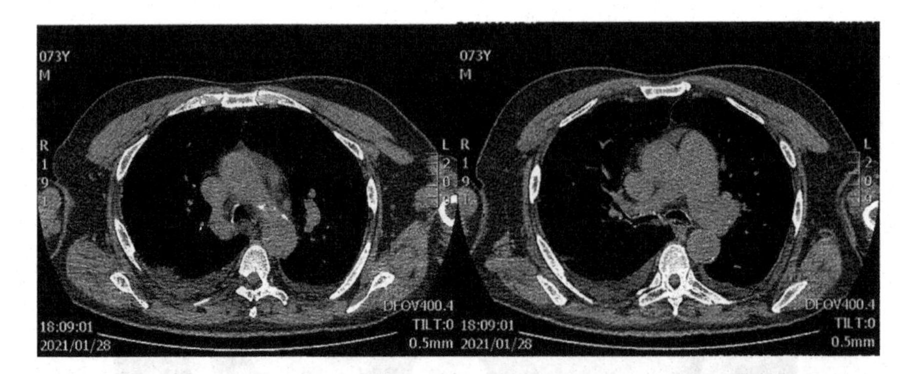

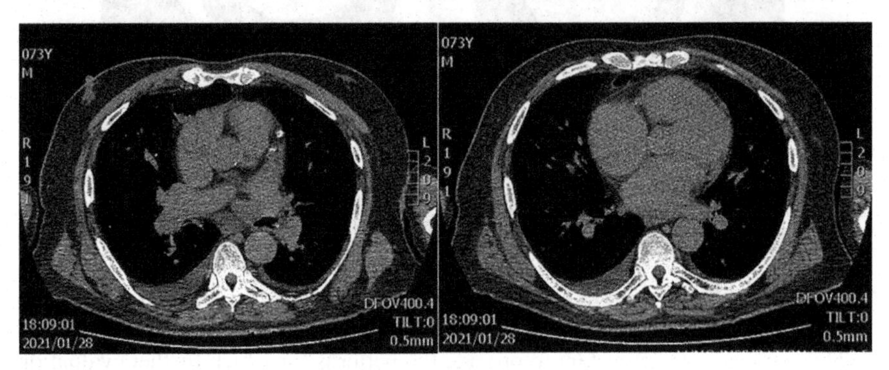

FIGURE 18.5 73-year-old male with COPD.

symmetrical, but are overinflated. When observing the lung fields, the anterior–posterior diameter appears increased. This could be attributed to COPD (Gupta et al., 2011). There is septal thickening indicating paraseptal emphysema and this occurs predominantly in the central area. There are small pleural effusions seen bilaterally and the right is slightly larger. CT is more sensitive for small pleural effusions than plain radiography as a small amount of fluid can be seen, whereas on a chest X-ray there would need to be excess of 250 mL/s of fluid for a pleural effusion to be visualised.

There are small calcifications seen in the first image in Figure 18.5; these are scattered granulomas and are probably an indication of previous resolved infection. In the third image, calcifications are again seen and these are calcifications of the coronary arteries. There is cardiomegaly seen in this patient and there is some dilation of the pulmonary artery.

The skeletal evaluation should observe all images to provide an overall interpretation. The ribs, scapula and sternum appear normal. The thoracic spine has the appearance of a scoliosis and degenerative changes, which would be in keeping with the age of the patient. There are no bony lesions seen. Figure 18.6 demonstrates a patient with bullae with underlying emphysema. Bulla are found most commonly in the apices of the lungs as seen here more predominantly in the right apical region. The term bulla refers to a focal region of emphysema over 1–2 cm. Something smaller

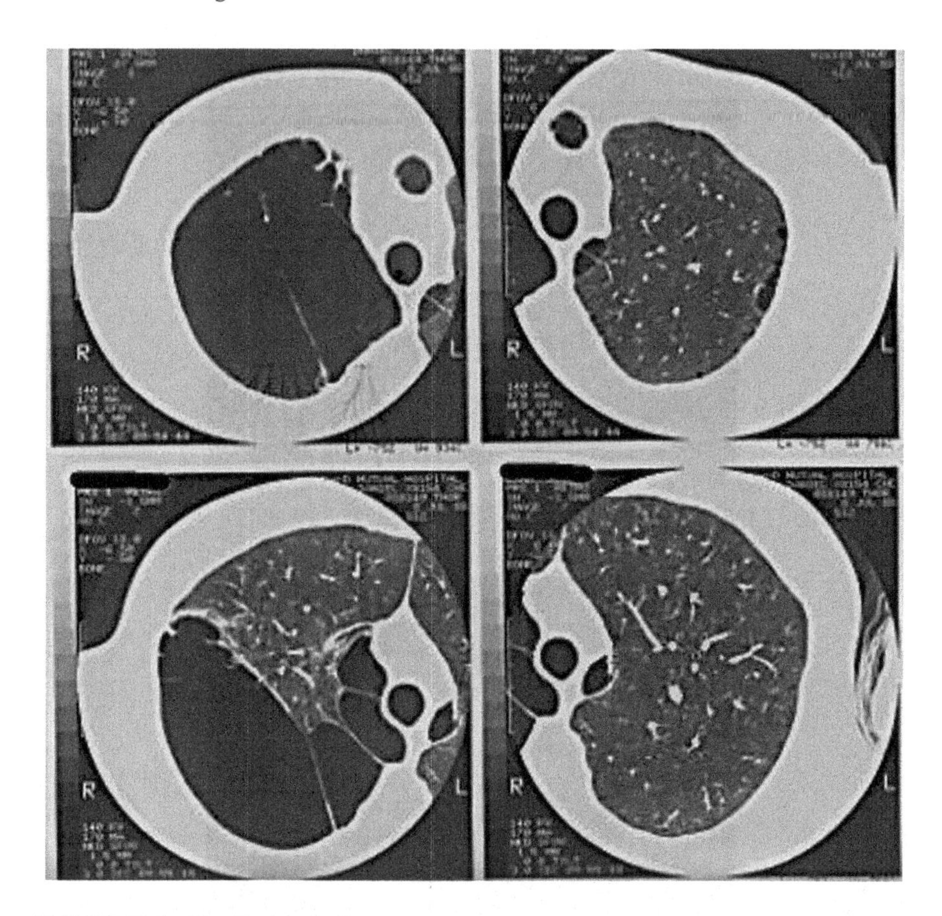

FIGURE 18.6 Emphysema bullae.

may be referred to as a pulmonary bleb which can be seen in the left lung. Sometimes when evaluating an image, it could be difficult to differentiate between a bulla and a pneumothorax (Aramini, Ruggiero, Stefani, and Morandi, 2019).

PULMONARY EMBOLISM

A pulmonary embolism (PE) is potentially a fatal condition, and therefore, recognition of an embolism and fast efficient treatment is essential (Eisenberg & Johnson, 2020). A CTPA Scan has become the examination of choice to detect a PE (Marchiori, 2014). The PE may be visualised either as a filling defect or a cut-off illustrating complete obstruction of the pulmonary vessel.

The following patient was referred for a CTPA in January 2021. The clinical history stated the patient was a 65-year-old female. The patient was Retro Virus Disease reactive, hypertensive and COVID negative. She presented with chest pain and query PE. Her D-dimer results were >17.6 and this is suggestive of a deep vein thrombosis.

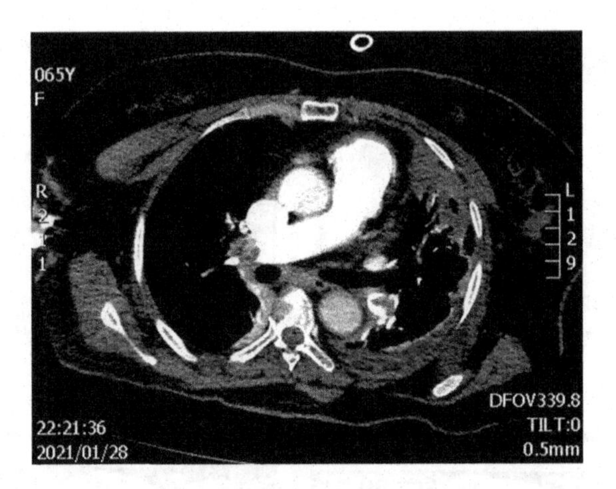

FIGURE 18.7 Pulmonary embolism: a filling defect of the right pulmonary artery.

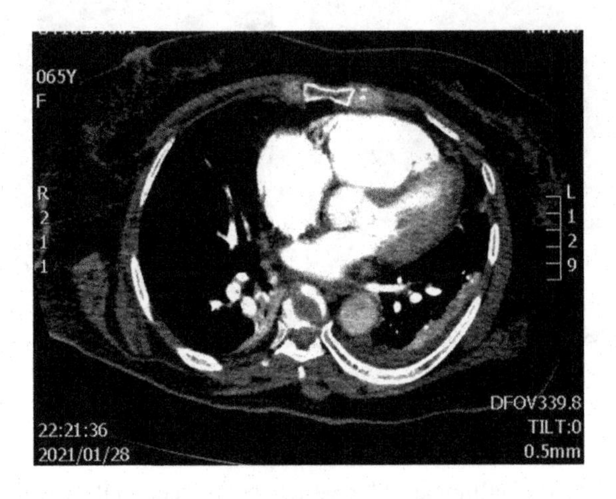

FIGURE 18.8 Right-sided heart failure: right atrial and ventricular enlargement.

The images for this patient are seen in Figures 18.6–18.8. The importance of a systematic evaluation of the images will be discussed. The adequacy of the images was acceptable and identification has been removed for publishing purposes. The anatomy of the thoracic cavity is well visualised with no movement unsharpness and all structures are included in the image.

For the evaluation of the airway, the right and left bronchi are visualised. The right bronchus is patent and round in appearance. The right main bronchus runs more vertical than the left, and therefore, the appearance is normal. The left main bronchus is also patent and can be seen running horizontally. Then, it follows with the evaluation of the breathing and the lung fields. There is a loss of symmetry between the right and left lungs. There is a loss of volume of the left lung in comparison with the right lung. On the periphery of the left lung, there are multiple wedge-shaped areas of consolidation possibly areas of infarction (Eisenberg & Johnson, 2020).

Pulmonary infarction is associated with pulmonary emboli and it is felt that this is more common in older patients with comorbidities, which would be supported by this patient's history (Eisenberg & Johnson, 2020). The patient also presented with chest pain which could be due to the areas of infarction as chest pain is rarely associated with PE. Most PE patients are asymptomatic (Eisenberg & Johnson, 2020).

In terms of circulation, in Figure 18.7, there is a low-density filling defect with an irregular appearance in the right pulmonary artery indicative of a PE (shown with the arrow). There is also a slight dilation of the pulmonary trunk seen. The aorta appears to have no filling defects or stenoses. If we now consider Figure 18.8, there is an enlargement of the right atrial and ventricular chambers in association with the cardiothoracic ratio being increased. The patient has right-sided heart failure and this is associated with pulmonary emboli due to the pulmonary hypertension (Eisenberg & Johnson, 2020).

As we consider the diaphragm, a collection of fluid can be seen on the posterior thoracic wall on the left lung. There is a left-sided pleural effusion. Pleural effusions are associated with a PE (Eisenberg & Johnson, 2020).

There are no extras seen in the patient. The skeletal structures all appear normal with no suspicious focal lesions and there are no soft tissue changes.

LUNG NEOPLASM AND PULMONARY METASTASES

Singular lesions found in the lungs can be difficult to evaluate whether they are benign or malignant (Eisenberg & Johnson, 2020). This is where age can aid in diagnosis; if the patient is under 30, then there is minimal risk of cancer if the lesion is solitary, well-defined and round; however, as age increases, so does the incidence of cancer (Eisenberg & Johnson, 2020). Once over the age of 50, the risk of the nodule being cancer increases to 50% (Eisenberg & Johnson, 2020). CT is then the best modality to assist in differentiating the nodule as it will provide the size and shape of the nodule and whether there are others possibly not seen on general radiography imaging. Also, it enables the assessment of other structures that may be affected by the lesion.

In Figure 18.9, the patient is a 56-year-old male and therefore in the more vulnerable population. The patient is a smoker, the patient had previous oral squamous cell carcinoma and completed surgery and radiotherapy and chemotherapy in 2019. The patient has returned in January 2021 with an asymptomatic lung mass previously seen on CT in June 2020. The mass is in the left lower lobe and the clinician is querying lung cancer.

The airways appear patent and the trachea is central. There is a small lesion in the upper lobe of the right lung measuring approximately 1.5 × 1.5 cm. The larger lesion is in the left lower lobe on the posterior aspect. The lesion appears lobulated and is 5.1 × 6.4 cm, and there is a slight increase in size since the previous CT scan. The lung fields have a ground glass appearance with some septal thickening. Ground glass is a term used when referring to increased diffuse lung opacities with a hazy appearance associated with inflammatory and infiltrative lung disorders (Infante et al., 2009). Ground glass appearances could be associated with malignant or benign pathologies (Infante et al., 2009).

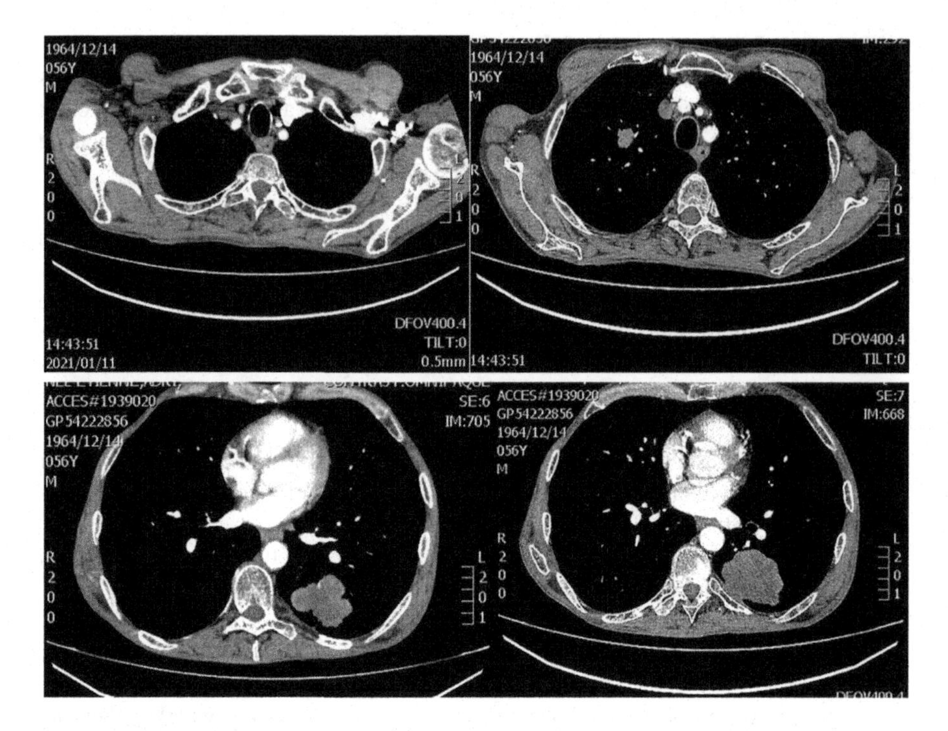

FIGURE 18.9 Lung lesions.

The circulation appears normal and the cardiothoracic ratio is within normal limits and the pulmonary vessels have no filling defects. The aorta is normal with no aneurysms or stenoses. There are some calcifications seen in the aorta. The skeletal structures have a generalised osteopaenic appearance. The density of the vertebra is decreased with the grey appearance rather than the white dense appearances normally seen, which can be observed in the other figures and cases. The bony trabecular pattern in the ribs is also demonstrating the thin cortices and expanded intertrabecular spaces associated with osteopaenia (Marchiori, 2014).

The increase in the size of the lesion may require further follow-up. The ground glass appearance on a CT chest has several differential diagnoses:

- Infectious processes;
- Chronic interstitial diseases and
- Acute alveolar diseases.

The osteopaenia may also require further consideration depending on the patient's symptoms. Pulmonary metastases occur in up to one-third of cancer patients and is often associated with breast, oesophagus or stomach cancer due to the close anatomical proximity (Marchiori, 2014). In the majority of cases, the metastases are confined to the lung fields. Hematogenous metastases will be seen throughout both lung fields and they will be multiple, well circumscribed and either round or oval in shape.

TUBERCULOSIS (TB)

Tuberculosis (TB) is caused by *Mycobacterium tuberculosis*. It is a rod-shaped bacterium, and the spread of the disease is by droplets in the air and a coughing patient will spread the disease by producing large numbers of bacteria dispersed into the atmosphere (Eisenberg & Johnson, 2020). Symptoms of TB are varied and diverse, and the most common would be productive cough, weight loss, haemoptysis, night sweats and fatigue (Nachiappan et al. 2017).

TB can have several appearances on CT: there may be enlarged hilar lymph nodes, and pleural effusions are often associated with primary TB, cavitation or abscess formation and fibrous changes and nodules (Nachiappan et al., 2017). Miliary TB would appear as multiple nodules and their distribution would be throughout both lung fields (Eisenberg & Johnson, 2020). HRCT is often the most relevant examination when looking for nodules related to military TB.

Lymphadenopathy would be seen in cases of primary pulmonary TB; when evaluating a CT scan, particular attention must be placed on the mediastinum to observe any lymph node enlargement. Also, it is important to look for the appearances of a unilateral pleural effusion seen in 25% of primary TB cases (Nachiappan et al., 2017). In active TB cases, the apical area and upper zones are the most common areas to see TB appearances such as cavitation and any distortion/deviation of the trachea.

An empyema can also be associated with TB. This is defined as pus in the pleural space (Eisenberg & Johnson, 2020). Initially, it may be difficult to distinguish an empyema from a pleural effusion. A CT will be able to differentiate between the empyema and the pleural effusion. A CT with contrast should be performed and possible imaging signs of an empyema would be pleural thickening (80%–100% of cases), pleural enhancement, bubbles where there is no chest tube and septation (Garvia & Paul, 2020).

Figure 18.10 is a HRCT of a 54-year-old male who had possibly been exposed to asbestos or dust and paint exposure and the clinician is querying post TB bronchiectasis.

The HRCT images demonstrate multiple cystic air spaces throughout both lung fields. There are also ground glass opacities bilaterally with the hazy and patchy appearances. There is an incidental finding of a right azygous lobe, which is important to recognise as a normal variant in the chest.

PLEURAL EFFUSION

A pleural effusion is the collection of fluid in the pleural space and it can be caused by many pathological conditions and is therefore non-specific (Marchiori, 2014:1186). The presence of pleural effusions in TB cases has been mentioned previously and this is often unilateral in such cases. Other common causes of pleural effusions are congestive heart disease, neoplastic disease and PE (Marchiori, 2014:1185). Pleural effusions can also be associated with abdominal pathologies such as ascites, subphrenic abscess and pancreatitis. They may also be associated with trauma.

The importance of CT when imaging pleural effusions is that a pleural effusion on conventional imaging may obscure other underlying pathology. A CT due to the

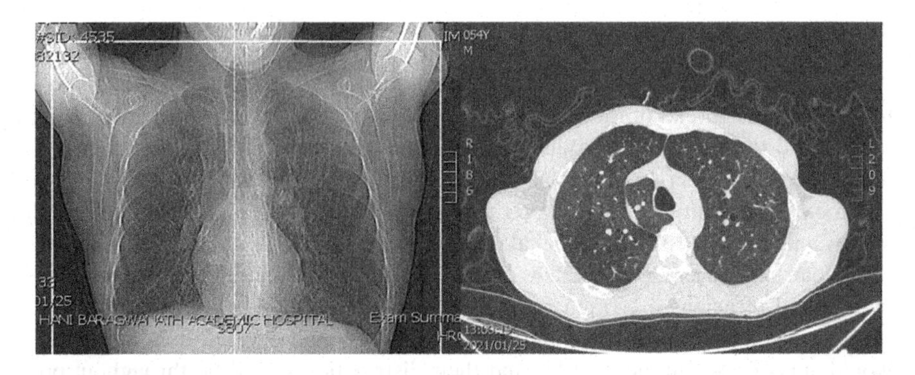

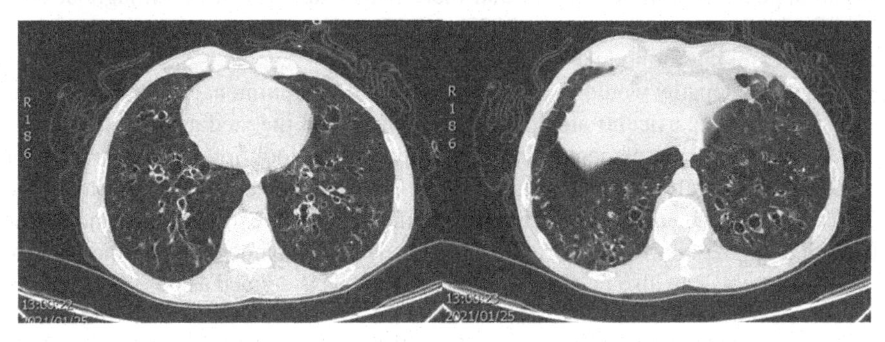

FIGURE 18.10 High-resolution CT chest.

ability to see the chest in different planes and reconstruct the images will identify any obscured pathology.

A 50-year-old male patient was in a pedestrian vehicle accident. The patient had bilateral tibia and fibula fractures, a haemopneumothorax with an intercostal drain inserted is present and the patient was in respiratory distress with chest pain. The CT findings indicate a large left pleural effusion with lower lobe collapse. A pericardial effusion and multiple fractures of the ribs, scapula and clavicle are seen in Figure 18.11. There is a comminuted fracture of the left scapula indicated with the arrows. There are also rib fractures on the left lateral aspect of the thorax the first, second, third and fourth ribs. Further drainage of the large effusion is indicated to relieve the pressure on the underlying lung.

PNEUMOTHORAX

Pneumothorax is the presence of air in the pleural cavity and can cause collapse of the lung either partially or total collapse (Marchiori, 2014:1238). Often a pneumothorax is associated with trauma or a procedure such as a biopsy may have caused the pneumothorax. However, pneumothorax may occur spontaneously in a patient and these patients are often young male patients (Marchiori, 2014:1238). The case shown in Figure 18.12 is a patient that has had trauma and has multiple rib fractures from the second to eighth ribs on the right side. The fractures are displaced and there is overlapping

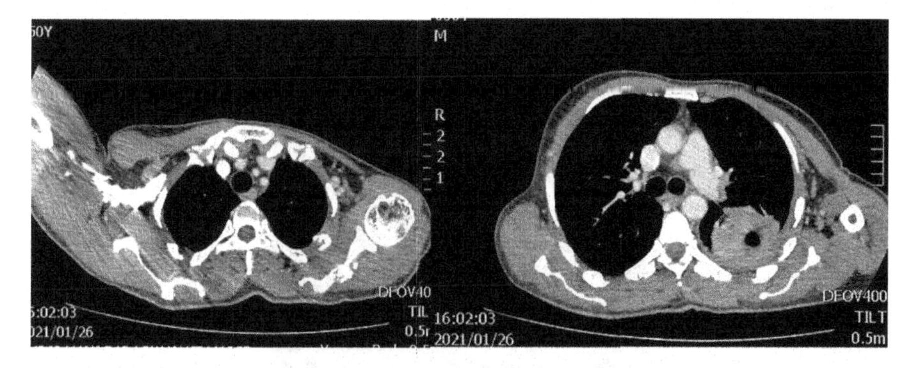

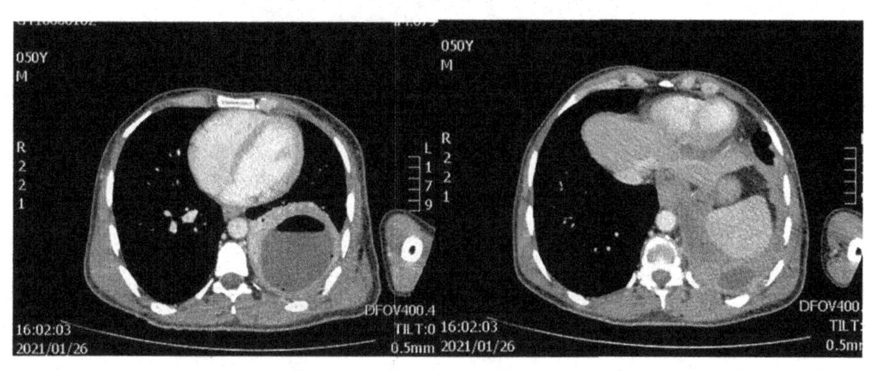

FIGURE 18.11 Trauma patient for CT chest.

of the fragments seen in image (a). Figure 18.12b demonstrates the right-sided anterior pneumothorax. There are no lung markings seen in the anterior space. There is a collapse of the right lung and then a collection of fluid in the posterior aspect. There is a large collection of fluid seen. The bronchi are seen and appear patent. There is an area of consolidation in the left lung on the posterior section of the lung field.

COVID-19

The coronavirus disease 19 is a novel coronavirus (Yao, 2020:2), the World Health Organization declared a Public Health Emergency of International Concern (PHEIC) on 30 January 2020 (https://www.who.int/emergencies/diseases/novel-coronavirus-2019/interactive-timeline). The first cases of COVID 19 were identified in the Wuhan province of China in December 2019 (Yao, 2020: 2), and as of April 2021, there are almost 3 million deaths worldwide. Radiology became an important diagnostic tool in the COVID-19 cases. In contrast with previous outbreaks such as the severe acute respiratory syndrome (SARS) where the chest radiograph was the imaging modality of choice, CT chest has been the modality most prevalent in COVID-19 cases (Ng et al., 2020).

A 62-year-old female patient was referred for a CTPA because she had an increased D-dimer test, she was COVID-19 positive and the clinician was querying

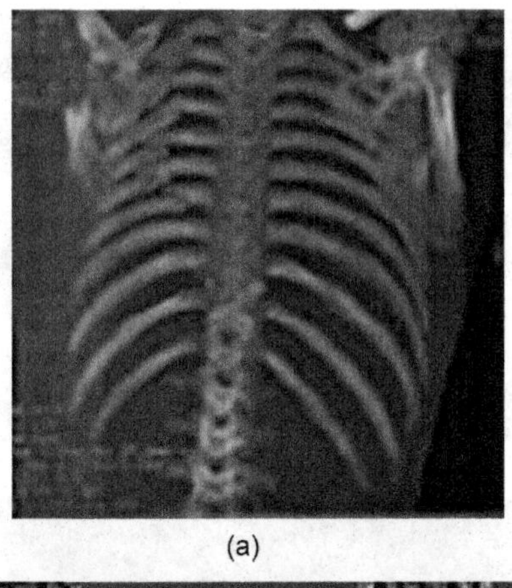

(a)

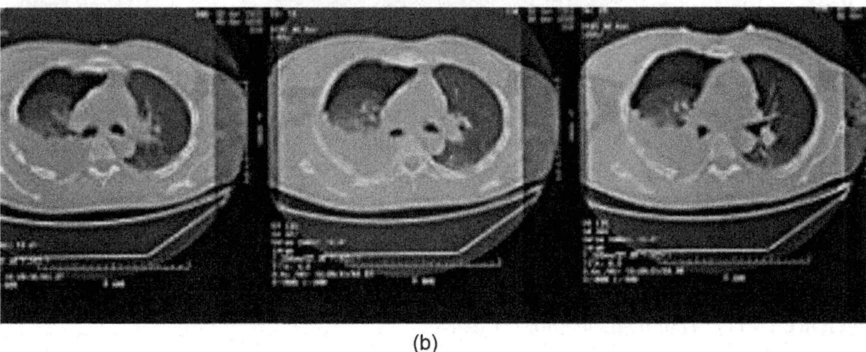

(b)

FIGURE 18.12 Pneumothorax: (a) 3D reconstruction of rib fractures and (b) axial CT chest of pneumothorax in the same patient.

fibrosis in the chest, post COVID-19 infection. A D-dimer test looks for D-dimer in blood; D-dimer is a protein fragment that's made when a blood clot dissolves in your body. Yao et al. (2020) found in their study that the elevated D-dimer levels are found in critical illness cases for COVID-19 and may be indicative of in-hospital mortality.

Figure 18.13 provides images from the CT scan, which demonstrate classic patterns of COVID-19 pneumonia. The airways were assessed and the trachea was patent and in a central position, and both bronchi were seen with no distortion.

The breathing was evaluated, and here, the typical bilateral multifocal opacities are seen with a reticular pattern. As can be seen in Figure 18.13, the abnormal patterns were seen located in the basal region of both lungs and the peripheral parts of the lungs. The right lung shows more involvement than the left, however, as mentioned previously, both lung fields are affected. The ground glass opacities are seen with the septal thickening and have formed denser areas of consolidation when they merge together (Infante et al., 2009).

The circulation was evaluated and there is an increased cardiothoracic ration seen. The thoracic aorta and major branches all appear normal. The pulmonary trunk is

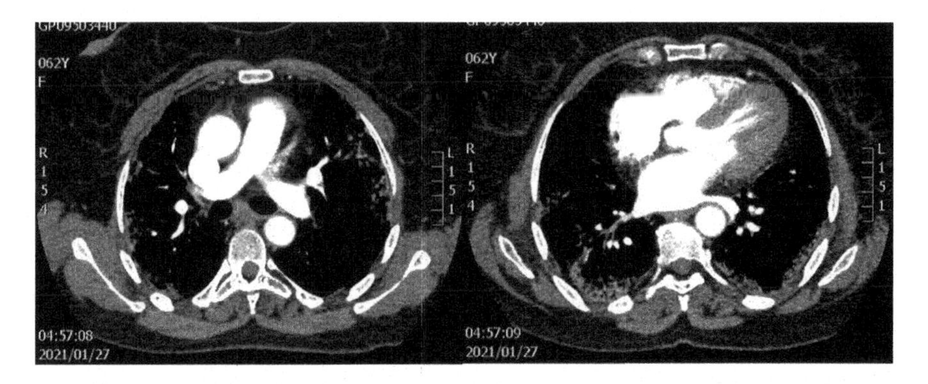

FIGURE 18.13 COVID-19 appearances.

also within normal limits with no filling defects visualised. The soft tissues appear normal and there are no skeletal abnormalities seen.

The CT demonstrates the bilateral, multifocal peripheral airspace opacities associated with COVID pneumonia (Parekh et al., 2020).

CONCLUSION

When evaluating a CT chest, it is important to always employ the same systematic method each time and ensure all regions of the thorax are assessed. Reconstruction of images to enable the visualisation of areas not well visualised or to confirm findings is an important factor in CT imaging. The findings are described in simple, clear terms and the location of an abnormality is always identified.

ACKNOWLEDGEMENT

I would like to thank the Radiology department at Chris Hani Baragwanath Academic Hospital for allowing me to use the anonymised CT images in this chapter and providing access to the reports on the images.

REFERENCES

Aramini, B. Ruggiero, C. Stefani, A. & Morandi, U. (2019). Giant bulla or pneumothorax: How to distinguish. *International Journal of Surgery Case Reports*. 62: 21–23.

Chan, O. (2013). *ABC of Emergency Radiology*. 3rd ed. BMJ Books.

Eisenberg, R.L. & Johnson, N.M. (2020). *Comprehensive Radiographic Pathology*. 7th ed. Mosby. St Louis, Missouri.

Garvia, V. & Paul, M. (2020). Empyema. StatPearls. Treasure Island (FL): StatPearls Publishing; Available from: https://www.ncbi.nlm.nih.gov/books/NBK459237/.

Gupta, N.K. Agrawal, R.K. Srivastav, A.B. & Ved, M.L. (2011). Echocardiographic evaluation of heart in chronic obstructive pulmonary disease and its co-relation with severity of disease. *Lung India*. 28: 105.

Infante et al. (2009). Differential diagnosis & management of focal ground-glass opacities. *European Respiratory Journal*. 33: 821–827.

Lynch et al. (2015). CT-definable subtypes of chronic obstructive pulmonary disease: A statement of the Fleischner society. *Radiology*. 277: 192–205.

Marchiori, D. (2014). *Clinical Imaging*. 3rd ed. MOSBY. St Louis, Missouri.

Nachiappan et al. (2017). Pulmonary tuberculosis: Role of radiology in diagnosis & management. *Radiographics*. 37: 52–72.

Ng et al. (2020). Imaging profile of the COVID 19 infection: Radiologic findings and literature review. *Radiology: Cardiothoracic Imaging*. 2: e200034.

Parekh, M., Donuru, A., Balasubramanya, R. & Kapur, S. (2020). Review of the chest CT differential diagnosis of ground glass opacities in the COVID era. *Radiology*. 297: E289–E302.

World Health Organization, (2020). Available from https://www.who.int/emergencies/diseases/novel-coronavirus-2019.

Yao et al. (2020). D-dimer as a biomarker for disease severity & mortality in COVID 19 patients: A case control study. *Journal of Intensive Care*. 8: 49.

19 CT Abdomen Image Evaluation

Lynne Hazell
University of Johannesburg

CONTENTS

INTRODUCTION

This chapter will consider the common pathologies seen on a CT Abdomen and the radiographic appearances. A systematic method should be used to ensure that the entire abdomen is evaluated. The abdomen requires an understanding of the abdominal organs, the bowel pattern and the skeletal structures of the abdomen. The objectives of this chapter are the following:

- Understand how to apply a systematic approach to image evaluation of the CT Abdomen;
- Understand the relationship of the organs and bowel in the CT Abdomen;
- Understand common pathologies and their appearances on a CT Abdomen.

CLINICAL HISTORY

A clinical history is always a requirement for any radiographic examination and one will be provided for the cases presented in this chapter. The cases presented have been reported on by a radiologist and the image evaluation in this chapter will be based on

DOI: 10.1201/9781003132554-25

the radiology report. Clinical history relevant to referral for CT Abdomen would be hypertension, jaundice, pancreatitis, cirrhosis, retroviral disease and ascites.

SYSTEMATIC METHOD

In line with the previous chapter, an ABCS method (Chan, 2013) will be incorporated when evaluating the CT images. The adequacy of the images should be established initially before undertaking the image interpretation. Adequacy has relevance to ensuring the area of interest has been included within both the field of view and in the entire abdominal cavity. This can be challenging with larger patients and those with a distended abdomen; as radiographers, we are required to ensure technically the image is adequate. The images used in this chapter have often been cropped due to the ethical requirement to remove any personal identification from the images. However, the size of the field of view for different patients is observed in the chapter.

When conducting a CT Abdomen and considering adequacy, the phases of contrast media observed need to be adequate to enable evaluation to take place. In one of the cases, the patient was given oral contrast media and then vomited as she was about to be scanned. The lack of oral contrast has a negative impact on the evaluation of the image as the position of the stomach and intestine cannot be assessed as it is not opacified. Any filling defects, wall thickening or masses will not be evaluated. If the intravenous contrast media is not captured in the correct phases, it will also impact image interpretation. The correct correlation between the phase and the normal blood flow is necessary for accurate interpretation. The comparison between a non-contrast, arterial and venous images is shown in Figure19.1. When providing an image evaluation, the ability to compare images is vital to identifying the pathology.

A – The anatomy and abdominal organs of the abdomen should be revised and the relationship of the organs to each other must be understood. In addition, the size and shape of the normal organs must be identified. The outline of normal organs will be smooth and well defined, and the loss of definition of the contour or a change in the shape needs further investigation. A change in the position of the organ should also be investigated. Thus, normal anatomy is essential for evaluation of the abdomen. In the context of the abdomen, the A will also consider air in the abdomen. Free air seen in the abdominal cavity is indicative of an abnormality.

B – This would evaluate air within the bowel and any air fluid levels seen that are normal or abnormal. Figure 19.2 demonstrates the normal fluid level seen in the stomach due to the patient being scanned in the supine position. There is also air seen within the large bowel indicative of a normal faecal pattern. Any abdominal distension should also be evaluated at this point.

C – Circulation and calcification would be assessed as C for the CT Abdomen. Circulation should evaluate the aorta, inferior vena cava (IVC) and the large vessels of the abdomen. They should be evaluated in terms of their calibre, any dilatation or narrowing which could be indicative of a filling defect or stenosis. The patency of the vessel would be assessed. Calcifications would be noted. For example, gall stones, renal and ureteric calculi or any calcification of the blood vessels.

Finally, **S** represents the soft tissue and the skeletal structures that should be evaluated.

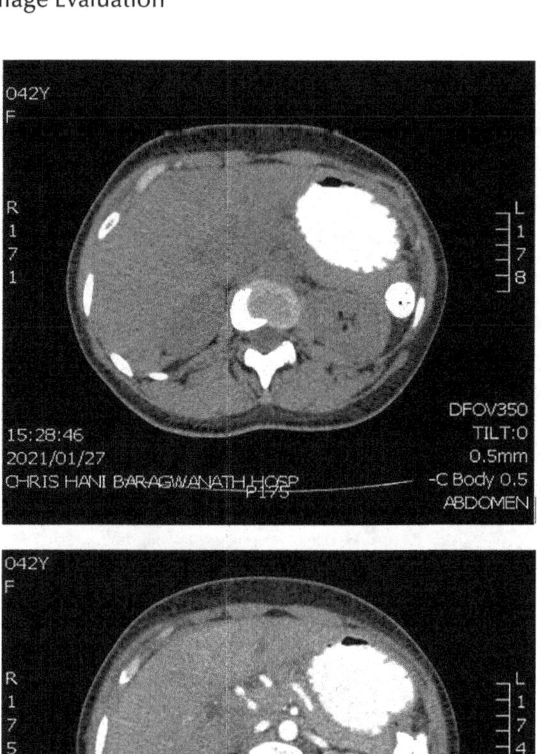

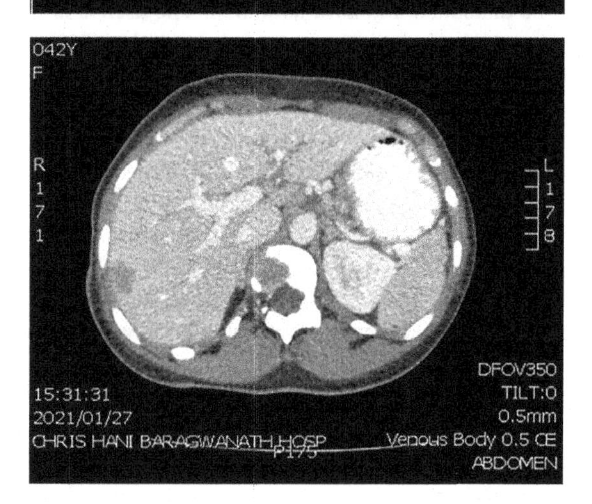

FIGURE 19.1 Demonstrating the phases of contrast enhancement during a CT Abdomen.

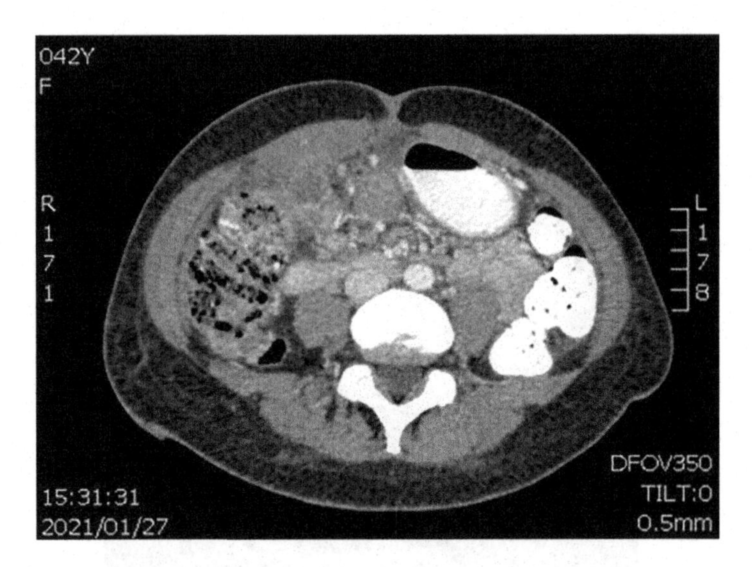

FIGURE 19.2 Air within the abdomen.

ASCITES

A 62-year-old male patient has hypertension and retroviral disease; he has been for ultrasound, and ascites was seen although there was no obvious pathology. The patient is referred for further imaging and a CT Abdomen was requested.

The patient had an unenhanced scan followed by a multiphasic contrast-enhanced CT imaging for the abdomen and pelvis. There was also oral contrast media given prior to the scan.

Ascites is the accumulation of fluid in the peritoneal cavity (Eisenberg & Johnson, 2020) and is easily visualised on CT Abdomen and ultrasound. The patient will often present with a distended and hard abdomen. The ascites is well demonstrated (Figure 19.3a). The abdominal distension can be noted and the fluid is encapsulated in this patient. The amount of fluid in this patient is large and complex. The Hounsfield unit for this area was 11 HU demonstrating a low attenuation value close to water/CSF.

In addition, the patient has bilateral pleural effusions. The one on the right is larger than the left (Figure 19.3b). On the right-hand side, it is also associated with atelectasis of the right lower lobe of the lung. Pleural effusion is a collection of fluid in the pleural cavity and can be associated with abdominal disease such as recent surgery, ascites, pancreatitis and subphrenic disease (Eisenberg & Johnson, 2020). The ascites was drained by paracentesis and the pleural effusions could be drained by a thoracentesis (Eisenberg & Johnson, 2020).

The liver appears normal (Figure 19.3c): there are no focal lesions seen and the parenchymal enhancement appears normal. It can be seen that the liver is displaced by the fluid in the abdomen, however, the liver has a smooth outline. The gall bladder has no evidence of calculi or distension of the ducts, and therefore, appears normal. The spleen can also be visualised with a smooth contour and is normal in size.

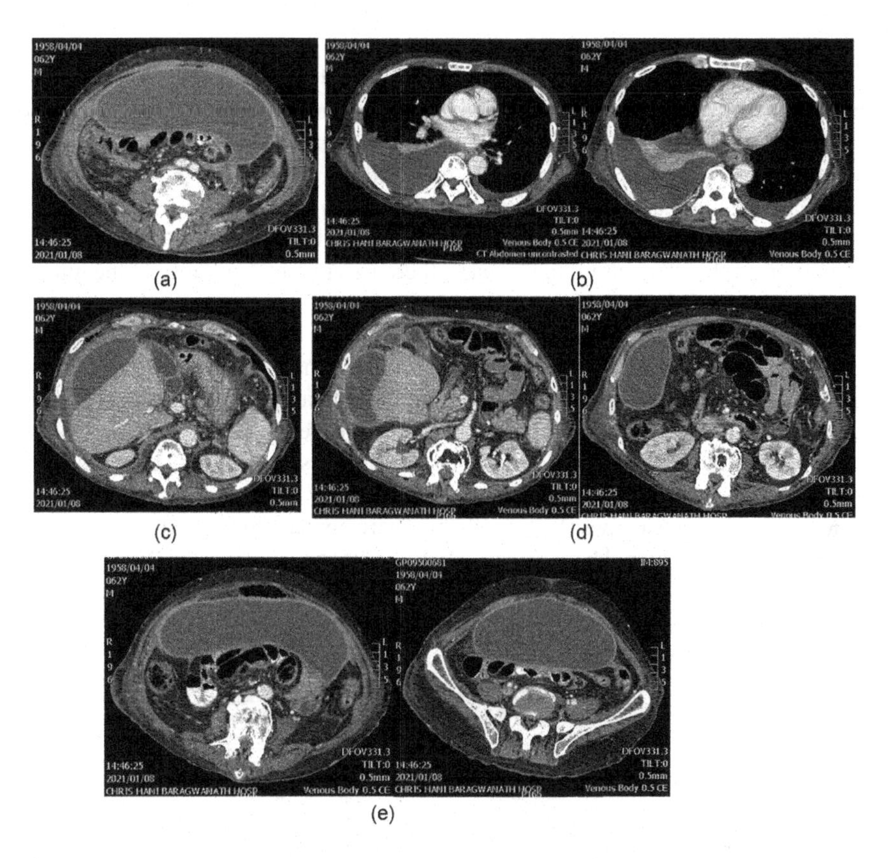

FIGURE 19.3 (a) Ascites, (b) pleural effusions and atelectasis, (c) liver, (d) kidneys and (e) encapsulated fluid.

The kidneys both have a smooth outline to them (Figure 19.3d), and there is normal cortical enhancement. There are no cysts or focal lesions seen. There is no evidence of hydronephrosis and the kidneys are excreting contrast media in a normal manner. There are no renal calculi seen.

The stomach, small and large intestine appear normal with no bowel wall thickening or masses visualised. The bladder is normally distended. The aorta, IVC and major branches are normal in size and they appear to have no filling defects or stenosis. The bony skeleton demonstrates chronic osteodegenerative changes with fusion of the lumbar vertebra (Figure 19.3e).

CHOLELITHIASIS

The patient is a 47-year-old female with severe acute pancreatitis. She also has respiratory dysfunction and an increased temperature. The patient has been referred for a CT Abdomen. An unenhanced scan was conducted followed by a multiphasic contrast-enhanced scan of the abdomen and pelvis. The patient was given oral contrast media before the examination, however, she vomited the contrast media before scanning, and therefore, there is no bowel opacification.

There are bilateral pleural effusions (Figure 19.4) which would explain the respiratory dysfunction noted in the clinical history. The right is larger being 51.4 mm and the left was 30.4 mm. There is associated atelectasis in the right and left lower lobes. Atelectasis is when there is incomplete air filling and when it is under expansion of the pulmonary tissue (Marchiori: 2014). It should be remembered that atelectasis is a radiographic sign that indicates another pathology. In the case of atelectasis, the air is not replaced by fluid, and therefore, results in total or partial collapse of the lung (Marchiori, 2014). Therefore, in this case, there is segmental collapse of the lungs on the right and the left sides.

The liver and spleen appear normal (Figure 19.4b). The kidneys also demonstrate normal size and contour with normal parenchymal enhancement. The pancreas does not have a normal appearance and there are multiple areas of hypoattenuation indicated by the yellow arrow. The pancreas appears to be ill-defined and there is fluid noted. The stomach, small and large intestine appears normal. With regard to calcifications, the gall bladder demonstrates multiple gallstones seen on two images indicated by the blue arrows (Figure 19.4b). There appears to be no thickening of the wall of the gall bladder. There are no renal or ureteric calculi seen. The circulation appears normal and there is no change in calibre or stenosis of the vessels. The soft tissue and skeletal structures appear normal.

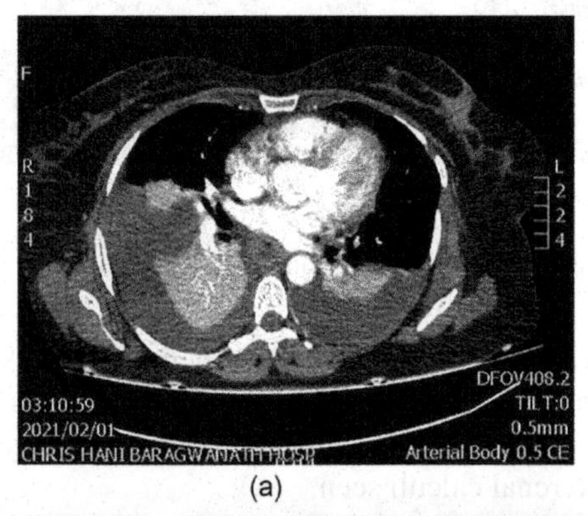

(a)

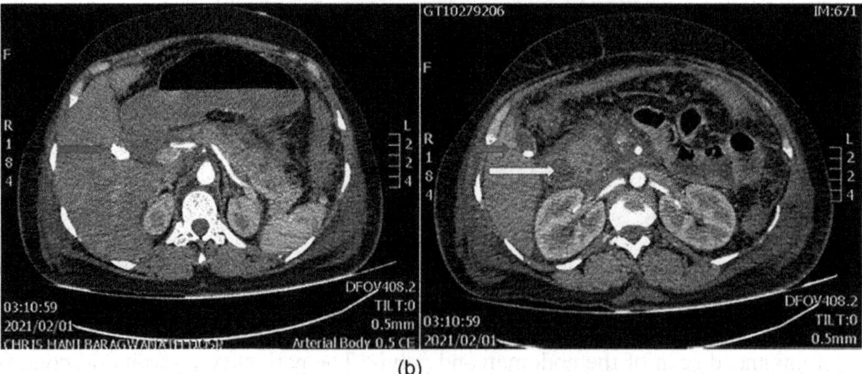

(b)

FIGURE 19.4 (a) Bilateral pleural effusions and (b) cholelithiasis,

HYDRONEPHROSIS

A 28-year-old female patient has been referred for a CT Abdomen. The patient is P3G4. This means that she has given birth three times to a foetus over 24 weeks and that she has been pregnant four times (https://teachmeobgyn.com/history-taking-examinations/history-taking/obstetric/). As a termination of pregnancy (TOP) is also indicated in the clinical history, this would correlate with the clinical history. The TOP was carried out at 12 weeks 4 days and the clinician is now querying for post-abortal sepsis and the patient has low blood pressure 94/53.

The liver demonstrates a normal parenchymal pattern. The right kidney demonstrates hydronephrosis with dilatation of both the major and minor calyces a Grade 2 hydronephrosis (Figure 19.5). The distal portion of the right ureter has been obstructed by the pelvic mass resulting in the hydronephrosis. Often for CT to demonstrate obstruction of the ureter by a renal calculus is not necessary to administer contrast media, however, in this case, with the history of TOP and possible uterine pathology, contrast media was required.

In a case where the ureter is obstructed, there may be delayed pelvicalyceal filling due to the elevated pressure created by the obstruction. The hydronephrosis was categorised as a Grade 2 hydronephrosis. There is a Radiology Grading System according to Onen et al. (2020):

Grade 1: Pelvic dilatation;

Grade 2: Calyces mildly dilated with renal pelvis dilatation;

Grade 3: Marked dilatation of the calyces;

Grade 4: Narrowing of the parenchyma;

Grade 5: Extreme hydronephrosis with thin membrane-like residual parenchymal rim.

There is a bulky uterus with a heterogeneously enhancing mass (Figure 19.5b). Due to the history of the patient, the intrauterine could be products of conception/lesion. The lesion is then causing the obstruction to the right ureter. The bones appear normal with no lytic or sclerotic lesions in keeping with a 28-year-old female. A second case of hydronephrosis is a 34-year-old male patient who has a history of alcohol abuse and has been binge drinking presents with cholestatic jaundice. The ultrasound demonstrated a moderate hydronephrosis of the right kidney. The patient is now referred for a CT intravenous pyelogram (IVP). Due to the history of the patient, an unenhanced and enhanced multiphasic scan was performed. A CT IVP is preferred to a conventional IVP as the other structures of the abdomen are included and assessed simultaneously. In addition, the relationship between the anatomical structures can be evaluated.

In Figure 19.6a, the liver can be seen and it is normal in size and there are no focal hepatic lesions seen. There were also no dilated intrahepatic bile ducts seen. The spleen also appears normal in size and shape.

The subsequent figures show a normal pancreas and gall bladder. There are no calculi seen in the gall bladder. The stomach, small and large bowel appears normal although no oral contrast media has been given to the patient. The aorta, IVC and major branches all appear of normal calibre and have no filling defects. The left kidney is 12 cm and has no renal calculi, obstruction; the ureter appears normal in calibre and flow (Figure 19.6b). The right kidney measures 10 cm. There is a

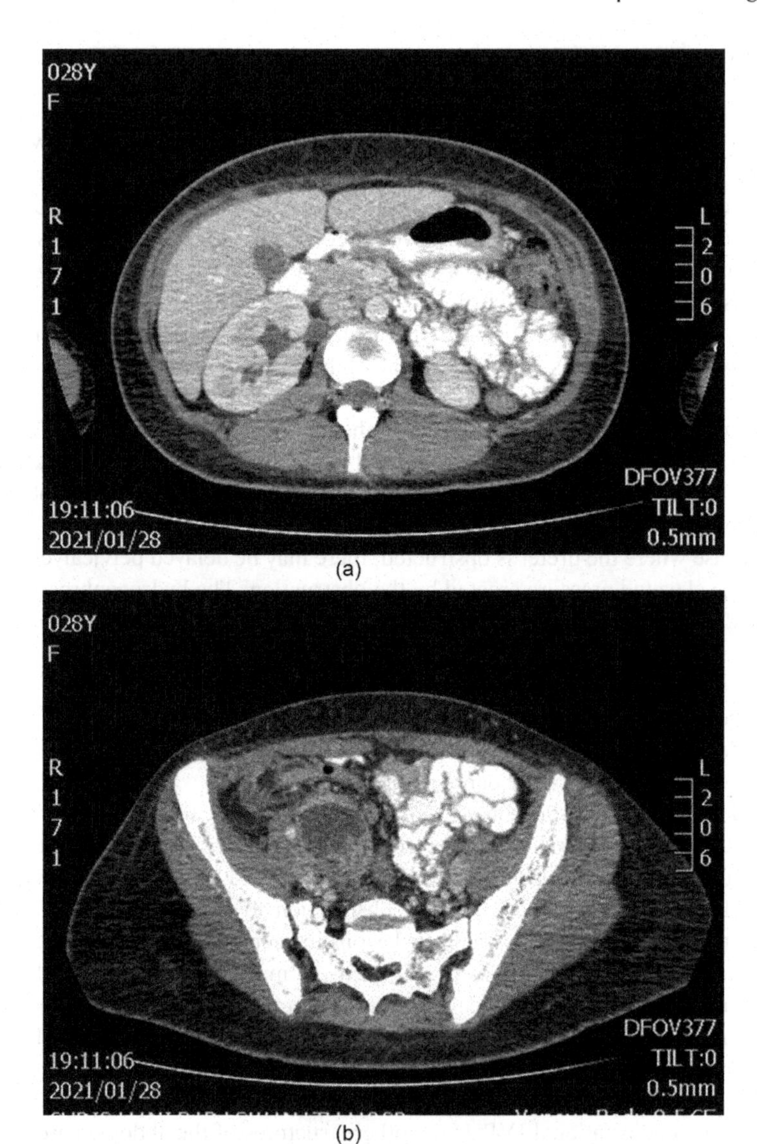

FIGURE 19.5 (a) Hydronephrosis and (b) intrauterine mass.

right hydroureteronephrosis and the dilation of the ureter can be seen in the images (Figure 19.6b). There is no obvious stone seen in the ureter. There will be delayed pelvicalyceal filling due to the dilatation and the elevated pressure in the collecting system. The cut-off of the ureter appears to be at lumbar vertebra 2. As there is no stone, it would be suggestive of a right proximal ureteric stricture. Figure 19.6c demonstrates a normal bladder with no wall thickening or masses visualised. The bony skeleton of the spine and pelvis appears normal.

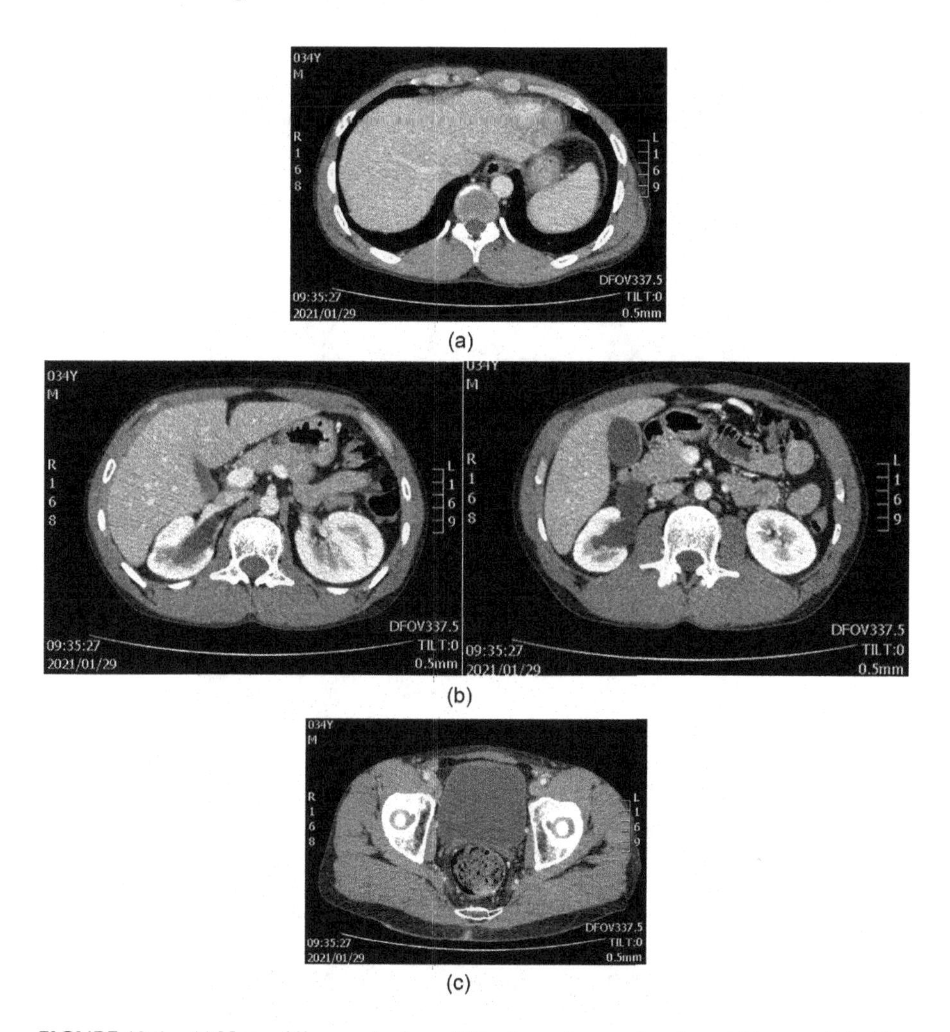

FIGURE 19.6 (a) Normal liver and spleen, (b) hydroureteronephrosis and (c) normal bladder.

JAUNDICE

A 65-year-old male patient with obstructive jaundice, suggestive of liver cirrhosis on ultrasound with dilated intrahepatic bile ducts, is referred for a CT Abdomen unenhanced and multiphasic with oral contrast media. The images are seen in Figure 19.7a–c. The dilated intrahepatic bile ducts indicate obstruction which would then lead to obstructive jaundice.

The initial image (Figure 19.7a) demonstrates the arterial phase and images 19.7b and c demonstrate the venous phase of the scan. In Figure 19.7a, both kidneys are demonstrated and their contour appears normal and the position and size are normal. The gall bladder is visualised with a loss of contour and multiple gallstones seen. The bowel has no wall thickening and appears normal. The calcifications seen are multiple gallstones. The bony structures also appear normal. In image 19.7b, the liver

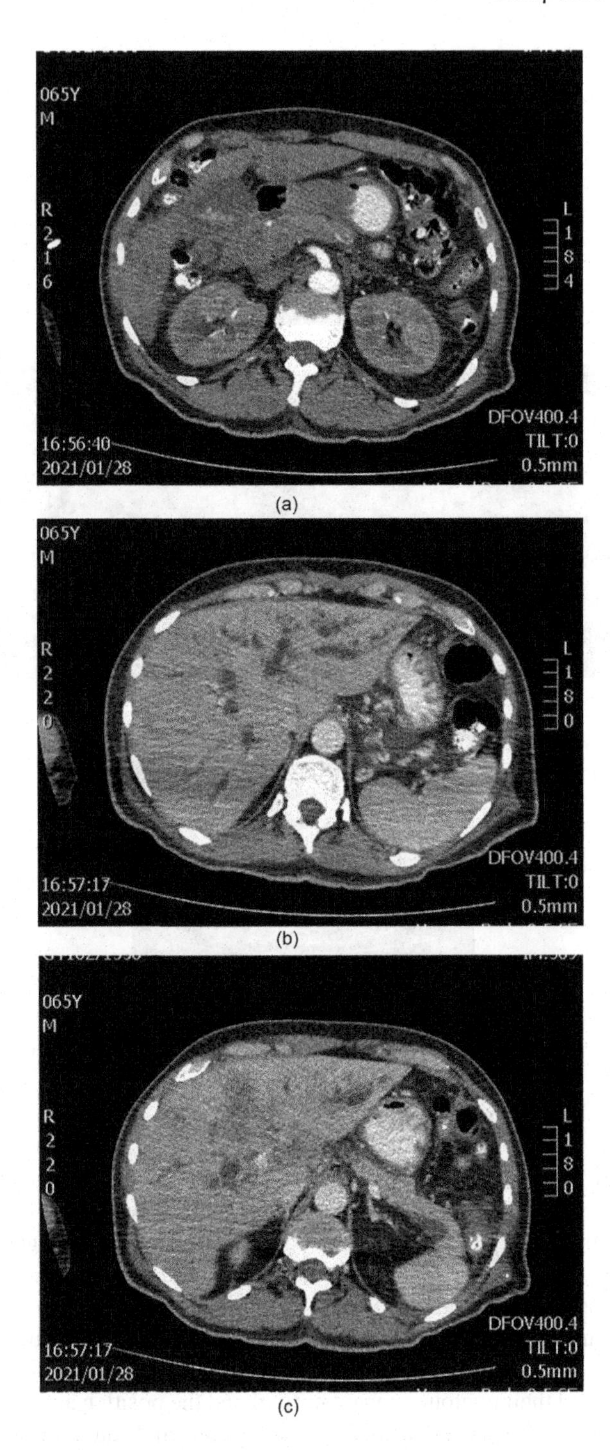

FIGURE 19.7 (a) Multiple gallstones, (b) dilated intrahepatic biliary ducts and (c) mass on liver.

is visualised and there are dilated intrahepatic ducts. The largest are seen centrally and measure 11 mm; the ducts at the periphery measure between 7 and 8 mm. The spleen is demonstrated and shows homogenous enhancement with no focal lesions. The stomach is seen with no masses or filling defects.

In image 19.7c, there is a mass seen infiltrating into the liver the mass has ill-defined margins and is suggestive of a gall bladder carcinoma infiltrating into the liver. This would cause the intrahepatic biliary obstruction seen in the previous image. Gallbladder carcinoma is the fifth most common cancer of the digestive system and gallstones are a risk factor for developing gallbladder carcinoma (Goetze, 2015). The lesion was referred to in the radiology report as T4N1 Mx. The TNM staging system is a common staging system for cancer: T refers to the size and extent of cancer; N refers to the lymph node involvement and M refers to the spread of the disease (https://www.cancer.gov/about-cancer/diagnosis-staging/staging). Therefore, for this patient, T4 indicates a large tumour; the size from the scan was 69 by 79 mm. N1 indicates that there is lymph node involvement and Mx indicates the spread cannot be measured and a number would suggest it had spread to other parts of the body.

PLACEMENT OF NASOGASTRIC TUBE

Figure 19.8a demonstrates the placement in the stomach of a nasogastric tube. The nasogastric tube is in situ in the gastric body. The gall bladder can be visualised and is normal, and the liver parenchyma appears normal in the image. The CTA was performed post-surgery as the patient had a clinical history of a gunshot wound and had no imaging before going to theatre. The kidneys appear normal in Figure 19.8b, but a large amount of air can be seen in the large bowel although there is no bowel wall thickening or any indication of obstruction. The air could be post-surgical.

COLOSTOMY

An 18-year-old male was referred for a CT Abdomen with contrast. He has a history of an appendectomy following a complicated case of appendicitis. Due to complications, a right hemicolectomy had to be performed with a resultant stoma. The patient had a previous CT in November 2020 which demonstrated multiple collections. Now, in January 2021, he is complaining of abdominal pain and vomiting. In Figure 19.9a, the image demonstrates a right abdominal colostomy from the previous surgery. There is evidence of the previous right hemicolectomy with the transverse colon connecting to the colostomy. A colostomy is when part of the colon, in this case, the transverse colon is brought to the outside through a surgical opening and a pouch is attached for the collection of faecal material (https://www.ostomy.org/colostomy/). Also seen in these images is the herniation of the bowel loops into the stoma. Although this herniation has occurred, it does not appear to have caused a proximal obstruction. Parastomal herniation is a common occurrence in stoma patients and is seen in 78% of patients usually within 2 years of the creation of ostomy (Aquina et al, 2014). Peristomal bulging can be seen in the images and this is caused by increased intra- abdominal pressure (Aquina et al, 2014). The colostomy bag can be seen on the right and is filled with the oral contrast media (Figure 19.9a). There are multiple

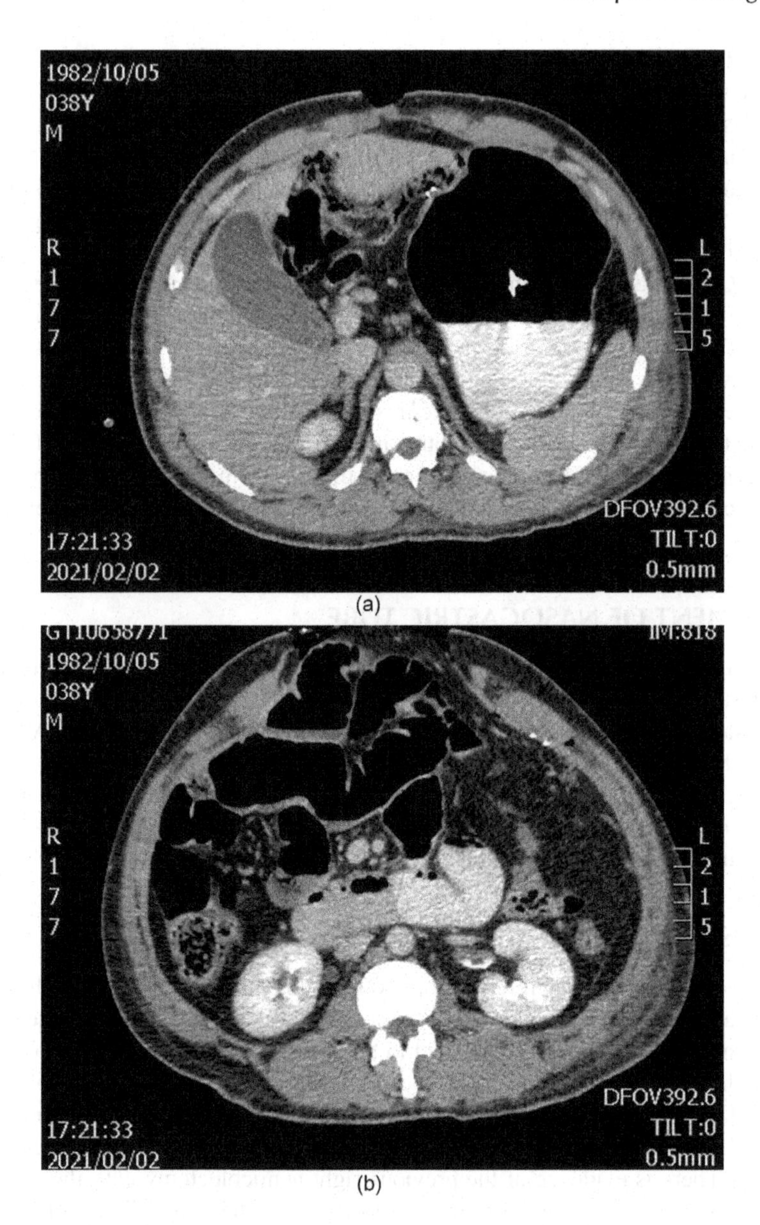

FIGURE 19.8 (a) Nasogastric tube and (b) normal kidneys.

small collections seen in the images with ring enhancement and they form an inflammatory mass. The largest diameter collection is 32 × 22 mm (Figure 19.9a and b).

There is no hepatomegaly, no focal lesions or dilation of the intrahepatic biliary ducts. The gallbladder, pancreas and spleen appear normal. The kidneys are normal in appearance with no hydronephrosis. Aorta, IVC and major branches are normal with no filling defects. The skeletal structures all appear normal.

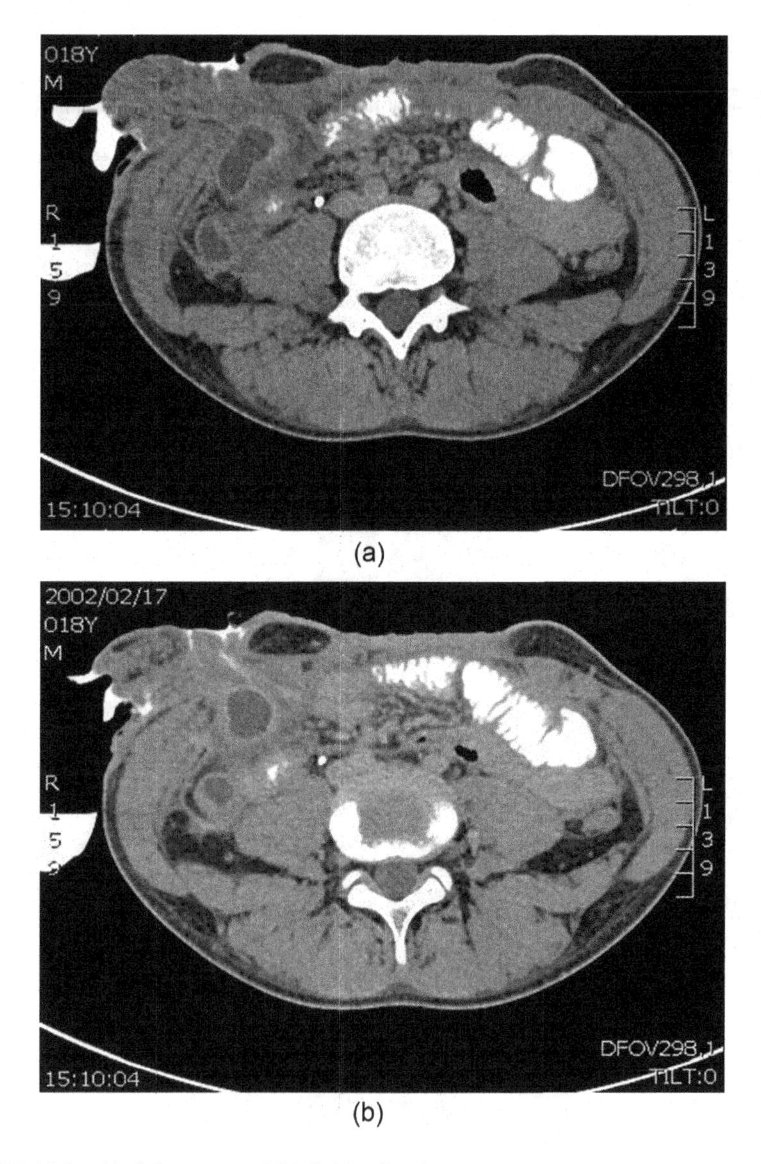

FIGURE 19.9 (a) Colostomy and (b) fluid collection.

PELVIC ABSCESS

A patient is referred for a CT Abdomen with a history of an ovarian mass and bilateral lung nodules. The patient has had previous a CT scan in 2017 and an MRI in 2020. The new CT is in January 2021. The liver appears to have a normal parenchyma and a smooth outline. There are no dilated intrahepatic bile ducts (Figure 19.10a). In Figure 19.10a, the kidneys are visualised: the right kidney demonstrates hydronephrosis and measures 125 mm and the left kidney is atrophic and

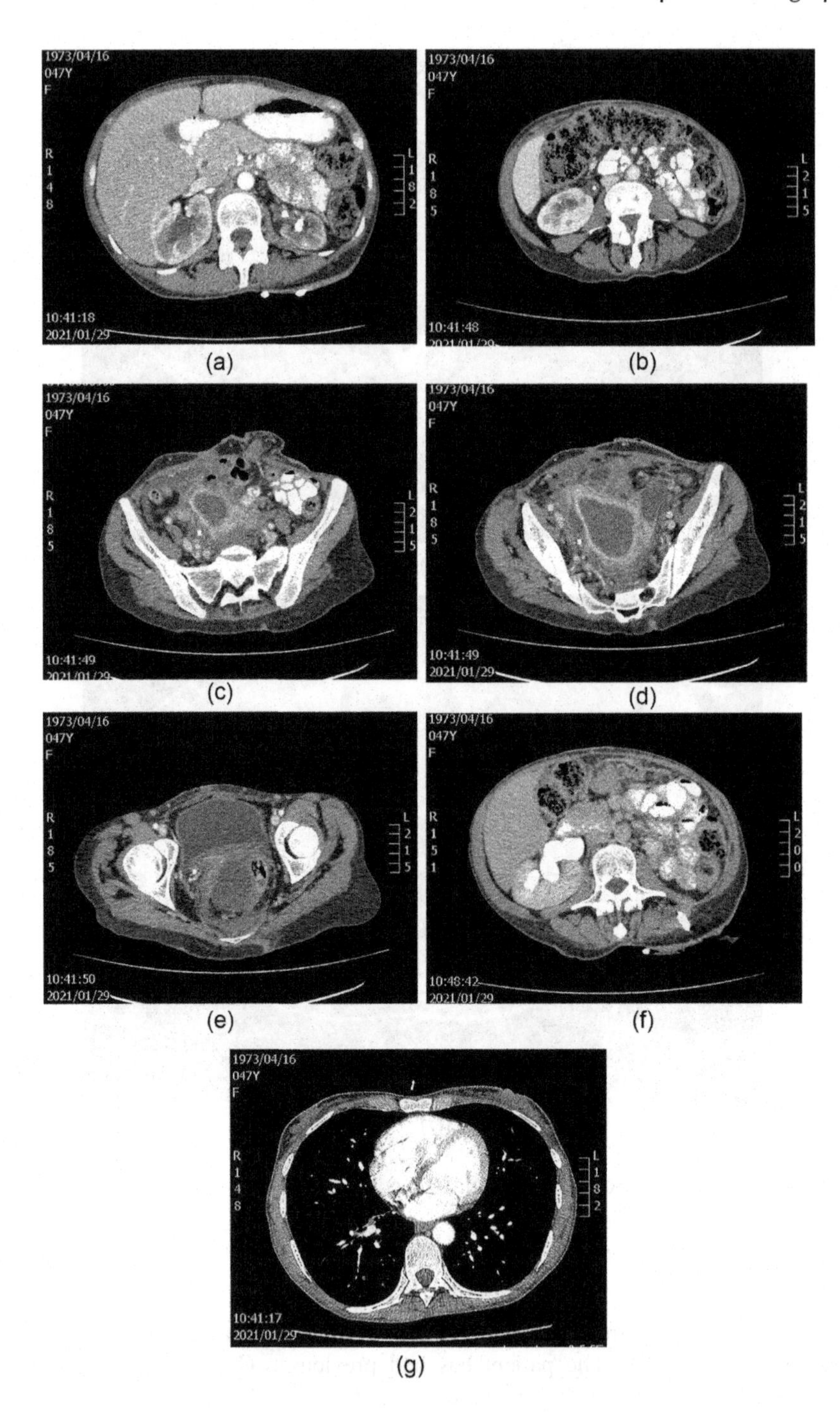

FIGURE 19.10 (a) Normal liver, hydronephrosis right kidney and atrophy left kidney; (b) hydronephrosis and stent right kidney; (c) pelvic mass and ileostomy; (d) enhancing pelvic mass and stent; (e) bladder; (f) right hydronephrosis with dilated ureter and (g) lung nodules.

measures only 79 mm. The normal size for the kidney is between 100 and 120 mm. A nephrostomy is in the mid calyx of the left kidney. A nephrostomy is an artificial opening between the kidney and the skin. The urine would then drain from the kidney via the nephrostomy.

Figure 19.10b demonstrates the DJ stent which is found in the right kidney: the tip is in the mid calx and the end is in the bladder. Faecal loading can also be seen in the image.

Figure 19.10c and d shows the ring enhancement of the abscess. The abscess is seen in the right lower quadrant and is presacral. The abscess demonstrates a mass effect and displaces the bowel and the rectum to the left. The patient also has an ileostomy demonstrated in Figure 19.10c in the left lower quadrant. The DJ stent is also seen in both images. The bladder appears normally distended and has no wall thickening (Figure 19.10e). In Figure 19.10f, the delayed image demonstrates the hydronephrosis of the right kidney and the dilated ureter.

The final image, Figure 19.10g, demonstrates the lung fields; as mentioned in the clinical history for the patient, she has multiple nodules bilaterally. The nodules are varying in size and are most likely metastatic.

ABDOMINAL AORTIC ANEURYSM

CT is considered the gold standard for abdominal aortic aneurysm imaging. Abdominal aortic aneurysms are defined as dilatation of the aorta greater than 3 cm or dilatation of more than 50% of the diameter (Kumar, 2017). The abdominal aortic aneurysm demonstrated in the axial plane in Figure 19.11a shows a contrast-enhanced lumen surrounded by mural thrombus. Figure 19.11b demonstrates the abdominal aortic aneurysm in the sagittal plane; this shows dilation of the aorta. The contrast-enhanced lumen and mural thrombus are again seen. There is no free fluid seen within the abdomen.

Abdominal aortic aneurysms are associated with atherosclerosis and are more common in men (Kumar, 2017). Most abdominal aortic aneurysms are asymptomatic; therefore, screening has been implemented in some countries using ultrasound as a non-invasive imaging modality without radiation (Hohneck, 2017).

CONCLUSION

In summary, it is important to understand the normal appearances of the abdominal organs and bowel to enable image interpretation. When undertaking image interpretation, it is essential to be systematic and provides a location for any abnormal structures seen. The description of the appearances can often be more important than the diagnosis. A diagnosis of a pathology must always be evaluated with reference to the clinical history.

ACKNOWLEDGEMENT

I would like to thank the Radiology department at Chris Hani Baragwanath Academic Hospital for allowing me to use the anonymised CT images in this chapter and providing access to the reports on the images.

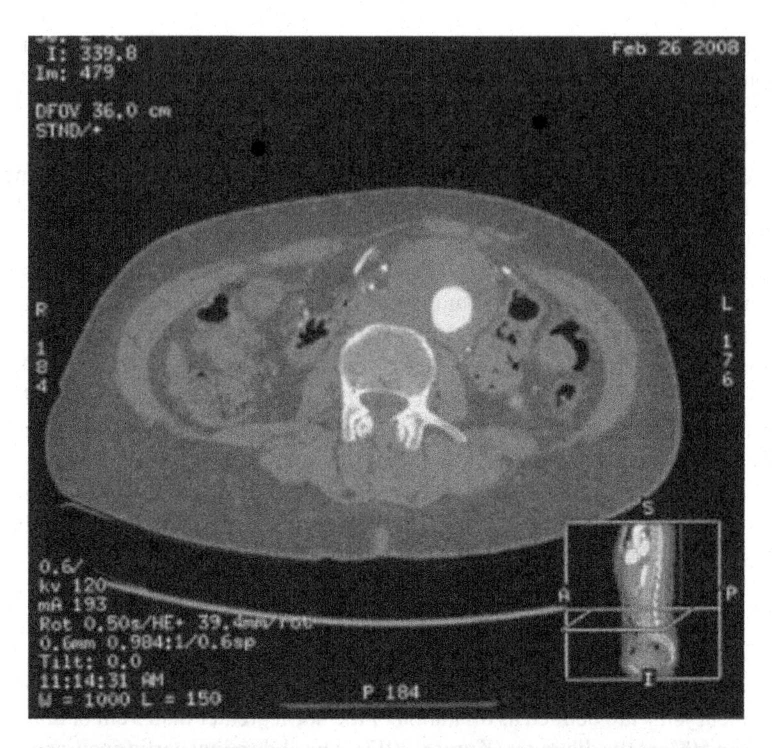

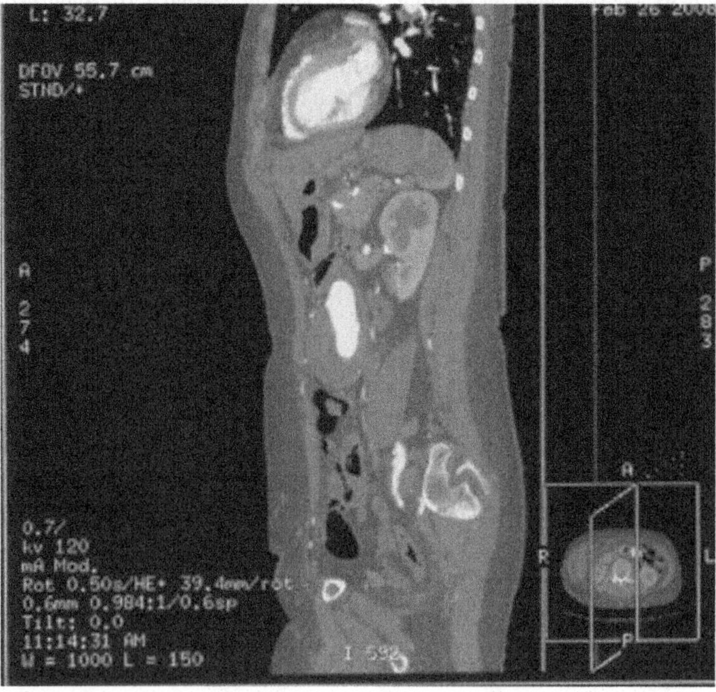

FIGURE 19.11 Abdominal aortic aneurysm: (a) axial and (b) sagittal.

REFERENCES

Aquina, C.T. Iannuzzi, J.C. Probst, C.P. Kelly, K.N. Noyes, K. Fleming, F.J.& Monson, J.R.T. (2014). Parastomal Hernia: A Growing Problem with New Solutions. *Digestive Surgery*. 31:366–376. doi:10.1159/000369279.

Cancer staging. Available from: https://www.cancer.gov/about-cancer/diagnosis-staging/staging.

Chan, O. (2013). *ABC of Emergency Radiology*. 3rd ed. BMJ Books.

Eisenberg, R.L. & Johnson, N. M. (2020). *Comprehensive Radiographic Pathology*. 7th ed. MOSBY. St Louis, Missouri.

Goetze, T.O. (2015). Gallbladder Carcinoma: Prognostic Factors and Therapeutic Options. *World Journal of Gastroenterology*. 21(43). doi:10.3748/wjg.v21.i43.12211.

Hohneck, A. Keese, M. Ruemenapf, G. Amendt, K. Muertz, H. Janda, K. Akin, I. Borggrefe, M. & Sigl, M. (2019). Prevalence of Abdominal Aortic Aneurysm & Associated Lower Extremity Artery Aneurysm in Men Hospitalized for Suspected or Known Cardiopulmonary Disease. *BMC Cardiovascular Disorders*. 19:284. doi:10.1186/s12872-019-1265-2.

https://teachmeobgyn.com/history-taking-examinations/history-taking/obstetric/

Kumar, Y. Hooda, K. Shuo, L. Goyal, P. Gupta, N. & Adeb, M. (2017). Abdominal Aortic Aneurysm Pictorial Review of Common Appearances and Complications. *Annals of Translational Medicine*. 5(12):256. doi: 10.21037/atm.2017.04.32

Marchiori, D. (2014). *Clinical Imaging*. 3rd ed. MOSBY. St Louis, Missouri.

Onen, A. (2020). Grading of Hydronephrosis: An Ongoing Challenge. *Frontiers in Paediatrics*. 458. doi:10.3389/fped.2020.00458.

Ostomy and colostomy. Available from: https://www.ostomy.org/colostomy.

20 CT Image Evaluation in Oncology

Matthew Jarvis
South Australia Medical Imaging

CONTENTS

DOI: 10.1201/9781003132554-26

INTRODUCTION

There were 135,133 new cancer diagnoses in Australia in 2016 and, due to improving diagnostic techniques, an ageing population and multiple other factors, incidence continues to rise, with an estimated 145,833 new cases in 2020 (Australian Institute of Health and Welfare (AIHW), 2020). Despite improving diagnostic and treatment options, 47,310 Australian cancer deaths were recorded in 2018 with an estimated 48,099 in 2020 (AIHW, 2020).

Oncology is "the study or science dealing with the physical, chemical, and biologic properties and features of neoplasms" (Stedman, 2006). In medicine, the specialty of Oncology encompasses the investigation, diagnosis and treatment of people with cancer or suspected cancer. Medical specialists, called Oncologists, oversee such treatment. The rapid and ongoing improvement of cancer diagnosis and treatment in addition to an ageing population means that individuals are surviving longer after their cancer diagnoses and now, not uncommonly, are being diagnosed with more than one different cancer (WHO, 2019).

Cancer is "the common term for all malignant tumours", which are neoplasms that have the potential to metastasise (spread) from the site of initial origin to other regions of the body (Kumar, Abbas and Aster, 2015). This includes spread to lymph nodes which drain lymph from nearly all body regions (lymphatic metastasis) and to distant organs via the bloodstream (haematogenous metastasis). Generally speaking, cancers arise in their primary site, where they grow larger and invade adjacent structures. Once cancer cells extend into small lymphatic channels, they may drain into regional (nearby) lymph nodes, then into more distant lymph nodes. In these sites, the cells continue to divide and replicate. Cells may also extend into blood vessels of the primary organ. Once in blood vessels, these cells can metastasise to virtually any other organ in the body, the brain, lungs, liver and bones being some of the more common organs of metastases.

CT

The high spatial resolution of CT in addition to its rapid acquisition time makes it a useful modality to assess the presence and burden of cancer (Seeram, 2016). It remains mainstay in the diagnosis, staging and surveillance of patients with all forms of malignant disease. It provides detailed information which allows Oncologists to prescribe targeted and/or systemic treatments, as well as effectively assesses the response to, and complications of, such treatments. These treatments may include surgery, radiotherapy, chemotherapy and other specialised treatments.

Despite the significant strengths of CT in oncology imaging, it is largely a static assessment, often requiring repeated imaging at differing time-points to "follow up" the cancer's progress or treatment response over time. Additionally, not all cancers are visible on CT, many being too small, located in structures beyond the capabilities of CT (particularly the skin or luminal structures such as the gut) or beyond the contrast resolution of CT. Nuclear Medicine techniques are a useful adjunct, which are often used in parallel with CT and, in fact, increasingly performed and interpreted together to provide structural information in conjunction with a more functional assessment of disease activity. Magnetic Resonance Imaging (MRI) is also a useful and increasingly utilised technique which is commonly used supplementary to CT in the assessment of cancer. It provides better soft tissue contrast resolution compared to CT (Allisy-Roberts and Williams, 2007). CT fluoroscopy is another useful adjunct, which can allow Interventional Radiologists to accurately target and obtain tissue samples of known or suspected cancer. CT is also the primary modality used by Radiation Oncologists to plan and target the delivery of radiotherapy.

Contrast

CT is most often performed with iodinated contrast media, which is a vital tool in optimising its performance in cancer assessment. The tissue properties of cancer generally differ from those of the tissue in which it has arisen. For example, tumours may have abnormally increased number of vascular channels, more than that of the background tissue (i.e., they may be hypervascular), and therefore, enhance more avidly than background tissues, particularly in the arterial phase. Common examples of such tumours include lung carcinoma, renal cell carcinoma, thyroid carcinoma, melanoma and neuroendocrine tumours. Conversely, tumours less rich in blood supply may enhance less than that of background tissue (i.e., they may be hypovascular). For example, the liver is a common site of metastasis and demonstrates hypoenhancing lesions in the arterial or portal venous (PV) phase in cases of colon, lung, breast and gastric carcinoma metastases.

Luminal Contrast

Iodinated contrast may be ingested orally to assess certain luminal malignancies, such as those in the gastrointestinal tract. CT colonography for the assessment of colorectal polyps is used as an adjunct screening tool to formal endoscopy in the assessment of pre-malignant disease. Negative oral contrast, typically water, is also often used to achieve gut distension and improve assessment.

THE TUMOUR, NODES, METASTASES (TNM) APPROACH

Cancer staging is the process of assessing the location and burden of cancer within the body. The American Joint Committee on Cancer (AJCC) framework uses the tumour, nodes, metastases (TNM) system, which is recognised globally in the staging of cancer (Amin and Edge, 2020). There are clinical, pathologic and re-staging criteria and the specific staging criteria vary between different organs, but this is beyond the scope of this chapter. When assessing the primary tumour, it may be obvious which structure is giving rise to cancer, though there are some factors which can make this more confusing. For example, large tumours that invade multiple structures.

The primary consideration of lymph node involvement from cancer is that of abnormal enlargement of the node. Typically, a measurement of 10 mm (short-axis diameter) is utilised as a cut-off, with nodes larger than that being considered "pathologically enlarged" (Van den Brekel et al, 1990). However, other criteria, such as abnormal rounded morphology, loss of the fatty hilum, eccentric thickening or irregular borders are some other factors which may indicate lymph node involvement. There are also different size criteria utilised for different body regions, beyond the scope of this chapter. These features, however, are not specific for malignant lymphadenopathy and can be caused by many other pathologies, most commonly infective, inflammatory and autoimmune causes (Figure 20.1).

Even when the primary aim of imaging is not formal cancer staging, using a "TNM" style approach to reviewing CT images provides a systematic method for interpretation. For example, one could consider the following mental framework when approaching CT interpretation:

- Tumour:
    - Can I see the primary tumour?
    - What size is it?
    - What does it look like?

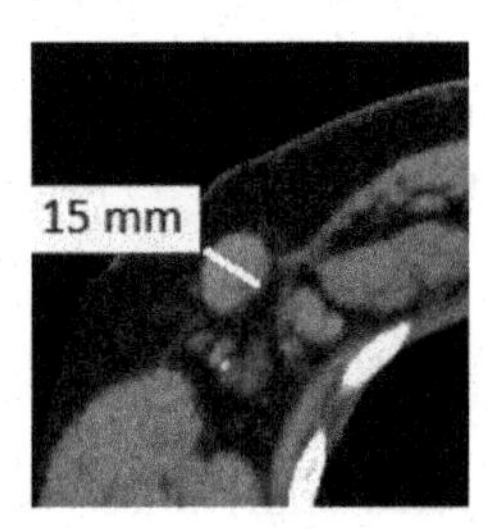

FIGURE 20.1 An example of how to measure the short-axis diameter. This case of lymphoma demonstrates a pathologically enlarged lymph node located in the right axilla. It also appears abnormally rounded in morphology.

    - Density – fat, calcification, soft tissue
    - Does it enhance post-contrast?
    - What do its borders look like?
  - What structure is it arising from?
  - What structures does it invade or compress?
- Nodes:
  - Are there enlarged or abnormal regional lymph nodes?
  - Are there enlarged or abnormal distant lymph nodes?
  - How many?
- Metastases:
  - Has it spread beyond primary and lymphatic sites?
  - If so, where to? Most common sites:
    - Bones,
    - Lungs,
    - Liver,
    - Brain,
    - Kidneys, soft tissues, etc.

NB. NOT ALL MASSES ARE CANCER AND NOT ALL CANCERS ARE SOLITARY

- The TNM approach helps exclude mimics (benign entities mimicking cancer).
- Also, being aware of the characteristics of different primary cancers can help one consider if multiple masses represent one disease process or if there may be a second cancer occurring in synchrony.

INITIAL DIAGNOSIS AND STAGING OF COMMON CANCERS

There is a broad range of cancers for which CT is utilised in the diagnosis and/or staging. To discuss all of them would be beyond the scope of a single book chapter. This section covers the TNM framework applied to a few common cancer examples. This includes how they may present on initial CT or CT performed for staging when a clinical or histological diagnosis has already been made. Whilst the list is far from exhaustive, the behaviours of the cancers discussed also provides a good basis for diagnosing and staging other cancers.

Lung Carcinoma

Many processes affect the lungs, not just neoplastic pathologies. Inflammatory, infective, traumatic and vascular pathologies can occur within the lungs and at times mimic cancer. Infection, for example, can present as a solitary mass, a diffuse process or even rarely invade adjacent structures. Infection can also spread from elsewhere in the body, such as septic embolic spread in *Staphylococcus aureus* bacteraemia.

With rates of smoking remaining high globally, the lung remains a common site of primary cancer. Additionally, the lung is one of the favoured sites for metastasis from many extrathoracic sites. There are multiple different histological sub-types of primary lung cancer, which may behave differently.

Therefore, one must first consider when viewing a lesion in the lung:

- Is it likely to be neoplastic or non-neoplastic?
- If neoplastic, is it more likely to be benign or malignant?
- If malignant, is it arising from the lung (i.e., a primary "T" lesion) or has it spread from elsewhere (i.e., "M" lesion)?

T

See Figure 20.2.

- Location:
  - May be a clue to subtype – primary squamous cell carcinoma more commonly central, adenocarcinoma more commonly peripheral.
- Size
- Shape/composition/morphology:
  - Characteristically enhancing "spiculated" mass of soft tissue density.
  - May have cavitation.
- Localised or diffuse:
  - May present as a nodule, mass or diffuse consolidation.
  - Diffuse consolidative appearance, such as in adenocarcinoma can mimic pneumonia, however, infection can also appear as a focal nodule or mass.
- Invasion present or absent:
  - Pleura, chest wall, oesophagus, pericardium.

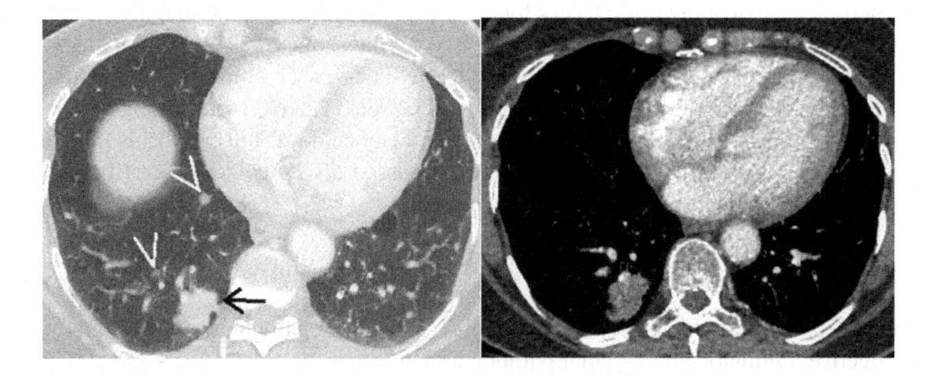

FIGURE 20.2 Soft tissue and lung windows, contrast-enhanced CT chest demonstrating a heterogenous, soft tissue density nodule (black arrow) within the right lower lobe consistent with a primary lung cancer. The nodule appears ovoid, irregular and lobulated and extends to the pleura at its posteromedial aspect. Separate tumour nodules (white arrowheads) are also present within the adjacent right lower lobe.

- Mass effect:
  - May obstruct central or smaller airways leading to collapse.
  - Lung cancer is a common cause of lobar collapse in adults.

N

See Figure 20.3.

- Regional lymph nodes – intrapulmonary, hilar, mediastinal, supraclavicular.
- Which ones? How many?
- Extrathoracic (non-regional) lymph nodes – though these are considered metastasis by the AJCC.

M

- Bone – typically lytic but a minority are mixed lytic/sclerotic,
- Contralateral lung,
- Pleura (+/– pleural effusion),
- Extrathoracic viscera (esp. adrenal and liver).

Colorectal Carcinoma

Colorectal carcinomas arise from the luminal (inner) surface of the large bowel. They spread locally, which may appear as protrusion into the bowel lumen with or without extension into (and beyond) the deeper layers of the bowel wall.

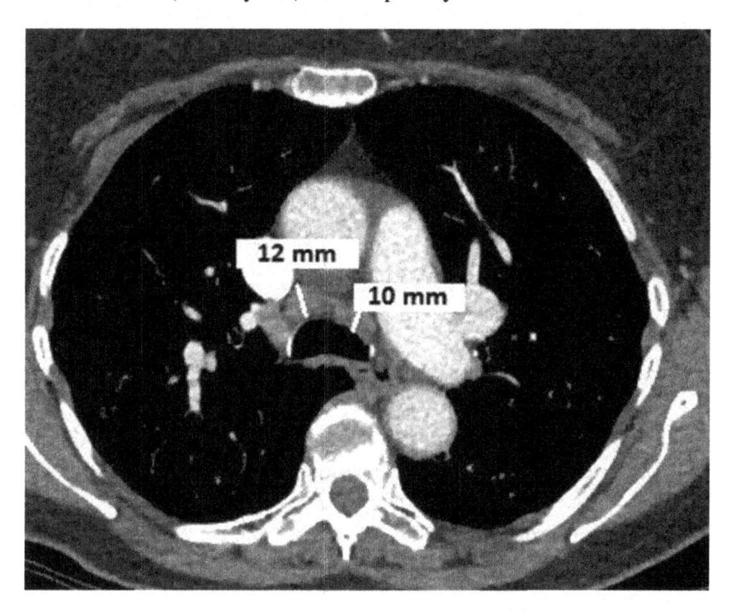

FIGURE 20.3 Enlarged and borderline enlarged mediastinal (pretracheal) lymph nodes, suggesting lymphatic spread.

The large bowel is a dynamic structure making it difficult to accurately assess a static modality such as CT. This is, at least partly, due to the imperfect temporal resolution of CT and physiological gut contractions (peristalsis). This can result in such luminal masses being obscured within segments of temporarily collapsed bowel. These cancers can therefore be difficult to detect, unless present as a large mass or there is extracolonic spread. Colonoscopy is the investigation of choice for colorectal cancer. If there is concern about a potential colonic mass on CT, colonoscopy is the preferred method to further investigate. In some settings, dedicated CT colonography can be used to evaluate the colon. This attempts to overcome these limitations by insufflating the bowel with air or carbon dioxide, improving the detection of smaller cancers or precancerous polyps.

The diagnosis of bowel cancer may already be made on colonoscopic biopsy in which case CT is being performed more to assess the extent of local and distant spread.

Clues

- Luminal mass.
- Obstructing mass with upstream bowel dilatation.
- Focal/short segment wall thickening – often asymmetric:
  - pple core" lesion.
- Stranding or nodular appearance in the pericolonic fat.
- Enlarged regional lymph nodes.

Mimics

- Inflammation – also causes wall thickening which may be diffuse or focal:
  - Diverticulitis,
  - Inflammatory bowel disease.
- Infection:
  - Bacteria, parasites or viral.
- Vascular:
  - Ischaemic colitis.

T

See Figure 20.4.

- Location:
  - Which part of the colon is involved?
    - Caecum, ascending colon, hepatic flexure, transverse colon, splenic flexure, descending colon, sigmoid or rectum.
- Size
- Shape/composition/morphology:
  - Typically, irregular, noncalcified, soft tissue masses.
- Invasion present or absent:
  - Pericolonic fat;

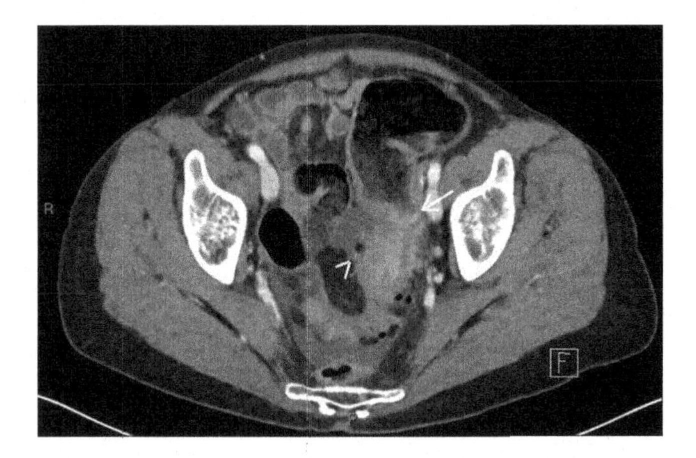

FIGURE 20.4 Marked short segment irregular, eccentric/semi-annular bowel wall thickening located within the distal sigmoid colon (white arrow) compatible with primary bowel cancer. Note – extra-colonic extension and fluid into the adjacent mesenteric fat, in keeping with mesenteric invasion. (Note – a number of other causes of bowel wall thickening are listed below.)

    - Adjacent organs, such as bladder or small bowel;
    - Other less common sites include liver, stomach, colon and abdominal wall.
- Mass effect:
    - May present as bowel obstruction.

N

See Figure 20.5.

- Adjacent to tumour along the mesentery (look along vessels),
- Retroperitoneal.

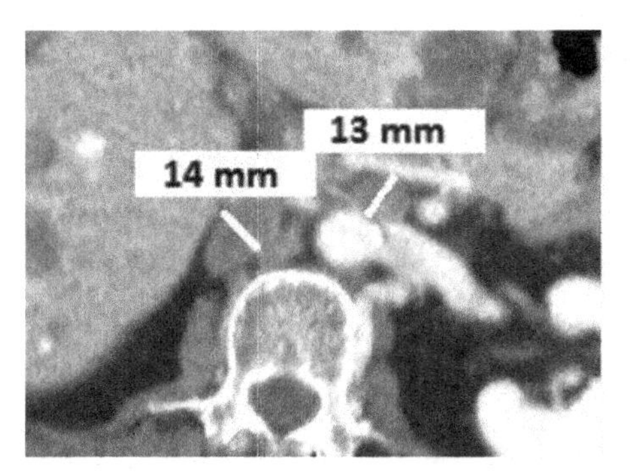

FIGURE 20.5 Enlarged retroperitoneal lymph nodes, suggesting lymphatic spread.

M

See Figure 20.6.

- Liver:
  - Common site for colorectal cancer to spread.
  - Typically causes hypoenhancing liver lesions in PV phase.
- Lung:
  - Look at lung bases in lung windows, even on abdominal scans.
- Brain:
  - Pre- and post-contrast imaging best.
- Bone:
  - Look on bone and soft tissue windows for any bone lesions.
  - May be either lytic, sclerotic or mixed.

Breast Cancer

The breast is comprised of a combination of glandular tissue, ducts which converge on the nipple, fat and other supporting tissues. Cancers of the breast predominantly arise from the glandular and ductal tissue and more commonly occur in middle aged to older females. They progress locally and can metastasise to varied body tissues.

CT is not the optimal modality for assessment of primary cancer of the breast, due to the high spatial resolution required to detect subtle tissue density differences between breast tissue and cancers. Clinical examination, mammography, ultrasound and biopsy therefore form the basis for investigation of most primary breast cancers. As with other cancers, however, CT may be performed to assess for extent of spread of distant disease. The breast is an uncommon location for metastases to occur.

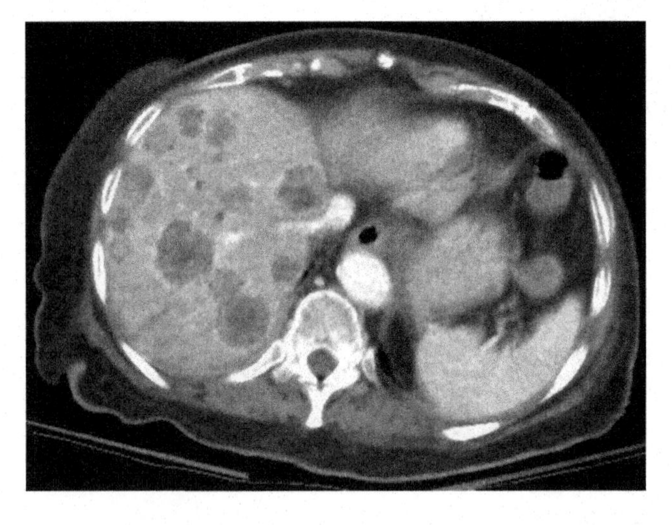

FIGURE 20.6 Multiple sizeable hepatic metastasis, demonstrating heterogenous, hypoenhancement, relative to background liver. (Note – the enhancing "capsule" relates to displacement/compression of the adjacent liver tissue, rather than part of the metastasis itself.)

Advanced primary breast cancers may grow into large masses and invade the skin, subcutaneous tissues, underlying pectoralis/intercostal muscles, adjacent ribs and/or pleura. All of these changes may be seen on CT as areas of abnormal soft tissue density and enhancement extending from a mass within the breast. One may see skin thickening or distortion of the breast contour, destruction of the ribs or mass-like soft tissue extending into the pleura and extra-pleural tissues of the thoracic cavity.

In patients with a more remote history of breast cancer who may be undergoing CT for re-staging purposes, or any number of other clinical reasons, one should look for evidence of prior disease and treatment. This may be demonstrated by prior mastectomy, localised breast resection and/or surgical clips within the axilla, indicating past lymph node resection. One may also see evidence of prior radiotherapy, such as skin and subcutaneous thickening and scarring, or scarring/fibrosis of the underlying lung (Figures 20.7 and 20.8).

Clues

- Breast mass +/−calcifications (best assessed mammographically);
- Architectural distortion (best assessed mammographically);
- Skin thickening (nonspecific);
- Muscle or chest wall invasion;
- Evidence of prior surgery or radiotherapy in the breast and/or axilla.

Important Mimics

- Mastitis – may be infective or non-infective:
  - Diffuse or localised with or without abscess formation.
  - May also cause lymph node enlargement.
  - Can look similar to the inflammatory subtype of breast cancer.
- Breast metastases:
- Breast involvement of lymphoma.

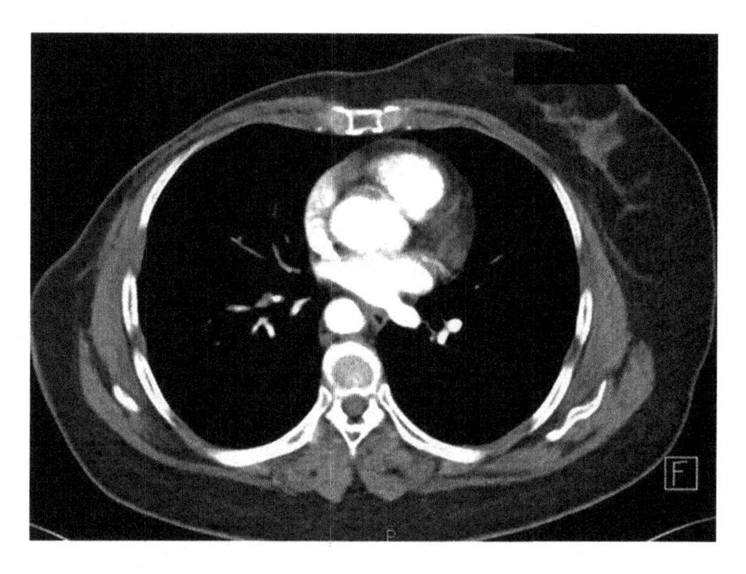

FIGURE 20.7 Prior right mastectomy, performed for breast cancer.

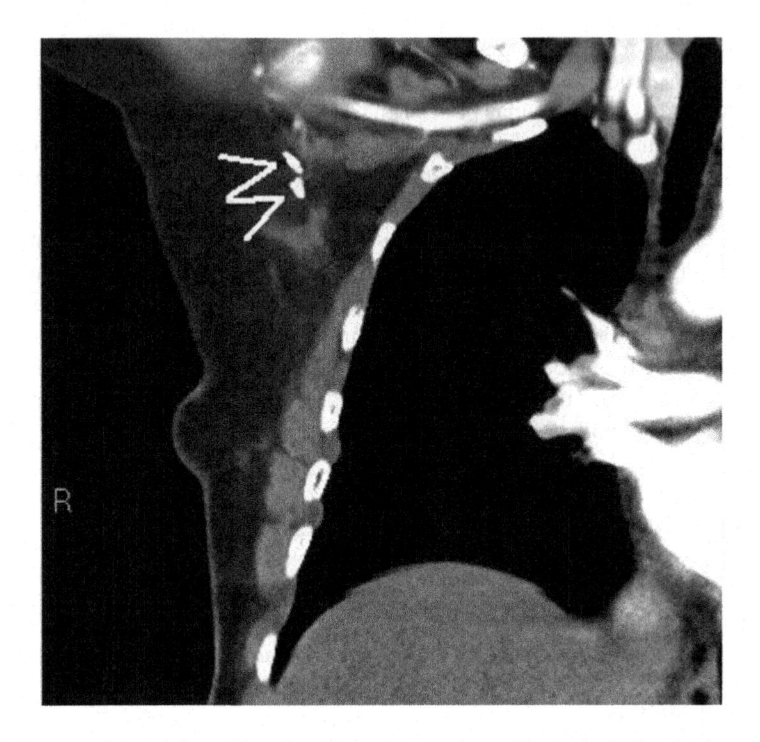

FIGURE 20.8 Prior right axillary lymph node resection with surgical clips in situ.

T

See Figure 20.9.

- Location:
  - Which side?
  - Which breast quadrant(s) are involved?
- Size
- Shape/composition/morphology
- Invasion present or absent:
  - For example, pectoralis muscle, muscular or bony chest wall, underlying pleura.
  - Skin thickening or eruption through skin.
- Mass effect:
  - Distortion of breast contour.

N

See Figure 20.10.

- Regional – intramammary, axillary, internal mammary, infra- or supraclavicular.

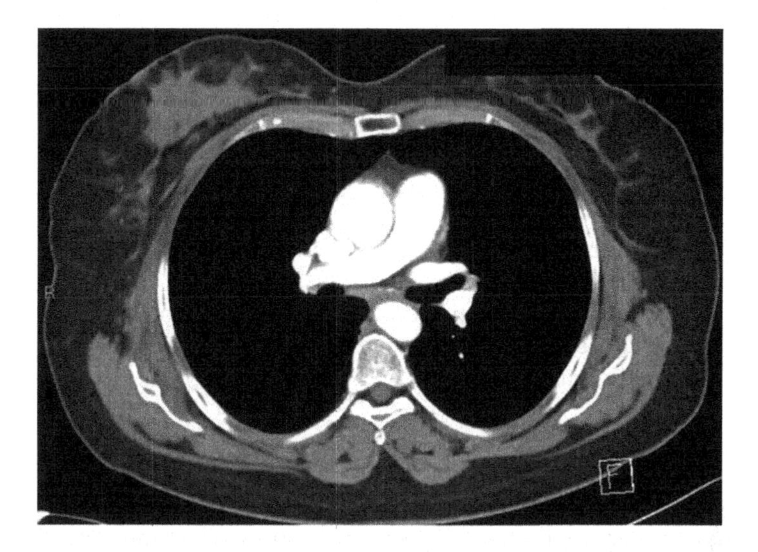

FIGURE 20.9 Earlier photo of Figures 2.7 and 2.8, showing a large, irregular, infiltrative mass of soft tissue attenuation within the right breast, compatible with primary breast cancer. Some spicules extend to the subcutaneous tissues and skin, without significant skin thickening. No chest wall extension (i.e., no rib or muscle involvement) seen.

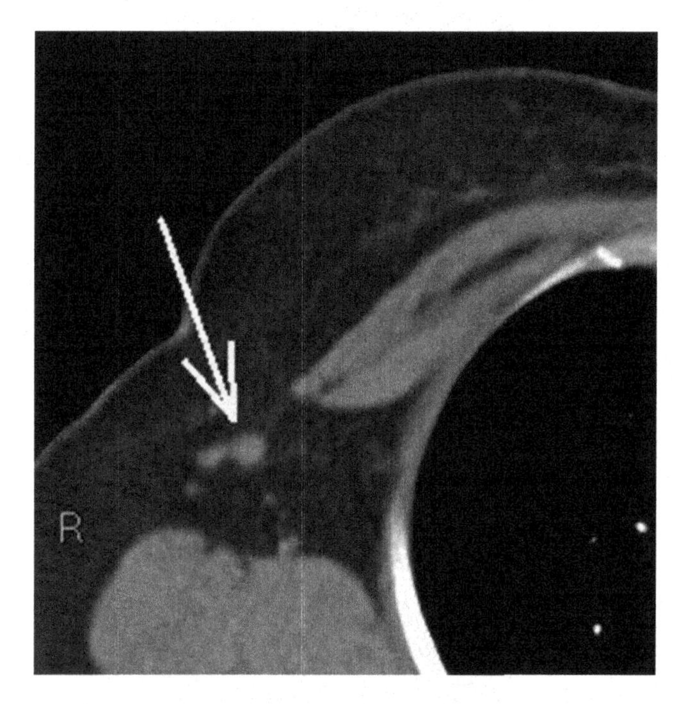

FIGURE 20.10 No pathologically enlarged axillary or intrathoracic lymph nodes are seen, however, one right axillary lymph node is eccentrically thickened and may therefore be suspicious for nodal metastasis. Metastatic involvement was demonstrated on histology.

M

See Figure 20.11.

- Liver:
  - Typically, hypoenhancing in PV phase.
- Lung:
  - Look at lungs in lung windows.
- Bone:
  - Look on bone and soft tissue windows for bone lesions.
  - Typically, sclerotic but some are mixed lytic/sclerotic.
  - May have pathological fractures.

Prostate Carcinoma

Carcinomas of the prostate are another common malignancy in older male populations. They arise within the prostate gland, which surrounds the prostatic urethra and is closely associated with the bladder neck, the rectum posteriorly and the seminal vesicles.

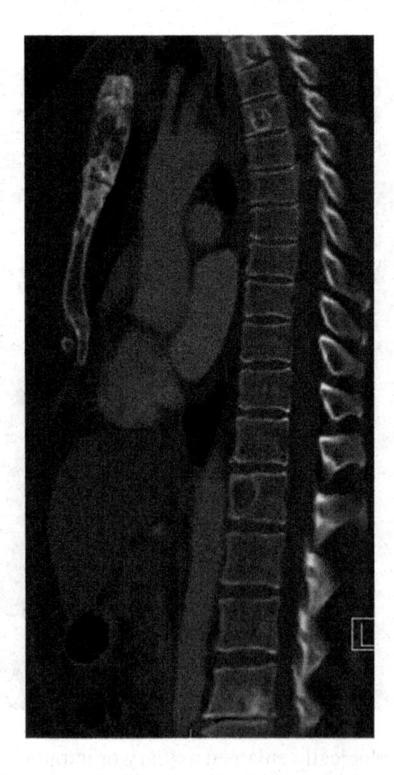

FIGURE 20.11 Extensive mixed lytic and sclerotic lesions throughout the skeleton, visualised here within vertebral bodies and within the sternal body and manubrium, compatible with osseous metastatic spread.

The prostate in most individuals, particularly those in the age demographic being investigated for prostate cancer, is commonly heterogenous and/or enlarged, secondary to benign prostatic hyperplasia. CT therefore has little to no role in the initial diagnosis of primary disease in small to moderate-sized lesions. In fact, unless the disease has infiltrated beyond the prostate capsule and into adjacent structures, even more advanced cancers can be difficult to assess on CT.

The diagnosis is typically made on clinical and histological grounds, increasingly complemented by improving MRI and nuclear medicine techniques, particularly PET-CT and/or bone scans, which may detect smaller metabolically active metastatic and primary disease. The utility of CT in this setting is therefore in staging and re-staging of disease.

Mimics

- Benign prostatic hyperplasia:
  - Very common cause of enlarged prostate.
- Prostatitis/prostatic abscess:
  - Clinical diagnosis, but CT can detect invasion of peri-prostatic tissues.
  - May be rim enhancing with central non-enhancing component (exudative/necrotic core).
- Bladder or urethral carcinoma.

Clues

- Solid areas of increased enhancement involving prostate.
- Bulging or distortion of prostate contour.
- Periprostatic invasion – especially seminal vesicles.
- Presence of enlarged pelvic lymph nodes.
- Sclerotic bone lesions in older men.

T

See Figure 20.12.

- Location:
  - Mass within the prostate.
  - Bulging, asymmetry or distortion of the prostate capsule.
- Size
- Periprostatic invasion present or absent:
  - Especially seminal vesicles, bladder, pelvic floor.
- Mass effect:
  - Is there evidence of bladder outlet obstruction such as excessively distended or thick-walled bladder?

N

See Figure 20.13.

- Regional – Pelvic or para-aortic.

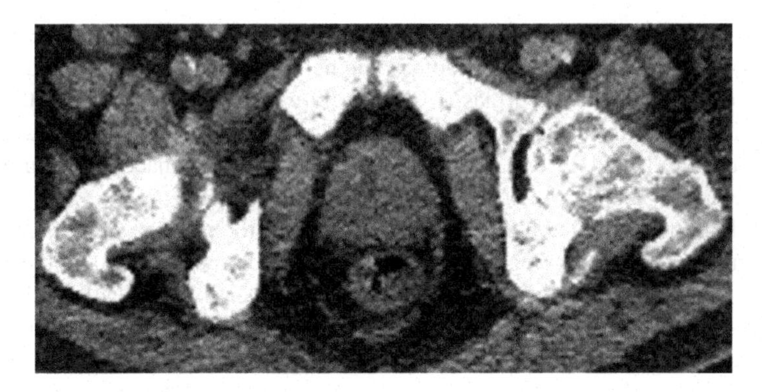

FIGURE 20.12 Note the limited soft tissue resolution of CT in assessing prostate cancer, particularly on this low-dose, non-contrast CT, performed as part of a PET-CT. There may, however, be extraprostatic extension in this case, noting some irregularity about the posterior prostatic capsule. This would be best assessed with MRI.

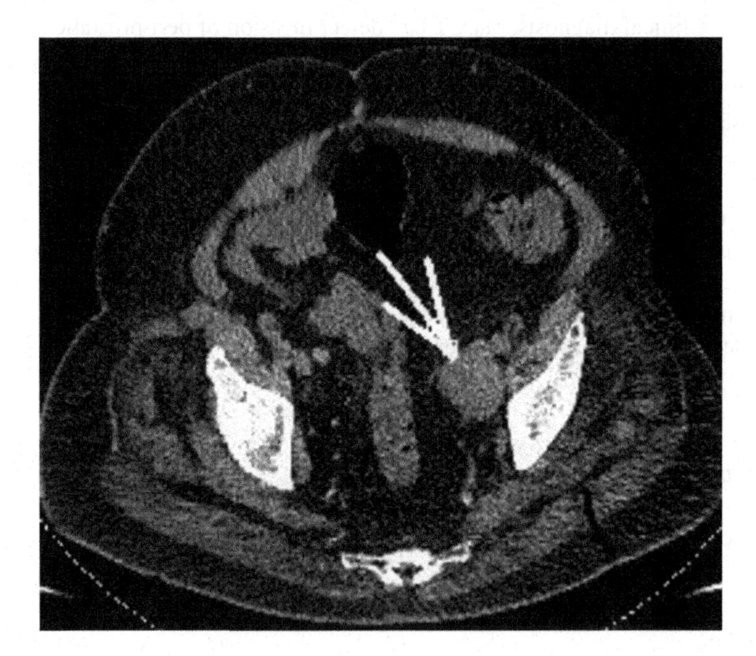

FIGURE 20.13 Large pathologically involved left iliac lymph node. There was no other metastatic disease in this case.

M

- Bone:
  - Look on bone and soft tissue windows for bone lesions.
  - Vast majority are sclerotic.
  - Favour lumbar and sacral spine.

- Lung:
  - Look at lungs in lung windows.
- Liver:
  - Typically, hypoenhancing in PV phase.

Melanoma

Melanoma is a primary malignancy that arises from melanocytes, most often within the skin; however, a number of non-cutaneous sites can also give rise to primary melanoma. CT has little to no role in T staging of primary cutaneous melanomas, which may be small or even clinically occult at presentation. MRI or ultrasound may be used to locate "satellite" nodules or "in-transit" metastases. CT is used in the assessment of lymph node and distant metastases. Of note, metastatic melanoma deposits often occur in organs which commonly see metastases from other cancers, but interestingly may also occur in more unusual sites, such as the wall of the small bowel.

Mimics – Other Hypervascular Metastases

- Renal cell carcinoma,
- Choriocarcinoma,
- Thyroid carcinoma,
- Neuroendocrine tumours.

Mimics

- Malignant:
  - Other primary skin malignancies,
  - Lymphoma,
  - Sarcomas,
  - Metastasis from other primary cancer (uncommon).
- Benign/non-neoplastic – many other skin/subcutaneous lesions which are always best assessed by direct clinical examination:
  - Traumatic – haematoma;
  - Inflammatory/infective – abscess;
  - Lipoma – well-circumscribed and fat density;
  - Sebaceous cyst – well-circumscribed, density approaches water;
  - Benign naevi, warts, keratoses.

Clues

- Melanoma metastases may be hypervascular, especially in the liver, and therefore, may be avidly enhancing with contrast-enhanced CT, particularly in the arterial phase.
- Metastases may be haemorrhagic and may occur in more unusual locations, such as the small bowel.
- Cerebral metastases are often dense on pre-contrast CT – relating to intralesional haemorrhage (Ginaldi et al., 1981).

T

- Limited role unless very large and deeply infiltrating.
- Similar density to skeletal muscle.

N

See Figure 20.14.

- Regional or distant lymph nodes (common).

M

See Figure 20.15.

- Skin and subcutaneous tissues;
- Lung;
- Brain;
- Unusual locations, e.g., small bowel.

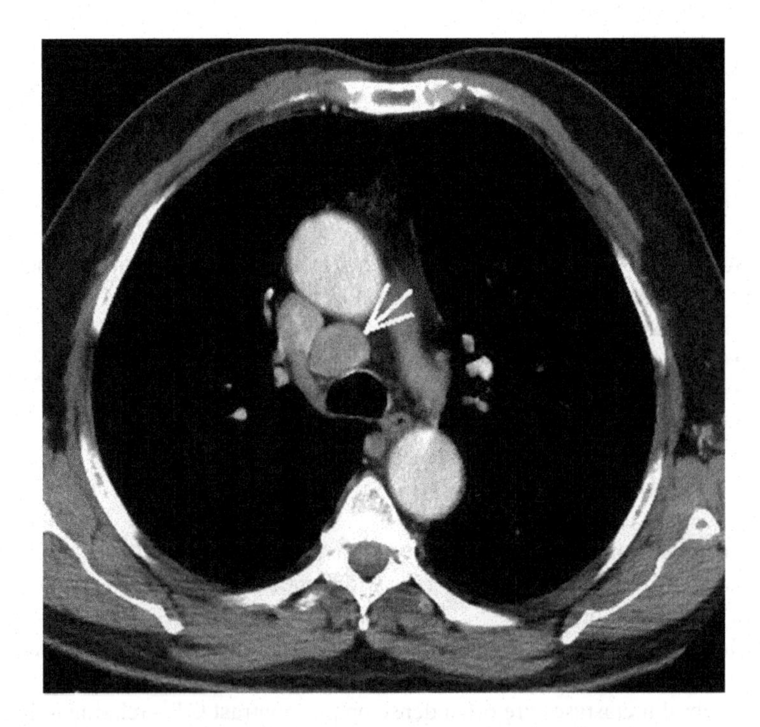

FIGURE 20.14 Large melanoma metastasis to a pretracheal lymph node.

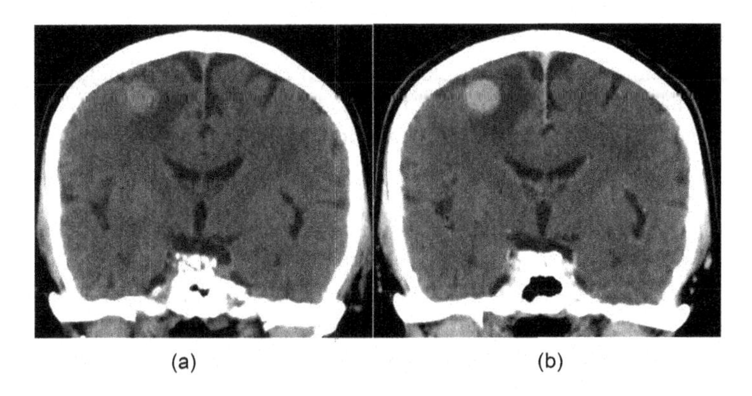

FIGURE 20.15 (a) and (b) Pre- and post-contrast CT brain demonstrating a common site for melanoma metastasis. Note the increased density on pre-contrast CT, suggesting intralesional blood products. Also note the rind of perilesional vasogenic oedema, which preserves the grey–white matter interface. Avid post-contrast enhancement.

Tumours of the Brain

This section has been structured a little differently as primary malignant tumours of the brain are less common, when considered as a proportion of all intra-cranial masses. CT of the brain not infrequently demonstrates both symptomatic and incidental masses. These may be subtle on non-contrast CT, as they are often of similar density to the adjacent grey matter. A helpful clue to the presence of a mass is adjacent cerebral oedema, which typically involves the surrounding white matter but spares the grey matter, known as "vasogenic oedema". This is in contrast to the "cytotoxic oedema" caused by cell death from ischaemic strokes, which characteristically involves the cortical grey matter and subjacent white matter, with loss of normal differentiation between the two differing densities.

Another helpful clue is the presence of mass effect. Tumours outside of the brain (extra-axial tumours) may displace the cerebral cortex, blood vessels and CSF. Tumours may also compress the ventricles causing hydrocephalus. These secondary features help one suspect the presence of an underlying mass for which contrast can be given to further assess and confirm these suspicions.

It is worthwhile noting that the brain is a particularly common site of metastasis from many primary cancers (especially breast, colon, lung and melanoma). In addition, there are a number of primary malignant neoplasms which arise in the brain. Brain malignancies progress locally and can be very aggressive but, in contrast to primary cancers elsewhere, they typically do not metastasise. This makes use of the "TNM" approach difficult for primary brain lesions.

CT is a vital tool in assessing brain masses, however, MRI is the optimal modality to characterise such lesions and is commonly performed as the next step once CT detects a mass in the brain.

Neoplastic causes of a mass can be thought of in terms of their location. Firstly, is the mass "in the brain" (intra-axial) or "outside the brain" (extra-axial)?

Examples of Intra and Extra-Axial Masses Include

- Malignant intra-axial (e.g., glioblastoma, metastases, lymphoma);
- Malignant extra-axial (most are metastases);
- Benign extra-axial (e.g., most meningiomas).

Mimics

- Infection (incl abscess)
- Ischaemia – cerebral infarction:
  - May cause mass effect and oedema, but this is of cytotoxic type.
  - Look for loss of grey–white matter differentiation.
  - Involves vascular territory or territories, often wedge-shaped.
- Inflammatory:
  - Including autoimmune.
- Haemorrhage
- Vascular – including cerebral aneurysms.

Clues

See Figures 20.16 and 20.17.

These clues are by no means specific for malignant disease and many benign entities can also have similar appearances, especially if large.

- Brain oedema or brain involvement.
- Mass effect – e.g., loss of sulcal pattern, obstruction to CSF drainage → ventricular dilatation.
- Haemorrhage – may be seen in metastatic or primary tumours.

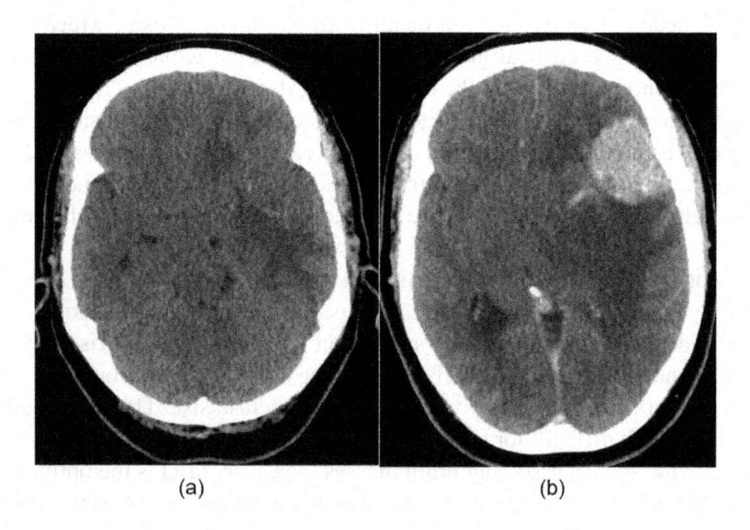

FIGURE 20.16 (a) and (b) Pre-contrast CT brain showing extensive left frontal and temporal vasogenic oedema (again note the preserved grey–white matter differentiation). The extra-axial mass is strikingly isodense to the cerebral cortex making it hard to see on pre-contrast imaging, but for a subtle rind of hyperdense material, likely tumoural calcification, and the secondary mass effect and oedema. Avid and homogenous contrast enhancement is present.

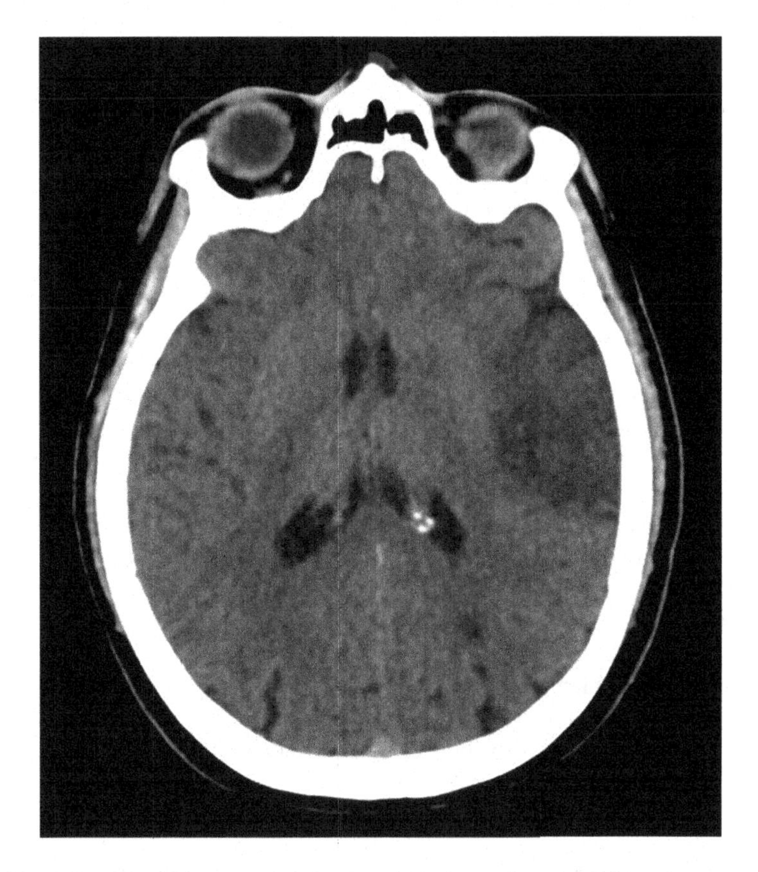

FIGURE 20.17 Note this example of cytotoxic oedema, for comparison, in a case of left middle cerebral artery territory infarction. The grey–white matter differentiation is lost which would not be compatible with the peri-tumoural oedema demonstrated in Figure 20.16a, even if there were regions of enhancement, which can occur post cerebral infarction.

ADDITIONAL ROLES FOR CT IN CANCER DIAGNOSIS

- Procedural:
  - CT fluoroscopy plays a role in the tissue diagnosis of malignant disease. As well as ultrasound, CT can allow a Radiologist to carefully target a suspicious abnormality, allowing tissue biopsy or needle aspiration for histopathological or cytological analysis to allow accurate diagnosis.
  - Examples of sites commonly targeted for CT biopsy:
  - Lung lesions;
  - Liver lesions;
  - Lymph nodes, particularly in the abdomen or chest;
  - Bone lesions.
- Follow-up and surveillance:
  - Patients who have had treated malignancies who may be in remission often undergo surveillance imaging to ensure malignant disease remains in remission.

    - This is performed to assess previously treated primary, nodal and metastatic lesions as well as to evaluate for new potential metastatic deposits.
- Screening:
    - CT colonography for colorectal carcinoma.
    - Potential future of low dose CT chest for lung carcinoma screening, already performed in some parts of the world.
- Dual Energy:
    - Improves lesion detection and characterisation (American Journal of Roentgenology, 2021).
- Nuclear Medicine:
    - Nuclear medicine studies generally provide limited anatomical information.
    - By fusing nuclear medicine studies with CT for anatomical localisation and attenuation correction, assessment of the functional information obtained can be combined with the spatial information of CT.
    - Increasingly utilised for PET and SPECT (Single-photon emission computed tomography).

See Figure 20.18.

- Radiotherapy planning:
    - CT is utilised by Radiation Oncologists to localise and accurately target malignant disease to allow delivery of radiation treatment.

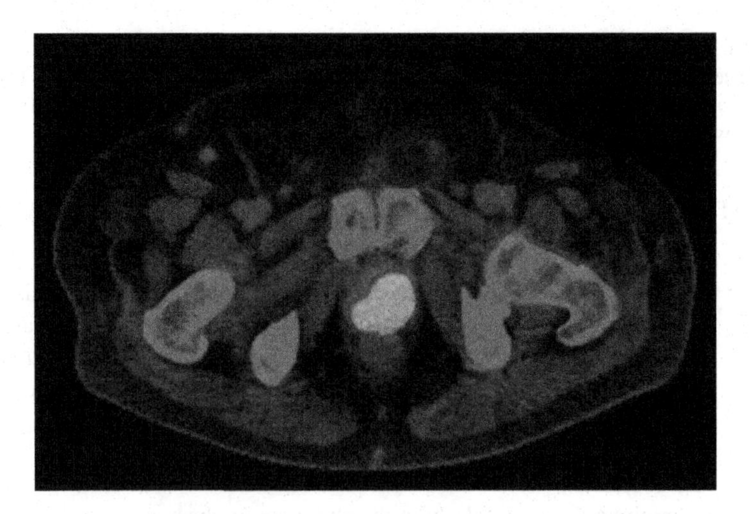

FIGURE 20.18 Example of prostate-specific membrane antigen PET-CT with functional PET information being "fused" with the low dose CT data, demonstrating increased tracer uptake in prostate cancer, in the same case pictured in Figures 20.13 and 20.14.

ACKNOWLEDGEMENTS

Note all images obtained from South Australian Medical Imaging (SAMI) PACS and have been deidentified. SAMI will need to be acknowledged.

REFERENCES

Allisy-Roberts, P. and Williams, J. (2007) Farr's Physics for Medical Imaging. W.B. Saunders Company.

Amin, M. and Edge, S. (2020) AJCC Cancer Staging System. Chicago, IL: American College of Surgeons.

Australian Institute of Health and Welfare (AIHW), 2020. Cancer Data in Australia. Canberra: Australian Government.

Dual-Energy CT: Oncologic Applications : American Journal of Roentgenology: Vol. 199, No. 5_supplement (AJR) (2021).

Ginaldi, S. et al. (1981) "Cranial computed tomography of malignant melanoma", *American Journal of Roentgenology*, 136(1), pp. 145–149. doi: 10.2214/ajr.136.1.145.

Seeram, E. (2016) Computed tomography. St. Louis Mo.: Saunders Elsevier.

Stedman, T. (2006) Stedman's medical dictionary. 28th edn. Baltimore, Md.: Lippincott Williams & Wilkins, p. 1365.

Van den Brekel, M.W.M., Stel, H.V., Castelijns, J.A., Nauta, J.J., Van der Waal, I., Valk, J., Meyer, C.J. and Snow, G.B., 1990. Cervical lymph node metastasis: assessment of radiologic criteria. *Radiology*, 177(2), pp.379–384.

World Health Organisation (WHO) (2019) Health and healthcare in the fourth industrial revolution. Global Future Council on the Future of health and healthcare 2016–2018. Coligny: World Economic Forum.

Index

Printed in the United States
by Baker & Taylor Publisher Services

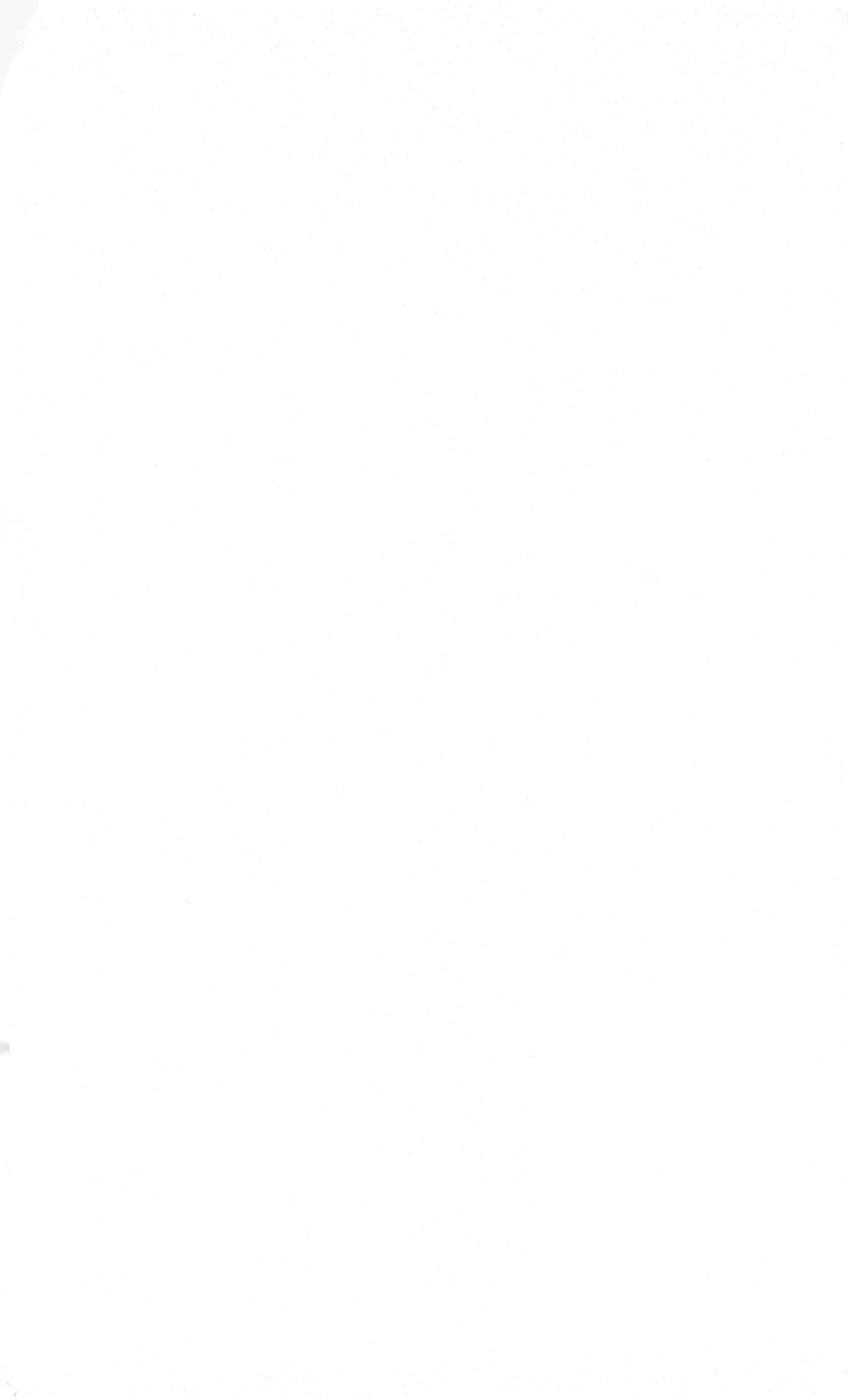